Handbook of
Acute Coronary Syndromes

REMEDICA
publishing

LONDON • CHICAGO

Published by Remedica Publishing
32–38 Osnaburgh Street, London, NW1 3ND, UK
Remedica Inc, Civic Opera Building, 20 North Wacker Drive,
Suite 1642, Chicago, IL, 60606, USA

Tel: +44 20 7388 7677
Fax: +44 20 7388 7457
Email: books@remedica.com
www.remedica.com/books

Publisher: Andrew Ward
In-house editor: Thomas Moberly

First edition: ISBN 1 901346 65 X
First edition with expanded index 2004

British Library Cataloguing in-Publication Data

A catalogue record for this book is available from the British Library.

Handbook of
Acute Coronary Syndromes

Deepak L Bhatt & Marcus D Flather, Editors

Editors

Deepak L Bhatt, MD, FACC, FSCAI, FESC
Director, Interventional Cardiovascular Fellowship
Associate Director, Cardiovascular Medicine Fellowship
Staff, Cardiac, Peripheral, and Cerebrovascular Intervention
Cleveland Clinic Foundation
Department of Cardiovascular Medicine
9500 Euclid Avenue, Desk F25
Cleveland, OH 44195
USA

Marcus D Flather, BSc, MBBS, FRCP
Director, Clinical Trials & Evaluation Unit
Royal Brompton Hospital
Sydney Street
London
SW3 6NP
UK

Contributors

Jeroen J Bax, MD, PhD
Leiden University Medical Center
Leiden, The Netherlands

Eric Boersma, PhD
Academisch Ziekenhuis Rotterdam–Dijkzigt
Kamer H 541, Postbus 2040
NL–3000 CA Rotterdam, The Netherlands

Christopher P Cannon, MD
Associate Professor of Medicine
Cardiovascular Division, Department of Medicine
Brigham and Women's Hospital and Harvard Medical School,
Boston, MA 02115, USA

Michael S Chen, MD
Cleveland Clinic Foundation
Department of Cardiovascular Medicine
9500 Euclid Avenue, Desk F25, Cleveland, OH 44195, USA

Derek P Chew, MBBS, MPH, FRACP
Department of Cardiovascular Medicine
Flinders Medical Centre
Flinders Way, Bedford Park, South Australia 5042, Australia

Mauricio G Cohen, MD
Assistant Professor of Medicine
Division of Cardiology, Department of Medicine
The University of North Carolina at Chapel Hill
CB #7075, Bioinformatics Building, Suite 4128
130 Mason Farm Road, Chapel Hill, NC 27599, USA

Nicholas LM Cruden, BSc (Hons), MB, ChB, MRCP
Research Fellow, Cardiovascular Research
University of Edinburgh, Chancellor's Building,
51 Little France Crescent, Edinburgh EH16 4SB, UK

Keith AA Fox, BSc (Hons), MB, ChB, FRCP, FESC
Duke of Edinburgh Professor of Cardiology
Cardiovascular Research, University of Edinburgh
Chancellor's Building, 51 Little France Crescent
Edinburgh EH16 4SB, UK

Chrisopher B Granger, MD
Associate Professor of Medicine, Director, CCU
Duke Clinical Research Institute, 2400 Pratt St.
Room 0311 Terrace Level, Durham NC 27705, USA

Umair Mallick, MD
Clinical Research Fellow (Cardiology)
Royal Brompton Hospital, Sydney Street, London SW3 6NP, UK

E Magnus Ohman, MD, FRCPI, FACC
Ernest and Hazel Craige Professor of Cardiovascular Medicine
Chief, Division of Cardiology
Director, UNC Heart Center
The University of North Carolina at Chapel Hill
CB #7075, Bioinformatics Building, Suite 4128
130 Mason Farm Road, Chapel Hill, NC 27599, USA

Jonas Oldgren MD, PhD
Senior Consultant, Head of CCU
Department of Cardiology
Uppsala University Hospital
SE-75185 Uppsala, Sweden

Don Poldermans, MD, PhD
Department of Vascular Surgery
Erasmus Medical Center, Room BA 300
Dr Molewaterplein 40, 3015 GD Rotterdam, The Netherlands

Ravish Sachar, MD
Cleveland Clinic Foundation
Department of Cardiovascular Medicine, 9500 Euclid Avenue,
Desk F25, Cleveland, OH 44195, USA

Peter Sinnaeve, MD, PhD
Department of Cardiology
University Hospital Gasthuisberg,
Herestraat 49, 3000 Leuven, Belgium

Anil K Taneja, BSc, MBBS, MRCP(UK), MRCP(Ire), MSc (Card)
Clinical Trials & Evaluation Unit
Britten Street Wing, Royal Brompton Hospital, Sydney Street
London SW3 6NP, UK

Eric J Topol, MD
Provost and Chief Academic Officer
Chairman, Department of Cardiovascular Medicine
Cleveland Clinic Foundation, 9500 Euclid Avenue, Cleveland,
OH 44195, USA

Frans Van de Werf, MD
Professor, Department of Cardiology,
University Hospital Gasthuisberg,
Herestraat 49, 3000 Leuven, Belgium

Lars Wallentin, MD, PhD
Professor of Cardiology, Director of Uppsala Clinical Research Center
Department of Medical Sciences, Cardiology
and Uppsala Clinical Research Center
Uppsala University Hospital, SE-75185 Uppsala, Sweden

Harvey D White, DSc
Professor, Director of Coronary Care and Cardiovascular Research
Green Lane Hospital, Green Lane Road West
Auckland 1003, New Zealand

Preface

Acute coronary syndromes (ACS) represent a global epidemic. While the prevalence of risk factors such as diabetes and obesity increase worldwide, there has been a parallel increase in acute coronary ischemia. As the leading cause of morbidity and mortality, ACS is a major public health problem. Research has propelled the field from one driven by anecdote to one guided by scientific evidence. The real challenge is to translate advances in treatment into improvements in healthcare.

This book provides the reader with an overview of state of the art management of ACS. A distinguished international panel of authors assembled from throughout the world has provided a global view of the treatment of ACS. Furthermore, the authors provide their insights into future developments in the field. The full spectrum of ACS, including both classical ST-segment-elevation myocardial infarction and non-ST segment-elevation myocardial infarction, as well as unstable angina, are covered in a comprehensive, evidence-based format. The latest clinical trials are incorporated into current guidelines to provide concrete recommendations for the optimal management of ACS.

The book is aimed at the wide range of health care professionals (including physicians, nurses, pharmacists, and managers) who treat ACS patients in busy hospitals throughout the world. A broad range of chapters cover pathophysiology, risk stratification, treatment, and future directions.

We are grateful to the contributors for distilling an enormous amount of data into succinct chapters that focus on the essential elements of treating patients with ACS. We are thankful to Remedica Publishing for producing this book. It is our sincere hope that readers of our book will obtain a deeper understanding of ACS that will directly benefit their patients.

Deepak L Bhatt & Marcus D Flather

To my wife Shanthala, and to my sons Vinayak and Arjun

DLB

To Ruth, Hannah, and Alex, and my colleagues in the
Clinical Trials and Evaluation Unit

MDF

Contents

1

Pathophysiology, classification, and clinical features

Derek P Chew & Harvey D White

Introduction

As further insights into the underlying pathophysiology have enhanced our understanding of acute coronary syndromes (ACS), the management paradigms used in the daily clinical care of patients have also evolved:

- Vascular inflammation has emerged as a key factor in the initiation and progression of atheroma, as well as in plaque instability.

- Assessment of inflammation has proved valuable for risk stratification with respect to both short- and long-term adverse outcomes.

- Appreciation of the importance of distal embolization from unstable epicardial lesions has led to the adoption of an early invasive approach of angiography and revascularization within the context of potent antithrombotic therapy.

This chapter explores some of the recent developments in our understanding of the pathophysiology of ACS, in particular, the roles of inflammation, thrombosis, and distal embolization. We describe the evolving definition of myocardial infarction (MI), with particular focus on the importance of troponins, and explain the nomenclature used in the clinical management of patients presenting with ACS. Finally, we suggest a diagnostic paradigm useful for daily clinical practice.

Atheroma formation and the vulnerable plaque

Plaque rupture

It has long been appreciated that ACS is the manifestation of sudden plaque rupture with subsequent occlusive or subocclusive thrombus formation, leading to distal myocardial ischemia or myonecrosis [1]. However, it is now recognized that high-grade stenoses demonstrated at angiography do not account for the bulk of acute ischemic events. Most ACS cases appear to arise from non-flow-limiting lesions, with diameter stenoses of <70% [2].

The risk of future ischemic events is, therefore, largely dependent on the presence of small, unstable, or "vulnerable plaque" (rather than high-grade) lesions assessed by angiography. This brings into question the ability of the angiogram to predict future cardiac events. Further, plaque rupture may often occur without clinical manifestation. This is evidenced by the presence of several ruptured plaques within the same individual, supporting a diffuse, underlying, pathogenic process [3–5]. It is likely that such a cycle of subclinical plaque rupture and healing underlies the process of atheroma progression [6].

Anatomic characterization of vulnerable plaque

More recently, the anatomic characterization of vulnerable plaque has been possible [6–9]. Postmortem and intravascular ultrasound studies have demonstrated a greater lipid core, thinner fibrous cap, and a high density of inflammatory cells in complex ruptured plaques (see **Box 1**) [10]. These lesions are not initially associated with high-grade angiographic stenoses due to outward expansion (positive remodeling) of the adventitia to accommodate the increased plaque volume [11].

Interestingly, models using Laplace's Law suggest that positive remodeling associated with active plaques is linked to greater shear stress favoring plaque rupture [12]. Studies also describe endothelial erosions of fibrous plaques with low lipid content. These lesions appear to be more prevalent among younger patients and suggest that a mechanism beyond shear stress is impacting a thin fibrous cap [3].

Functional factors contributing to plaque instability

Recent studies have focused on the functional factors contributing to plaque instability (such as inflammatory activity resident in the "at-risk" plaque, compromising the integrity of the endothelium and intima) and the contribution of hemostatic factors to the propensity for and pathogenesis of coronary thrombus formation.

It is likely that an increase in prothrombotic factors (fibrinogen, F1.2, von Willebrand factor, factor VII, and plasminogen activator inhibitor type 1) and a reduction in fibrinolytic factors (tissue plasminogen activator and urokinase-type plasminogen activator) also explain this propensity for thrombosis [13].

Such changes have been linked to traditional risk factors for coronary artery disease, such as diabetes, smoking, hypercholesterolemia, and

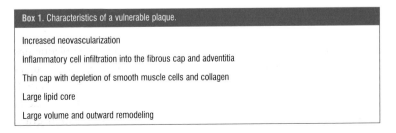

Box 1. Characteristics of a vulnerable plaque.

Increased neovascularization

Inflammatory cell infiltration into the fibrous cap and adventitia

Thin cap with depletion of smooth muscle cells and collagen

Large lipid core

Large volume and outward remodeling

increased homocysteine levels. Like vulnerable plaque, coronary thrombosis may also be multifocal, with several sites of thrombus seen within the same vessel, lending further support to the notion that a diffuse process is at play.

Insights into the underlying process

Inflammation

The contribution of inflammatory activity to the pathogenesis of ACS is well established. Atherectomy specimens of patients presenting with ACS demonstrate an increased presence of macrophages within active plaques, particularly in the fibrous cap [10]. These cells are an important source of inflammatory cytokines and are key regulators of several processes that lead to the compromise of the blood–vascular wall interface. These processes include:

- up-regulation of degradative enzymes that promote loss of collagen within the fibrous cap
- triggering of endothelial and smooth muscle cell apoptosis, contributing to both endothelial cell desquamation and plaque vulnerability
- increased expression of adhesion molecules and chemotactic factors promoting inflammatory cell adhesion molecule migration and the generation of a prothrombotic milieu within the blood (see **Table 1**) [7,9]

A correlation between C-reactive protein (CRP) and lesion morphology observed on angiography provides further evidence of the inflammatory nature of unstable coronary plaques [14,15]. Studies of neutrophil transit through the coronary circulation among patients with unstable angina show neutrophil activation even in the vessel contralateral to the culprit lesion, supporting the multifocal nature of the inflammatory process [16–19].

At the bedside, clinical appreciation of this inflammatory activation is reflected in detectable increases in CRP by high-sensitivity assays and with simple measures such as the white cell count [20]. Interestingly, while the correlation between inflammation and late mortality is robust, no relationship has been observed between inflammation and recurrent MI [21]. This observation suggests that CRP provides insights into pathophysiologic processes above and beyond that of thromboembolism, as provided by the electrocardiogram (ECG) and troponin levels.

Table 1. Mediators of vascular inflammation. NF: nuclear factor.

Mediator	Cellular origin	Process
Interferon-gamma	Inflammatory cells	Inhibition of collagen synthesis by smooth muscle cells
Matrix metalloproteinases	Macrophages	Weakening of collagen fibrils in the fibrous cap. Reduced integrity of endothelial–intimal adherence leading to desquamation of endothelial cells
Elastolytic cathepsins	Macrophages	Degrade elastin in the fibrous cap
Fas ligand	–	Endothelial and smooth muscle cell apoptosis
Plasminogen activator inhibitor 1	Endothelial cells	Promotion of thrombosis
Reduced nitric oxide production	Endothelial cells	Impaired vasodilatory response and decreased inhibition of NF-kappa B, a key proinflammatory transcription factor
NF-kappa B	Endothelial cells	Increased expression of adhesion molecules (intercellular adhesion molecule-1, vascular cell adhesion molecule-1, and E-selectin)
Tissue factor	Macrophages	Increased expression in unstable plaque (macrophages), leading to increased thrombogenicity
C-reactive protein	Hepatic cells	Increased endothelial cell adhesion molecules
CD40 ligand	Platelets	Binds CD40 on inflammatory cells leading to up-regulation of inflammatory cytokine production, adhesion molecule expression, and cellular apoptosis

Nevertheless, the factors regulating the waxing and waning of this inflammatory coronary process require further elucidation [22].

Vessel occlusion versus distal embolization

Platelet thrombus fragmentation and embolization into the microvasculature has emerged as an important concept. Distal impaction of activated platelets and platelet–leukocyte aggregates sets up new foci of microvascular inflammation, leading to further adhesion-molecule activation, inflammatory cell egress, and, eventually, focal myonecrosis [2,23].

Autopsy studies have provided important insights into this process and demonstrated a high prevalence of platelet microemboli among patients who have died from ACS. Among patients experiencing unstable angina before death, platelet emboli were present in 44.4% of patients, observed as multifocal loci of necrosis distributed throughout the ventricular wall supplied by the epicardial vessel with the culprit lesion [24]. An even higher prevalence (79%) of this phenomenon has been reported among patients presenting with acute MI and sudden death [25].

Further evidence suggesting the intermittent nature of this thrombotic and embolic process comes from the finding of layered thrombus of differing ages within the epicardial thrombus of patients with dynamic coronary thrombosis leading to MI or sudden death [26]. Finally, these lesions may be associated with an increased propensity for ventricular fibrillation and sudden death [27,28].

Insights from the measurement of troponin levels

Troponins are proteins specific to the contractile apparatus of the cardiac myocyte. As sensitive and specific markers of cardiac myonecrosis, elevation in serum troponin levels correlates with the presence of visible thrombus at the culprit lesion, reduced TIMI grade flow in the culprit vessel, increased lesion complexity and tighter stenoses at the culprit lesion, and a higher prevalence of TIMI myocardial perfusion grade 0–1, suggesting a closed microvasculature [29–31]. These findings suggest a strong correlation between troponin release and embolization of platelet–inflammatory cell aggregates into the distal microcirculation with subsequent local inflammation and myonecrosis [32]. Elevations in troponin levels are associated with an increased risk of both mortality and recurrent MI, though the relationship with MI appears to only hold below a certain threshold – beyond a certain level of troponin, greater elevations are not associated with a greater risk of recurrent MI, probably reflecting the complete infarction of an "at-risk area" [33]. Newer biomarkers have provided insights into the pathophysiology of ACS, and a rationale for the adoption of early invasive strategies in the context of potent antithrombotic therapies.

The diagnosis of myocardial infarction

MI can be defined as myocardial necrosis resulting from subtotal or total occlusion of an epicardial coronary vessel. Conceptually, the diagnosis of MI appears straightforward. Clinically, however, the definition of MI is often more complex, since confirmation of myocardial necrosis is often delayed and ECG criteria evolve over time. Consequently, the nomenclature or classification of ACS develops from those used as an initial working diagnosis (guiding the initial management of patients presenting with chest pain or angina equivalents) to those used as a final or established diagnosis with pathological, prognostic, and social significance (see **Table 2**).

The development of sensitive assays for myocardial necrosis, namely those for troponins I and T, has enabled the clinical diagnosis of MI to be made with greater sensitivity. The recent European Society of Cardiology (ESC)/American College of Cardiology (ACC) definition of MI has evolved to embrace troponins as the preferred biomarker [34]. This definition focuses on a "typical rise and gradual fall in troponin" or a "rise and more rapid fall in CK-MB [creatine kinase isoenzyme MB]" within the context of a clinical presentation consistent with coronary occlusion (see **Box 2**) [34]. However, this definition has little utility for those presenting with ischemic cardiac arrest, and the criteria also warrant several other comments [35].

Utility and prognostic considerations

With the incorporation of a sensitive threshold for the diagnosis of MI, such a definition has great utility for identifying patients with ACS who may benefit from specific therapies. Conversely, the prognosis and social implications of MI are dependent on the degree of myocardial injury; that is, the prognostic implications of troponin elevation differ within various clinical scenarios (see **Figure 1**). Consequently, for prognostic considerations, the degree of injury needs to be further qualified, either biochemically (absolute level of marker elevation) or by cardiac imaging (eg, echocardiography, magnetic resonance imaging, positron emission tomography).

Table 2. Potential causes of troponin elevation, other than acute coronary syndromes.

Disease state	Iatrogenic	False positive
Pericarditis	Cardiac surgery	Heterophile antibodies
Pulmonary embolism	Electrophysiological ablation	
Sepsis and shock	Cardiotoxic drugs	
Acute left ventricular failure	Cardioversion	
Drug toxicity	Percutaneous coronary intervention	
Hypertension/hypotension		
Trauma		

Clinical context

The clinical context remains important. Several disease processes beyond coronary occlusion may be associated with elevations in cardiac markers. Thus, the presence of CK-MB or troponin elevation without a clinical presentation suggestive of transient or persistent coronary occlusion does not necessarily constitute ACS (see **Table 3**).

Assay specificity

When using CK-MB (mass assay), any increase above normal (above the 99th percentile of a reference control group) is defined as MI. With troponin, a value above the 99th percentile of a normal population is considered elevated. Current standards require that this level be measurable with <10% coefficient of variation. However, current assays are unable to meet this level of accuracy at such low concentrations. Consequently, some commentators have suggested adopting the diagnostic concentration where <10% coefficient of variation is achievable (this value varies among the assays) [36]. The diagnosis of MI is, therefore, assay specific.

Ischemic cardiac arrest

This definition has little utility for those presenting with ischemic cardiac arrest.

Box 2. The European Society of Cardiology/American College of Cardiology definition of myocardial infarction. CK-MB: creatine kinase isoenzyme MB; ECG: electrocardiogram.

The presentation with either a typical rise and gradual fall (troponin) or more rapid rise and fall (CK-MB) of biochemical markers of myonecrosis with at least one of the following:

- ischemic symptoms
- development of pathological Q waves on ECG
- ECG evidence indicative of ischemia (ST-segment elevation or depression)
- coronary intervention
- pathological findings of myocardial infarction

Classifications and nomenclature of ACS

Establishing a working diagnosis

Reflecting the fact that definitive evidence of myonecrosis with cardiac markers is often delayed, the initial ECG is used to establish a working diagnosis and provide guidance for when time-dependent therapy, namely reperfusion therapy, should be instituted.

Figure 1. Significance of troponin elevation by clinical context. ACS: acute coronary syndromes; CABG: coronary artery bypass graft; LAD: left anterior descending; LV: left ventricular; MI: myocardial infarction; PCI: percutaneous coronary intervention; ULRR: upper limit of reference range.

ST-segment elevation ACS

There is a strong correlation between ST-segment elevation and an occluded epicardial vessel [37,38]. Included within this subset of patients are those presenting with a bundle branch block (BBB) pattern on the initial ECG. Thus, the presence of ST-segment elevation or a BBB identifies those patients who are

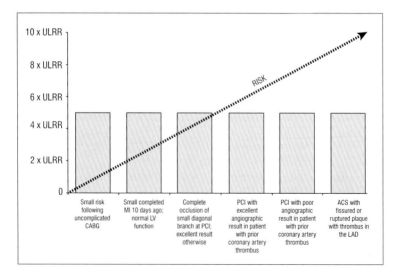

likely to benefit from either pharmacologic or catheter-based reperfusion.

Non-ST-segment elevation ACS

In the absence of persistent ST-segment elevation, ACS patients represent a relatively heterogeneous population of patients, spanning transient ST-segment elevation and depression, T-wave inversion, and the absence of ECG changes. From the perspective of a working diagnosis, benefit from emergent reperfusion therapy has not been demonstrated collectively among these patients. Nevertheless, the presenting ECG provides important diagnostic and prognostic information. For example, an analysis of the GUSTO-IIa study observed a better

Table 3. Classifications of myocardial infarction (MI) used in clinical trials. ACS: acute coronary syndromes; BBB: bundle branch block; CABG: coronary artery bypass graft; CK-MB: creatine kinase isoenzyme MB; ECG: electrocardiogram; PCI: percutaneous coronary intervention; STEMI: ST-segment elevation myocardial infarction.

Working diagnosis	Established diagnosis
ST-segment elevation ACS: • new or presumed new ST-segment elevation at the J point in two or more contiguous leads with the cut-off ≥ 0.2 mV (in leads V1, V2, or V3) or ≥ 0.1 mV (in other leads) Non-ST-segment elevation ACS: • ST-segment depression or T-wave abnormalities in the absence of ST-segment elevation (although these patients may have no ECG changes on admission) BBB/uncertain-type MI: • left BBB (old or new) or paced rhythm that obscures assessment of ST-segment elevation or Q waves (if definite new ST-segment elevation can be identified compared with an old ECG, then STEMI should be the classification)	Q-wave MI: • development of any Q wave in leads V1 through V3, or the development of a Q wave ≥ 30 ms in leads I, II, aVL, aVF, V4, V5, V6 (Q-wave changes must be present in any of two contiguous leads and be ≥ 1 mm in depth) Non-Q-wave MI: • the absence of Q waves (see above definition) on ECG performed at least 12 hours after the event MI following coronary revascularization: • post-PCI: CK-MB >3 times the upper limit of normal (on at least one occasion), with or without ECG changes • post-CABG: CK-MB >5 times the upper limit of normal (with the development of new Q waves) or >10 times the upper limit of normal (without the development of Q waves)

prognosis for patients presenting with only T-wave inversion as opposed to either ST-segment elevation or depression [39]. Furthermore, among patients presenting with non-ST-segment elevation ACS, the magnitude of ST-segment depression and the number of leads involved appear to provide clear independent prognostic information [21].

Diagnosis of established MI

With time, the detection of a characteristic rise and fall in either troponin or CK-MB levels provides confirmatory evidence for the diagnosis of MI [34]. Evolution of the ECG, with respect to the development of Q waves, provides a further subclassification of patients with established MI. The development of Q waves (Q-wave MI) in the territory of ischemia correlates with full-thickness ventricular wall necrosis (transmural MI), and the absence of Q waves on the ECG of patients experiencing MI (non-Q-wave MI) implies the presence of viable myocardial tissue in the area of infarction (subendocardial MI). However, while some evidence suggests that the lack of Q-wave development confers a prognostic advantage, other evidence suggests that there is little difference between Q-wave and non-Q-wave MI with respect to in-hospital clinical outcomes [40,41].

Working diagnosis versus established diagnosis

While commonly observed, the progression of ST-segment elevation ACS to Q-wave MI is not a clinical certainty. Often, especially with effective reperfusion, the development of Q waves does not occur and a non-Q-wave MI results. Similarly, the converse applies. Patients initially presenting with non-ST-segment elevation ACS often do not develop Q waves, but occasionally they do. Rarely, with both ST-segment elevation and non-ST-segment elevation ACS, rapid resolution of ECG changes occurs and there is no evidence of cardiac marker elevation; thus, the diagnosis of MI cannot be made (see **Figure 2**).

Postrevascularization MI

Adding to the complexity of classifying MI, thresholds of myonecrosis used for defining MI following revascularization have differed from those used for spontaneous MI. These definitions have focused on postprocedural CK–MB elevations, and are largely independent of the development of ECG changes and clinical symptoms. Nevertheless, the degree of myonecrosis occurring as the result of coronary revascularization appears to confer the same magnitude of risk as seen in spontaneous infarction [42]. The ESC/ACC consensus group recommends that the same definition be used for PCI–related MI as for spontaneous MI.

Some clinical trials have sought to use a common definition of MI for both spontaneous and postrevascularization MI [49]. Emerging work with postprocedural troponin elevation suggests that this

Figure 2. Classification of acute coronary syndromes (ACS): evolution from working diagnosis to established diagnosis. ECG: electrocardiogram; MI: myocardial infarction.

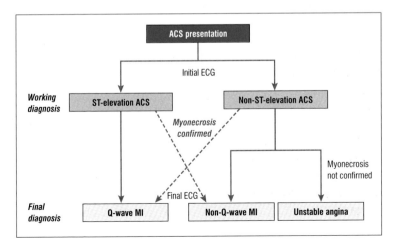

13

marker may also be useful for defining patients with an increased risk of future adverse outcomes, but specific levels have not yet reached widespread acceptance [43–46].

Pathophysiology, diagnosis, risk stratification, and management: an integrated paradigm

An integrated strategy (including an evaluation of the clinical history and examination, ECG, and cardiac markers and an assessment of markers of inflammation and left ventricular dysfunction) provides not only improved utility for the diagnosis of ACS, but also insights into the underlying pathophysiology, providing a rationale for the management of patients across the entire continuum of ACS presentations. Such an integrated approach appears to provide insights into coronary vessel patency, coronary lesion morphology, distal embolization, and left ventricular dysfunction.

Chest pain or discomfort

Chest pain or discomfort remains the principal clinical manifestation of ACS. Its location is classically central with radiation to the jaw or left shoulder and arm, with a dull or heavy, ill-defined nature, and may be associated with shortness of breath. Its onset is usually related to exertion (with a lower exercise threshold among patients with pre-existing stable angina) with increasing frequency and severity. Often the onset of discomfort is at rest. Clinical examination is often nonspecific, though an S4 or a new mitral regurgitant murmur may be suggestive of ischemia-induced diastolic dysfunction or papillary muscle dysfunction, respectively. Evidence of pulmonary edema provides evidence of left ventricular dysfunction (ischemia is one cause of this). However, caution must be used when relying on a classical clinical presentation for the diagnosis of ACS. Specifically, while the presence of a classical description is highly suggestive of coronary pathology, its absence does not exclude the diagnosis.

Electrocardiogram

The ECG remains a simple, effective, and low-cost investigation for initial diagnosis and risk stratification. The ECG manifestations of ACS are diverse, covering BBB and ST-segment elevation, through to ST-segment depression and T-wave inversion. In general, criteria used for inclusion within clinical trials have been more stringent than the wider spectrum of changes observed in clinical practice. Nevertheless, these criteria provide a useful guideline for assisting in the immediate diagnosis of ACS in everyday practice (see **Table 3**):

- Initial ST-segment elevation or a BBB pattern is strongly correlated with an acute occlusive obstruction of an epicardial vessel and suggests potential benefit from reperfusion therapy [47,48].

- The absence of ST-segment elevation or a BBB pattern does not preclude the presence of complete epicardial occlusion (often seen with circumflex artery occlusion). However, the benefit of pharmacologic reperfusion (fibrinolysis) has not been demonstrated among these patients. Nevertheless, compared with patients with normal ECGs, ECG changes consistent with ischemia portend an increased risk of recurrent ischemic events, suggesting the need for potent antiplatelet therapies and early invasive investigation and management [18,49].

Myonecrosis

Evidence of myonecrosis with elevations in either CK-MB or troponin levels suggests coronary occlusion and distal embolization. These offer strong supportive evidence for the diagnosis of ACS. Within an appropriate clinical context, robust data link elevations in cardiac markers to the presence of a high-risk lesion, and to early and late adverse outcomes among patients with ACS, making troponins important tools in early risk stratification. Furthermore several trials within the context of glycoprotein IIb/IIIa inhibition and an early invasive management strategy have demonstrated that troponin elevation is clinically useful in guiding the use of these therapeutic options [50–54].

Inflammation

CRP levels and white cell counts appear to reflect the inflammatory activity in the vascular wall and offer prognostic information that is independent of that offered by the ECG and troponin elevation. Among patients presenting with ACS, an increased inflammatory response is associated with an increase in mortality but not recurrent MI. Furthermore, a strategy of early revascularization appears to mitigate this risk [55,56].

B-natriuretic peptide

Elevation of B-natriuretic peptide portends increased risk of mortality, MI, and heart failure [57]. As a sensitive marker of left ventricular dysfunction or stretch, this serum marker is a useful tool for identifying patients who may benefit from therapies aimed at preventing or treating cardiac failure.

Multimarker approach

A multimarker approach (troponin, CRP, and B-natriuretic peptide) may provide the most accurate risk assessment of patients presenting with ACS [58].

New methods for assessing plaque instability

Improved understanding of the vulnerable plaque has led to the search for tools offering early detection, and thus the ability for the early institution of preventative interventions. Several imaging tools with potential utility in this area have focused on the delineation of plaque content, in particular the lipid core content and thickness of the fibrous cap [59,60]. Such tools include:

- magnetic resonance imaging with gadolinium derivatives for plaque morphology or ferrous oxide for macrophage density
- contrast computed tomography for plaque volume or calcium scoring
- intravascular ultrasound and optical coherence tomography
- positron emission tomography with 18 fluoro-deoxy-glucose for disease burden

The future of screening strategies

Currently, these modalities are costly and in some cases invasive, making them suboptimal as an alternative to imaging studies and serological measures of inflammatory activity. Among these, CRP appears the most promising [20]. Interestingly, studies have suggested that not all MI incidents are preceded by the same degree of inflammatory activation, underlining the fact that inflammation is just one component in the process of atherothrombosis [22]. Thus, before widespread screening for vulnerable plaque is embarked upon, it is valuable to reflect on the goals of such an endeavor. Specifically, the aim of screening is to identify patients at increased risk (beyond the risk defined by established risk factors) in whom a different management strategy would be considered, with evidence that such therapies reduce subsequent risk. Further validation of these screening strategies is therefore awaited [61].

Summary

Novel insights into the pathophysiology of ACS have evolved beyond the simple model of coronary thrombosis. Assays of a variety of inflammatory markers and mediators indicate that inflammation frequently underlies the atherothrombotic process, underscoring the multifocal nature of the disease and its involvement of both the vascular wall and blood components. Furthermore, as a sensitive

Figure 3. An integrated conceptual approach to acute coronary syndromes (ACS), linking clinical diagnosis, risk stratification, and management to the underlying pathophysiology. Risk stratification in **bold**; pathophysiology in *italics*. BNP: B-natriuretic peptide; CRP: C-reactive protein; LV: left ventricular.

marker of myonecrosis, troponins improve the noninvasive prediction of distal embolization and the presence of high-risk coronary lesions. This forms the rationale for an invasive management strategy combined with potent antithrombotic therapies validated in clinical trials. Often, the diagnosis among patients presenting with chest pain requires the adoption of a working diagnosis, with the final diagnosis only emerging after some time. An integrated approach incorporating clinical, ECG, and biochemical factors enables an adaptive management strategy that is cognizant of the evolving information regarding the individual patient's risk (see **Figure 3**). Such an approach merges the

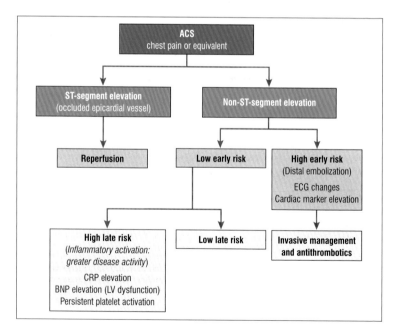

concepts of diagnosis and short- and long-term prognosis, with optimization of the utilization of invasive and often costly therapies.

References

1.   Ambrose JA, Winters SL, Arora RR, et al. Coronary angiographic morphology in myocardial infarction: a link between the pathogenesis of unstable angina and myocardial infarction. *J Am Coll Cardiol* 1985;6:1233–8.
2.   Ambrose JA, Tannenbaum MA, Alexopoulos D, et al. Angiographic progression of coronary artery disease and the development of myocardial infarction. *J Am Coll Cardiol* 1988;12:56–62.
3.   Davies MJ. Stability and instability: two faces of coronary atherosclerosis. The Paul Dudley White Lecture 1995. *Circulation* 1996;94:2013–20.
4.   Goldstein JA, Demetriou D, Grines CL, et al. Multiple complex coronary plaques in patients with acute myocardial infarction. *N Engl J Med* 2000;343:915–22.
5.   Zairis MN, Papadaki OA, Manousakis SJ, et al. C-reactive protein and multiple complex coronary artery plaques in patients with primary unstable angina. *Atherosclerosis* 2002;164:355–9.
6.   Corti R, Fuster V, Badimon JJ. Pathogenetic concepts of acute coronary syndromes. *J Am Coll Cardiol* 2003;41:7S–14S.
7.   Shah PK. Mechanisms of plaque vulnerability and rupture. *J Am Coll Cardiol* 2003;41:15S–22S.
8.   Shah PK. Plaque disruption and coronary thrombosis: new insight into pathogenesis and prevention. *Clin Cardiol* 1997;20:II-38–44.
9.   Libby P. Current concepts of the pathogenesis of the acute coronary syndromes. *Circulation* 2001;104:365–72.
10. Moreno PR, Falk E, Palacios IF, et al. Macrophage infiltration in acute coronary syndromes. Implications for plaque rupture. *Circulation* 1994;90:775–8.
11. Schoenhagen P, Ziada KM, Kapadia SR, et al. Extent and direction of arterial remodeling in stable versus unstable coronary syndromes: an intravascular ultrasound study. *Circulation* 2000;101:598–603.
12. Loree HM, Kamm RD, Stringfellow RG, et al. Effects of fibrous cap thickness on peak circumferential stress in model atherosclerotic vessels. *Circ Res* 1992;71:850–8.
13. Rauch U, Osende JI, Fuster V, et al. Thrombus formation on atherosclerotic plaques: pathogenesis and clinical consequences. *Ann Intern Med* 2001;134:224–38.
14. Burke AP, Tracy RP, Kolodgie F, et al. Elevated C-reactive protein values and atherosclerosis in sudden coronary death: association with different pathologies. *Circulation* 2002;105:2019–23.
15. Sano T, Tanaka A, Namba M, et al. C-reactive protein and lesion morphology in patients with acute myocardial infarction. *Circulation* 2003;108:282–5.
16. Buffon A, Biasucci LM, Liuzzo G, et al. Widespread coronary inflammation in unstable angina. *N Engl J Med* 2002;347:5–12.
17. Sabatine MS, Morrow DA, Cannon CP, et al. Relationship between baseline white blood cell count and degree of coronary artery disease and mortality in patients with acute coronary syndromes: a TACTICS-TIMI 18 (Treat Angina with Aggrastat and determine Cost of Therapy with an Invasive or Conservative Strategy-Thrombolysis in Myocardial Infarction 18 trial) substudy. *J Am Coll Cardiol* 2002;40:1761–8.

18. Cannon CP, McCabe CH, Wilcox RG, et al. Association of white blood cell count with increased mortality in acute myocardial infarction and unstable angina pectoris. OPUS-TIMI 16 Investigators. *Am J Cardiol* 2001;87:636–9, A10.

19. Barron HV, Cannon CP, Murphy SA, et al. Association between white blood cell count, epicardial blood flow, myocardial perfusion, and clinical outcomes in the setting of acute myocardial infarction: a thrombolysis in myocardial infarction 10 substudy. *Circulation* 2000;102:2329–34.

20. Yen MH, Bhatt DL, Chew DP, et al. Association between admission white blood cell count and one-year mortality in patients with acute coronary syndromes. *Am J Med* 2003;115:318–21.

21. James SK, Armstrong P, Barnathan E, et al. Troponin and C-reactive protein have different relations to subsequent mortality and myocardial infarction after acute coronary syndrome: a GUSTO-IV substudy. *J Am Coll Cardiol* 2003;41:916–24.

22. Maseri A, Fuster V. Is there a vulnerable plaque? *Circulation* 2003;107:2068–71.

23. Ambrose JA, Hjemdahl-Monsen CE, Borrico S, et al. Angiographic demonstration of a common link between unstable angina pectoris and non-Q-wave acute myocardial infarction. *Am J Cardiol* 1988;61:244–7.

24. Davies MJ, Thomas AC, Knapman PA, et al. Intramyocardial platelet aggregation in patients with unstable angina suffering sudden ischemic cardiac death. *Circulation* 1986;73:418–27.

25. Frink RJ, Rooney PA Jr, Trowbridge JO, et al. Coronary thrombosis and platelet/fibrin microemboli in death associated with acute myocardial infarction. *Br Heart J* 1988;59:196–200.

26. Falk E. Unstable angina with fatal outcome: dynamic coronary thrombosis leading to infarction and/or sudden death. Autopsy evidence of recurrent mural thrombosis with peripheral embolization culminating in total vascular occlusion. *Circulation* 1985;71:699–708.

27. Mehta P, Mehta J. Platelet function studies in coronary artery disease. V. Evidence for enhanced platelet microthrombus formation activity in acute myocardial infarction. *Am J Cardiol* 1979;43:757–60.

28. El-Maraghi N, Genton E. The relevance of platelet and fibrin thromboembolism of the coronary microcirculation, with special reference to sudden cardiac death. *Circulation* 1980;62:936–44.

29. Wong GC, Morrow DA, Murphy S, et al. Elevations in troponin T and I are associated with abnormal tissue level perfusion: a TACTICS-TIMI 18 substudy. Treat Angina with Aggrastat and Determine Cost of Therapy with an Invasive or Conservative Strategy-Thrombolysis in Myocardial Infarction. *Circulation* 2002;106:202–7.

30. Heeschen C, van Den Brand MJ, Hamm CW, et al. Angiographic findings in patients with refractory unstable angina according to troponin T status. *Circulation* 1999;100:1509–14.

31. Giannitsis E, Muller-Bardorff M, Lehrke S, et al. Admission troponin T level predicts clinical outcomes, TIMI flow, and myocardial tissue perfusion after primary percutaneous intervention for acute ST-segment elevation myocardial infarction. *Circulation* 2001;104:630–5.

32. Lindahl B, Diderholm E, Lagerqvist B, et al. Mechanisms behind the prognostic value of troponin T in unstable coronary artery disease: a FRISC II substudy. *J Am Coll Cardiol* 2001;38:979–86.

33. Antman EM. Troponin measurements in ischemic heart disease: more than just a black and white picture. *J Am Coll Cardiol* 2001;38:987–90.

34. Myocardial infarction redefined – a consensus document of The Joint European Society of Cardiology/American College of Cardiology Committee for the redefinition of myocardial infarction. *Eur Heart J* 2000;21:1502–13.

35. White HD. Things ain't what they used to be: impact of a new definition of myocardial infarction. *Am Heart J* 2002;144:933–7.

36. Apple FS, Wu AH, Jaffe AS. European Society of Cardiology and American College of Cardiology guidelines for redefinition of myocardial infarction: how to use existing assays clinically and for clinical trials. *Am Heart J* 2002;144:981–6.

37. DeWood MA, Spores J, Notske R, et al. Prevalence of total coronary occlusion during the early hours of transmural myocardial infarction. *N Engl J Med* 1980;303:897–902.

38. DeWood MA, Spores J, Hensley GR, et al. Coronary arteriographic findings in acute transmural myocardial infarction. *Circulation* 1983;68:I39–I49.

39. Savonitto S, Ardissino D, Granger CB, et al. Prognostic value of the admission electrocardiogram in acute coronary syndromes. *JAMA* 1999;281:707–13.

40. Furman MI, Dauerman HL, Goldberg RJ, et al. Twenty-two year (1975 to 1997) trends in the incidence, in-hospital and long-term case fatality rates from initial Q-wave and non-Q-wave myocardial infarction: a multi-hospital, community-wide perspective. *J Am Coll Cardiol* 2001;37:1571–80.

41. Murphy SA, Dauterman K, de Lemos JA, et al. Angiographic and clinical characteristics associated with the development of Q-wave and non-Q-wave myocardial infarction in the thrombolysis in myocardial infarction (TIMI) 14 trial. *Am Heart J* 2003;146:42–7.

42. Akkerhuis KM, Alexander JH, Tardiff BE, et al. Minor myocardial damage and prognosis: are spontaneous and percutaneous coronary intervention-related events different? *Circulation* 2002;105:554–6.

43. Januzzi JL, Lewandrowski K, MacGillivray TE, et al. A comparison of cardiac troponin T and creatine kinase-MB for patient evaluation after cardiac surgery. *J Am Coll Cardiol* 2002;39:1518–23.

44. Kizer JR, Muttrej MR, Matthai WH, et al. Role of cardiac troponin T in the long-term risk stratification of patients undergoing percutaneous coronary intervention. *Eur Heart J* 2003;24:1314–22.

45. Lasocki S, Provenchere S, Benessiano J, et al. Cardiac troponin I is an independent predictor of in-hospital death after adult cardiac surgery. *Anesthesiology* 2002;97:405–11.

46. Nallamothu BK, Chetcuti S, Mukherjee D, et al. Prognostic implication of troponin I elevation after percutaneous coronary intervention. *Am J Cardiol* 2003;91:1272–4.

47. Fibrinolytic Therapy Trialists' (FTT) Collaborative Group. Indications for fibrinolytic therapy in suspected acute myocardial infarction: collaborative overview of early mortality and major morbidity results from all randomised trials of more than 1000 patients. *Lancet* 1994;343:311–22.

48. Weaver WD, Simes RJ, Betriu A, et al. Comparison of primary coronary angioplasty and intravenous thrombolytic therapy for acute myocardial infarction: a quantitative review. *JAMA* 1997;278:2093–8.

49. Fox KA, Poole-Wilson PA, Henderson RA, et al. Interventional versus conservative treatment for patients with unstable angina or non-ST-elevation myocardial infarction: the British Heart Foundation RITA 3 randomised trial. Randomized Intervention Trial of unstable Angina. *Lancet* 2002;360:743–51.

50. Cannon CP, Weintraub WS, Demopoulos LA, et al. Comparison of early invasive and conservative strategies in patients with unstable coronary syndromes treated with the glycoprotein IIb/IIIa inhibitor tirofiban. *N Engl J Med* 2001;344:1879–87.

51. Hamm CW, Heeschen C, Goldmann B, et al. Benefit of abciximab in patients with refractory unstable angina in relation to serum troponin T levels. c7E3 Fab Antiplatelet Therapy in Unstable Refractory Angina (CAPTURE) Study Investigators. *N Engl J Med* 1999;340:1623–9.
52. Kleiman NS, Lakkis N, Cannon CP, et al. Prospective analysis of creatine kinase muscle-brain fraction and comparison with troponin T to predict cardiac risk and benefit of an invasive strategy in patients with non-ST-elevation acute coronary syndromes. *J Am Coll Cardiol* 2002;40:1044–50.
53. Heeschen C, Hamm CW, Goldmann B, et al. Troponin concentrations for stratification of patients with acute coronary syndromes in relation to therapeutic efficacy of tirofiban. PRISM Study Investigators. Platelet Receptor Inhibition in Ischemic Syndrome Management. *Lancet* 1999;354:1757–62.
54. Newby LK, Ohman EM, Christenson RH, et al. Benefit of glycoprotein IIb/IIIa inhibition in patients with acute coronary syndromes and troponin T-positive status: the paragon-B troponin T substudy. *Circulation* 2001;103:2891–6.
55. Lindahl B, Toss H, Siegbahn A, et al. Markers of myocardial damage and inflammation in relation to long-term mortality in unstable coronary artery disease. FRISC Study Group. Fragmin during Instability in Coronary Artery Disease. *N Engl J Med* 2000;343:1139–47.
56. Bhatt DL, Chew DP, Lincoff AM, et al. Effect of revascularization on mortality associated with an elevated white blood cell count in acute coronary syndromes. *Am J Cardiol* 2003;92:136–40.
57. de Lemos JA, Morrow DA, Bentley JH, et al. The prognostic value of B-type natriuretic peptide in patients with acute coronary syndromes. *N Engl J Med* 2001;345:1014–21.
58. Sabatine MS, Morrow DA, de Lemos JA, et al. Multimarker approach to risk stratification in non-ST elevation acute coronary syndromes: simultaneous assessment of troponin I, C-reactive protein, and B-type natriuretic peptide. *Circulation* 2002;105:1760–3.
59. Naghavi M, Madjid M, Khan MR, et al. New developments in the detection of vulnerable plaque. *Curr Atheroscler Rep* 2001;3:125–35.
60. Jang IK, Bouma BE, Kang DH, et al. Visualization of coronary atherosclerotic plaques in patients using optical coherence tomography: comparison with intravascular ultrasound. *J Am Coll Cardiol* 2002;39:604–9.
61. Bhatt DL, Topol EJ. Need to test the arterial inflammation hypothesis. *Circulation* 2002;106:136–40.

2

Epidemiology

Christopher B Granger

Introduction

The term "acute coronary syndromes" (ACS) covers the clinical spectrum of acute myocardial ischemia, including unstable angina, acute myocardial infarction (MI) without ST-segment elevation (non-ST-segment elevation MI [NSTEMI]), and ST-segment elevation MI (STEMI) [1,2]. This nomenclature is oriented towards the early classification of patients into categories that are useful for risk assessment and acute treatment. As additional information, such as serial cardiac markers, becomes available, patients may shift from one category to another.

This chapter describes the epidemiology of ACS, including the incidence of unstable angina and MI, the related outcomes, current international practice patterns, and sources of information about ACS (including national databases and registries).

In 2000, a consensus statement from the Joint European Society of Cardiology (ESC) and the American College of Cardiology (ACC) redefined MI in the context of widespread availability and recommended use of troponin testing [3].

The joint ESC/ACC definition of acute, evolving, or recent MI requires that either one of the following is present:

1. A typical rise and gradual fall (troponin) or more rapid rise and fall (creatine kinase-MB) of biochemical markers of myocardial necrosis with at least one of the following:

- ischemic symptoms
- development of pathologic Q waves
- electrocardiogram (ECG) changes of ischemia (ST-segment elevation or depression)
- coronary artery intervention

2. Pathologic findings of acute MI

The change meant that a substantial portion of patients who were previously classified as having unstable angina with elevated troponin were reclassified as having acute MI. Since then, a change has been taking place in how ACS patients are classified: a greater proportion of ACS patients are now classified as MI and there is a closer relationship between the diagnosis and the risk of hospital death [4].

Box 1. US coronary heart disease (CHD) death statistics (American Heart Association statistics, 2003)

- Single largest killer of males and females
- An American suffers a CHD event every 29 seconds, and dies of one every minute
- 47% of people having a CHD event will die from it that year
- 250,000 people die each year from a CHD event without being hospitalized, most from cardiac arrest
- From 1990 to 2000, the CHD death rate declined by 25%, but the actual number of deaths fell by <10%
- 84% of CHD deaths are among people aged ≥65 years

Incidence and outcomes

Coronary heart disease (CHD), and in its acute form ACS, is the number one cause of death worldwide [5]. In the US in 2003, an estimated 650,000 people will have a new CHD event (definite or probable MI or CHD death) and 450,000 people will have a recurrent event [6]. The estimated total number of MIs per year in the US is 540,000. The average age of patients suffering their first MI is 66 years for men and 70 years for women. There are over 2 million hospital discharges for CHD, and the total estimated cost of CHD is $130 billion per year [6]. Estimates of mortality from CHD in the US are shown in **Box 1**.

The incidence and outcomes of ACS depend on the strictness of criteria used for the definition. Clinical trials, and to a lesser extent registries, often only include patients with clear objective criteria for ACS and may exclude patients with confounding factors such as renal insufficiency that can make diagnosis more difficult and often relate to a much worse outcome [7].

Over the past 5 years, there has been a shift in the pattern of ACS, such that a smaller proportion of patients with acute MI have ST-segment elevation and a larger proportion have no ST-segment elevation (see **Figure 1**) [8]. Whilst patients with STEMI generally have higher in-hospital and 30-day mortality, patients presenting with ST-segment depression have higher mortality at 6 months and beyond, related to their older age and greater burden of underlying disease (see **Figure 1**) [9]. The risk of death and (re)infarction following ACS is highest in the first few days, and then declines over time (see **Figure 2**) [1,10].

Population studies show an age-adjusted decline in CHD over the past 20 years [6]. However, there is a misperception that mortality from acute MI has dramatically decreased. This has been fueled by results from highly selected populations from trials such as GUSTO-V, in which 30-day mortality was only 6% for a population of patients with STEMI treated with fibrinolytic-based reperfusion therapy [11], compared to over 10% mortality in the ISIS-2 trial [12]. It is likely that this misperception is also in part related to the exclusion of high-risk patients from trials, especially those conducted recently.

The HERO-2 trial provides a population of patients from countries in which very few patients were excluded, and 70% of the population was enrolled in Eastern Europe and Russia. There was a 10.7% 30-day mortality rate for patients with STEMI treated with streptokinase [13].

In the Swedish acute MI registry [14], which included the majority of patients admitted to coronary care units from 1995 to 1998 with acute MI in Sweden,

Figure 1. Six-month mortality by baseline electrocardiogram findings.

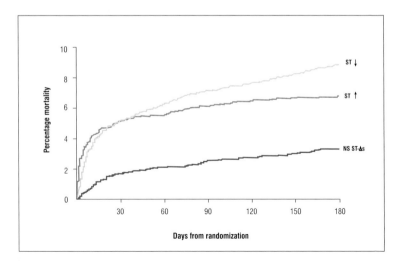

the 1-year mortality rate among those <80 years old was 17%. Moreover, for elderly patients (>75 years old) treated with reperfusion therapy, the 1-year mortality rate was 31.4%, but for those not treated with reperfusion therapy (generally due to late presentation or exclusion criteria) it was 41.8%.

Patients who fulfill exclusion criteria for thrombolysis have high mortality rates, especially if not treated with primary coronary angioplasty, in which case in-hospital mortality is ~30% [15]. Unselected elderly populations with acute MI (such as from the Cooperative Cardiovascular Project [16]) have especially high mortality, with 22% 1-year mortality among hospital survivors.

A major factor influencing the incidence, features, and outcomes of acute MI is the aging population

Figure 2. Timing of adverse events following presentation in non-ST-segment elevation acute coronary syndromes. MI: myocardial infarction.

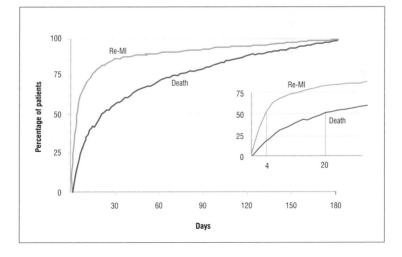

worldwide. In the US, there were approximately 5 million people aged 85 or older in 2000 – this figure is anticipated to increase to nearly 20 million by 2050 (US Census Bureau). Patients over the age of 75 years (even the healthier ones enrolled in clinical trials) have early mortality rates of >20%, as well as high stroke (3.4%) and bleeding (nearly 20%) rates [17].

Risk factors

Among the most important epidemiologic observations have been the relationships between risk factors and the development of CHD, especially modifiable risk factors [18]. Among patients experiencing CHD events, especially younger patients, most have treatable conventional risk factors such as cigarette smoking, diabetes, hyperlipidemia, or hypertension.

Although cigarette smoking has declined in the US, its impact on worldwide cardiovascular disease is projected to increase and it remains among the most important preventable causes of disease [19].

The incidence of obesity and diabetes are increasing at an alarming rate both in the US and worldwide [20–22]. The estimated lifetime risk of diabetes among people born in the US in the year 2000 is 32.8% for males and 38.5% for females [23].

Nearly 90% of patients aged ≤55 years who were enrolled in clinical trials of acute MI or ACS had at least one conventional risk factor [24]. The older the patients were at trial entry, the more likely they were to lack conventional factors (see **Figure 3**).

Cigarette smoking was strongly related to development of premature (~10 years early) CHD. The INTERHEART study, a large worldwide case-controlled study of MI, has shown that risk factors for acute MI appear to impart similar risks regardless of world geographic region and patient ethnicity [25].

Impaired glucose metabolism is more prevalent among patients presenting with ACS than is generally appreciated.

In a study of consecutive patients presenting with acute MI in Sweden, careful assessment of diabetes status among patients without known diabetes found that 40% had impaired glucose tolerance and 25% had undiagnosed diabetes [26].

Figure 3. Temporal changes in acute myocardial infarction presentation: National Registry of Myocardial Infarction. LBBB: left bundle branch block; NSTE: non-ST-segment elevation; STE: ST-segment elevation.

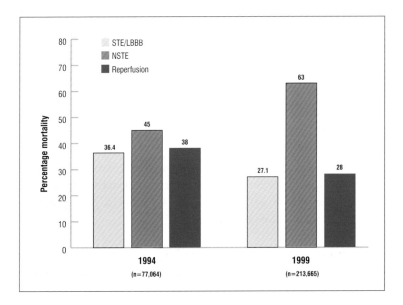

Registries

As effective therapies for ACS have emerged over the past 20 years, the need for systematic collection of data on the use of therapies at hospital, national, and international levels has led researchers to conduct several large, high-quality registries that provide rich insights into the epidemiology of ACS. Selected registry and database studies and their key features are listed in **Table 1**. Such registries have redefined the demographics and outcomes of patients with ACS.

Although clinical trial databases have provided important sources of information for understanding populations of patients with ACS, they are a selected population that is less ill and has better outcomes than general practice [27]. As expected, compared to patients enrolled in clinical trials, registry patients are older, with an average age of ST-segment elevation patients of 63–66 years, and age of patients without ST-segment elevation of 66–73 years.

Women comprise approximately 40% of the ACS population. Women have higher mortality rates, with in-hospital mortality rates for ST-segment elevation ranging from 8% to 12% (and non-ST-segment elevation rates of 3%–5%).

Both clinical trial and registry studies provide information on international difference in process of care and outcomes [28–30]. In addition to major differences in use of interventional procedures and related use of glycoprotein IIb/IIIa inhibitors (with higher use in the US) there are also major differences in use of heparins and in-hospital length of stay.

Registries and claims database studies have also allowed assessment of changes in ACS presentation and management over time. The most extreme hemodynamic complication, cardiogenic shock following acute MI, has not decreased in incidence over the past decade, nor have the number of resultant fatalities [31].

	NRMI 4 [39]	CCP [16]	GRACE [30]	EHS-ACS [36]	CRUSADE [38]
Patient eligibility	STEMI	MI, hospital survivors aged ≥65 years	ACS with and without ST-segment elevation	STEMI/ NSTEMI	High risk UA/NSTEMI
Hospitals	US	US non-governmental	Regional population-based clusters of hospitals representing the full spectrum from community to tertiary facilities	Hospital clusters representing academic and nonacademic hospitals and those with/ without specialist cardiac services	Diverse group of hospitals (geographic, number of beds, hospital type)
Number of hospitals	1,247	All	106	103	Over 400
Countries	US only	US only	International	European	US and Canada
Main funding source	Industry	Government	Industry	ESC/industry	Industry
Cardiac catheterization laboratory	–	–	67%	77%	88%
Enrolment period	July 1990 to June 1994	1994–1995	April 1999 and ongoing	September 2000 to May 2001	July 2001 to present
Number of patients	240,989	115,015	31,068	10,484 (of 14,271 logged)	27,768
Follow-up	In-hospital	1 year	6 months	30 days	In-hospital
Age (years)	63–73	≥65	64–68	63–66	68
Female	37%–44%	50%	28%–38%	28%–35%	40%
Mortality	12%	22%	3%–7%	3.5%–8.4%	4.6%

Table 1. Characteristics of the large registries of acute coronary syndromes (ACS). CCP: Cardiac Cooperative Project; ESC: European Society of Cardiology; MI: myocardial infarction; STEMI: ST-segment elevation myocardial infarction; UA: unstable angina.

Following the evidence from clinical trials, appropriate medication use and intervention appears to be increasing in incidence over time [8,32]. Beta-blocker use at discharge following MI has improved from 72% to 79% between 1999 and 2001 in US Medicare beneficiaries [33].

Quality improvement programs

Epidemiologic studies have shown a clear relationship between use of proven, guideline-indicated therapies and better patient outcomes [34]. While this is not surprising, it provides evidence to support the use of programs to improve patient outcomes. In one of the largest quality improvement programs ever established for patient care, the US Joint Commission on Accreditation of Healthcare Organizations (JCAHO) established ORYX® to integrate performance measurement into the hospital accreditation process [35].

As of July 2002, US hospitals have been expected to begin collection on the first set of ORYX core performance indicators:

- aspirin and beta blockers in the first 24 hours
- aspirin, beta blockers, angiotensin-converting enzyme inhibitors (in patients with left ventricular dysfunction/heart failure) at discharge
- time to fibrinolytic therapy and time to primary percutaneous coronary intervention
- smoking cessation advice
- mortality

Five of the nine core performance measures for acute MI deal with the use of evidence-based medicine in eligible patients. Each of these medication indications carries the strongest recommendation of the

ACC/American Heart Association (AHA) acute MI and unstable angina guidelines, a class IA indication.

Registries have also been used to quantify the gap between ideal evidence-based care and actual care [8,36–38] and to identify factors related to failure to use proven therapies, such as reperfusion therapy for STEMI. Analyses from two registries have found older age, lack of ongoing chest pain, bundle branch block, and congestive heart failure to be associated with failure to use reperfusion therapy [39,40].

The NRMI registry played a central role in identifying the problem of delay in administration of fibrinolytic therapy and in tracking its improvement during the 1990s [8]. Some studies have found that patients who are cared for in "better" hospitals [41], in teaching institutions [42], and by cardiologists [43] have improved outcomes. Ongoing programs in Europe [44] and the US will be important to correlate the collection of data that describes ACS patients and their care to improved treatment and ultimately better outcomes.

Specific programs to improve quality of care of patients with acute MI have included the Cooperative Cardiovascular Project [45] and the American College of Cardiology Guidelines Applied in Practice (GAP) Project [46], both of which have shown that targeted interventions are associated with improved care [47]. Large registries (such as NRMI, GRACE, and CRUSADE) have provided practitioners with feedback and have shown improved care over time [32]. Registries have shown that, in spite of better quantitative means of risk stratification, there is little evidence that even simple measures, such as troponin, are used in clinical practice to guide more aggressive treatment like cardiac catheterization [34].

Conclusions

ACS has become the most common cause of death worldwide. Understanding of its incidence, characteristics of the patient population, and patterns of treatment has greatly improved over the past several years. Ongoing studies are providing important information to further that understanding and opportunities to improve treatment and outcomes.

References

1. Braunwald E, Antman EM, Beasley JW, et al. ACC/AHA 2002 guideline update for the management of patients with unstable angina and non-ST-segment elevation myocardial infarction: a report of the American College of Cardiology/American Heart Association Task Force on Practice Guidelines (Committee on the Management of Patients with Unstable Angina). 2002. Available at: http://www.acc.org/clinical/guidelines/unstable/unstable.pdf. Accessed on October 2, 2003.
2. Bertrand ME, Simoons ML, Fox KA, et al. Task Force on the Management of Acute Coronary Syndromes of the European Society of Cardiology. Management of Acute Coronary Syndromes in patients presenting without persistent ST-segment elevation. *Eur Heart J* 2002;23:1809–40.
3. Alpert JS, Thygesen K, Antman E, et al. Myocardial infarction redefined – a consensus document of The Joint European Society of Cardiology/American College of Cardiology Committee for the redefinition of myocardial infarction. *J Am Coll Cardiol* 2000;36:959–69.
4. Goodman SG, Steg PG, Eagle KA, et al; GRACE Investigators. The diagnostic and prognostic impact of the new definition of acute myocardial infarction: Lessons from the Global Registry of Acute Coronary Events (GRACE). *Arch Intern Med* (in press).
5. Murray CJ, Lopez AD. Mortality by cause for eight regions of the world: Global Burden of Disease Study. *Lancet* 1997;349:1269–76.
6. American Heart Association. *Heart Disease and Stroke Statistics – 2003 Update*. Dallas, Texas, American Heart Association: 2002.
7. Santopinto JJ, Fox KA, Goldberg RJ, et al; GRACE Investigators. Creatinine clearance and adverse hospital outcomes in patients with acute coronary syndromes: findings from the global registry of acute coronary events (GRACE). *Heart* 2003;89:1003–8.
8. Rogers WJ, Canto JG, Lambrew CT, et al. Temporal trends in the treatment of over 1.5 million patients with myocardial infarction in the U. S. from 1990 through 1999: the National Registry of Myocardial Infarction 1, 2 and 3. *J Am Coll Cardiol* 2000;36:2056–63.
9. Savonitto S, Ardissino D, Granger CB, et al. Prognostic value of the admission electrocardiogram in acute coronary syndromes. *JAMA* 1999;281:707–13.
10. The PURSUIT Trial Investigators. Inhibition of platelet glycoprotein IIb/IIIa with eptifibatide in patients with acute coronary syndromes. *N Engl J Med* 1998;339:436–43.
11. Topol EJ. Reperfusion therapy for acute myocardial infarction with fibrinolytic therapy or combination reduced fibrinolytic therapy and platelet glycoprotein IIb/IIIa inhibition: the GUSTO V randomized trial. *Lancet* 2001;357:1905–14.

12. ISIS-2 (Second International Study of Infarct Survival) Collaborative Group. Randomised trial of intravenous streptokinase, oral aspirin, both, or neither among 17,187 cases of suspected acute myocardial infarction: ISIS-2. *Lancet* 1988;2:349–60.

13. White HD. Thrombin-specific anticoagulation with bivalirudin versus heparin in patients receiving fibrinolytic therapy for acute myocardial infarction: the HERO-2 randomized trial. *Lancet* 2001;358:1855–63

14. Stenestraud U, Wallentin L. Fibrinolytic therapy in patients 75 years and older with ST-segment elevation myocardial infarction. One-year follow-up of a large prospective cohort. *Arch Intern Med* 2003;163:965–71.

15. Grzybowski M, Clements EA, Parsons L, et al. Mortality benefit of immediate revascularization of acute ST-segment elevation myocardial infarction in patients with contraindications to thrombolytic therapy: a propensity analysis. *JAMA* 2003;290:1891–8

16. Krumholz HM, Chen J, Chen YT, et al. Predicting one-year mortality among elderly survivors of hospitalization for an acute myocardial infarction: results from the Cooperative Cardiovascular Project. *J Am Coll Cardiol* 2001;38:453–9.

17. White HD, Barbash GI, Califf RM, et al. Age and outcome with contemporary thrombolytic therapy. Results from the GUSTO-I trial. Global Utilization of Streptokinase and TPA for Occluded coronary arteries trial. *Circulation* 1996;94:1826–33.

18. Hennekens CH. Increasing burden of cardiovascular disease. Current knowledge and future directions for research on risk factors. *Circulation* 1998;97:1095–102.

19. Peto R, Lopez AD, Boreham J, et al. Mortality from smoking worldwide. *Br Med Bull* 1996;52:12–21.

20. Mokdad AH, Ford ES, Bowman BA, et al. Prevalence of obesity, diabetes, and obesity-related health risk factors, 2001. *JAMA* 2003;289:76–9

21. Mokdad AH, Ford ES, Bowman BA, et al. Diabetes trends in the US: 1990-1998. *Diabetes Care* 2000;23:1278–83.

22. Boyle JP, Honeycutt AA, Narayan KM, et al. Projection of diabetes burden through 2050: impact of changing demography and disease prevalence in the US. *Diabetes Care* 2001;24:1936–40.

23. Narayan KM, Boyle JP, Thompson TJ, et al. Lifetime risk for diabetes mellitus in the United States. *JAMA* 2003;290:1884–90.

24. Khot UN, Khot MB, Bajzer CT, et al. Prevalence of conventional risk factors in patients with coronary heart disease. *JAMA* 2003;290:898–904.

25. Jeffrey S. INTER-HEART: largest case-control study confirms similar impact of MI risk factors across the globe. Available at: http://www.theheart.org. Accessed May 17, 2002.

26. Norhammar A, Tenerz A, Nilsson G, et al. Glucose metabolism in patients with acute myocardial infarction and no previous diagnosis of diabetes mellitus: a prospective study. *Lancet* 2002;359:2140–4.

27. Jha P, Deboer D, Sykora K, et al. Characteristics and mortality outcomes of thrombolysis trial participants and nonparticipants: a population-based comparison. *J Am Coll Cardiol* 1996;27:1335–42.

28. Van de Werf F, Topol EJ, Lee KL, et al. Variations in patient management and outcomes for acute myocardial infarction in the United States and other countries. Results from the GUSTO trial. *JAMA* 1995;273:1586–91.

29. Yusuf S, Flather M, Pogue J, et al. Variations between countries in invasive cardiac procedures and outcomes in patients with suspected unstable angina or myocardial infarction without initial ST elevation. OASIS (Organisation to Assess Strategies for Ischaemic Syndromes) Registry Investigators. *Lancet* 1998;352:507–14.

30. Steg PG, Goldberg RJ, Gore JM, et al. Baseline characteristics, management practices, and in-hospital outcomes of patients hospitalized with acute coronary syndromes in the Global Registry of Acute Coronary Events (GRACE). *Am J Cardiol* 2002;90:358–63.

31. Goldberg RJ, Samad NA, Yarzebski J, et al. Temporal trends in cardiogenic shock complicating acute myocardial infarction. *N Engl J Med* 1999;340:1162–8.

32. Fox FA, Goodman SG, Anderson FA, et al. From guidelines to clinical practice: the impact of hospital and geographical characteristics on temporal trends in the management of acute coronary syndromes. The Global Registry of Acute Coronary Events (GRACE). *Eur Heart J* 2003;24:1414–24.

33. Jencks SF, Huff ED, Cuerdon T. Change in the quality of care delivered to Medicare beneficiaries, 1998–1999 to 2000–2001. *JAMA* 2003;289:305–12.

34. Parson LS, Pollack CU, Newby LK, et al. Variation in AMI care across 1247 hospitals and its association with hospital mortality. *Circulation* 2002;106:II–722.

35. Joint commission on accreditation of healthcare organizations. Available http://www.jcaho.org. Accessed on October 20, 2003.

36. Hasdai D, Behar S, Wallentin L, et al. A prospective survey of the characteristics, treatments and outcomes of patients with acute coronary syndromes in Europe and the Mediterranean basin; the Euro Heart Survey of Acute Coronary Syndromes (Euro Heart Survey ACS). *Eur Heart J* 2002;23:1190–201.

37. Rationale and design of the GRACE (Global Registry of Acute Coronary Events) Project: a multinational registry of patients hospitalized with acute coronary syndromes. *Am Heart J* 2001;141:190–9.

38. Hoekstra JW, Pollack CV Jr, Roe MT, et al. Improving the care of patients with non-ST-elevation acute coronary syndromes in the emergency department: the CRUSADE initiative. *Acad Emerg Med* 2002;9:1146–55.

39. Barron HV, Bowlby LJ, Breen T, et al. Use of reperfusion therapy for acute myocardial infarction in the United States: data from the National Registry of Myocardial Infaction 2. *Circulation* 1998;97:1150–6.

40. Eagle KA, Goodman SG, Avezum A et al; GRACE Investigators. Practice variation and missed opportunities for reperfusion in ST-segment-elevation myocardial infarction: findings from the Global Registry of Acute Coronary Events (GRACE). *Lancet* 2002;359:373–7.

41. Chen J, Radford M, Wabg Y, et al. Do "America's Best Hospitals" Perform Better for Acute Myocardial Infarction? *N Engl J Med* 1999;340:286–92.

42. Allison JJ, Kiefe CL, Weissman NW, et al. Relationship of hospital teaching status with quality of care and mortality for medicare patients with acute MI. *JAMA* 2000;284:1256–62.

43. Jollis JG, DeLong ER, Peterson ED, et al. Outcome of acute myocardial infarction according to the specialty of the admitting physician. *N Engl J Med* 1996;335:1880–7.

44. Simoons ML. The quality of care in acute coronary syndromes. *Eur Heart J* 2002;23:1141–2.

45. Marciniak TA, Ellerbeck EF, Radford MJ, et al. Improving the quality of care for Medicare patients with acute myocardial infarction: results from the Cooperative Cardiovascular Project. *JAMA* 1998;279:1351–7.

46. Mehta RH, Montoye CK, Gallogly M, et al. Improving quality of care for acute myocardial infarction: The Guidelines Applied in Practice (GAP) Initiative. *JAMA* 2002;287:1269–76.

47. Guidelines Applied in Practice. Available at: http://www.acc.org/gap/gap.htm. Accessed October 20, 2003.

3

Risk assessment

Nicholas LM Cruden & Keith AA Fox

Introduction

The risk of death or recurrent infarction varies widely amongst patients presenting with acute coronary syndromes (ACS). Accurately predicting an individual's risk within this continuum is essential for a number of reasons. It guides the physician in determining the most appropriate level of care for an individual patient, often facilitating the early discharge of those identified as being at low risk [1]. In addition, risk stratification may identify individuals who are most likely to benefit from specific therapeutic interventions [2]; in the current economic climate, the ability to target these expensive treatments has significant financial and resource benefits for health care providers. Finally, the value of providing patients and their relatives with an accurate and realistic expectation following an ischemic cardiac event should not be forgotten.

For risk stratification to be effective it should be both rapid and easy to use. Assessment should be performed at the time of diagnosis and continued until the patient's condition has stabilized. Risk stratification should focus on three principal areas: the extent of underlying vascular disease, the acute thrombotic event, and complications attributable to myocardial ischemia.

Underlying vascular risk

Analyses of large-scale clinical trials and cohort studies have identified a number of risk factors relating to the presence, severity, and distribution of underlying coronary disease that are predictive of short- and long-term cardiac events in patients with ACS (see **Box 1**) [3–5]. It is, perhaps, not surprising that a history of angina, recent myocardial infarction (MI), or previous coronary artery bypass grafting is strongly associated with a worse outcome [6–8]. More traditional prognostic factors include a family history of coronary disease and the presence of diabetes mellitus, hypertension, or hypercholesterolemia [7]. Coexisting peripheral or cerebral vascular disease, metabolic syndrome (characterized by the combination of insulin resistance, hypertension, obesity, and dyslipidemia), and renal dysfunction are also associated with a poor outcome in ACS [6,9,10].

Increasing age was identified early in clinical trials as a significant predictor of mortality and cardiac risk increases disproportionately with age [3]. This acceleration of risk is probably due, in part, to the greater prevalence

Box 1. Markers of vascular risk in patients with acute coronary syndromes. The evidence for items in brackets is less clear than for other factors.

Increasing age

History of:
- angina or myocardial infarction
- coronary artery bypass grafting

Presence of:
- peripheral or cerebral vascular disease
- diabetes mellitus
- hypertension
- hypercholesterolemia
- metabolic syndrome
- renal dysfunction

Family history of coronary disease
(Gender)
(Smoking habit)

and severity of underlying coronary artery disease, traditional risk factors, and comorbidity in elderly patients. It is important, therefore, when assessing risk in an elderly patient presenting with ACS that additional information is taken into account, including premorbid status, associated comorbidities, social issues, and the patient's expectations.

The influence of gender and smoking status on risk in ACS is less clear. Although men are more likely to develop atherosclerotic vascular disease, women appear to do less well following an acute MI [6,7,11,12]. Whether this reflects a true gender-based difference, older age at presentation, or simply recruitment bias associated with randomized clinical trials is not clear. Similarly, although cigarette smoking is associated with a greater risk of developing vascular disease, patients who smoke have a lower in-hospital mortality following ST-segment elevation MI (STEMI) [13]. This "smoker's paradox" is thought to reflect smoking-related imbalances in hemostasis that result in not only a greater propensity for intravascular thrombus formation, but also a better response to fibrinolytic therapy [14].

Acute thrombotic risk

The markers of thrombotic risk in patients with ACS are outlined in **Box 2**. Cardiac risk variables by which patients with ACS could

---

Box 2. Markers of thrombotic risk in patients with acute coronary syndromes. The evidence for the item in brackets is less clear than for other factors.

Tempo of angina

Response to medical therapy

Dynamic electrocardiogram changes

Elevated markers of myocardial damage

Intracoronary thrombus

(Elevated inflammatory markers)

---

potentially be stratified include appropriate clinical symptoms, electrocardiogram (ECG) findings, and markers of myocardial damage, inflammation, and hemostasis.

Symptoms

In the majority of cases, the hallmark of ACS is the presence of appropriate clinical symptoms. A classification system for unstable angina based on symptoms was first proposed by Braunwald in 1989 and has subsequently been validated in several large-scale clinical trials (see **Table 1**) [15]. The major limitation of risk assessment based on symptoms alone, however, is a lack of specificity [16]. As a result, a great deal of effort has been put into identifying additional variables that stratify patients with ACS on the basis of cardiac risk.

The electrocardiogram

In addition to its diagnostic potential, the ECG can provide valuable prognostic information in the setting of ACS. The presence of ST-segment deviation, be it elevation or depression, is associated with a significant increase in cardiac risk [17]. Additional prognostic information may be obtained from the vectorial sum

Table 1. Symptomatic presentation of angina and short-term cardiac risk. Adapted from *Circulation* 1989;80:410–4.

Cardiac risk	Presentation	Symptom description
Low	Increasing angina	Deterioration in previously stable angina (eg, increase in frequency, duration, or lower threshold)
Medium	New-onset angina	Recent onset angina markedly limiting daily activities
High	Rest angina	Anginal symptoms at rest, usually lasting >20 minutes

and distribution of ST–segment deviation, reflecting the volume and distribution of threatened myocardium [18]. Moreover, in patients presenting with acute MI receiving reperfusion therapy, the time taken for the ST-segment elevation to resolve correlates with mortality [19,20].

Silent myocardial ischemia occurs in as many as a third of patients with ACS. It may be identified by ST-segment shift during continuous ST monitoring and is associated with an increased risk of cardiovascular events [21,22]. In contrast, minor changes in T-wave morphology are of limited prognostic value [23]. Of note, patients with suspected ACS in whom the admission ECG pattern prevents ST-segment interpretation (due either to bundle branch block, left ventricular [LV] hypertrophy, or a paced rhythm) have the greatest risk of death [18,24].

Markers of myocardial damage

Arguably one of the single most important advances in the management of ACS in recent years has been the recognition that circulating markers of myocardial damage play a key role in the identification of intermediate- and high–risk patients [25,26]. Although creatine kinase MB remains an acceptable diagnostic marker of MI, the presence of creatine kinase MB in plasma, in both healthy individuals and those who have suffered skeletal muscle damage, limits its prognostic value. As a result, the use of creatine kinase as a prognostic marker in patients with ACS has largely been superseded by the measurement of cardiac troponin levels.

The troponins (T, I, and C), components of the troponin–tropomyosin complex, are involved in the regulation of striated muscle contraction. Antibody-based assays have been developed that are specific for the cardiac isoforms of troponin T and I. Elevated troponin levels, not normally detectable in the absence of recent myocardial necrosis, strongly predict death and recurrent infarction both in the short and long term in patients with ACS [27,28]. Moreover, a direct correlation exists between troponin elevation and the risk of death in these patients [28]. In the FRISC trial, which examined treatment with low molecular weight heparin (LMWH) in patients with ACS, peak troponin levels of <0.06 μg/L, 0.06–0.59 μg/L, and ≥ 0.6 μg/L in the 24 hours following enrolment in the study were associated with a cardiovascular mortality rate at 2 years of 1.2%, 8.7%, and 15.8%, respectively [2]. Moreover, this prognostic information appears to be both independent of, and additive to, information obtained from other biochemical markers or ECG changes [29].

Although elevated troponin levels have been reported in patients with renal insufficiency in the absence of significant myocardial ischemia [30], analysis of the recent GUSTO-IV ACS trial has confirmed that troponin levels remain a powerful prognostic marker in patients with ACS and impaired renal function [31]. Indeed, the presence of these two risk markers in combination was associated with the greatest risk of death or MI [31].

Markers of inflammation

Evidence of a role for inflammation in the pathophysiology of atherosclerosis has led to the investigation of a number of acute phase inflammatory proteins as prognostic markers in ACS [32]. There is substantial evidence that serum levels of C-reactive protein provide prognostic information in ACS that is independent of, and additive to, information supplied by troponin estimation [2,33–36]. However, C–reactive protein is a general marker of inflammation and is not cardiac specific.

Whether the results of population-based studies can be applied at an individual level is not yet clear. Additional inflammatory markers that may be of prognostic value in ACS include tumor necrosis factor-α, interleukin-6, serum amyloid protein, and, more recently, soluble CD40 ligand, a marker of platelet activation [37–41].

Markers of hemostasis

The presence of intracoronary thrombus in the setting of ACS is associated with a poor clinical outcome [26]. A number of surrogate markers of activation of the coagulation and fibrinolytic cascades, including fibrinogen [2], have been associated with increased cardiac risk. However, current guidelines do not recommend the use of hemostatic markers for risk assessment in ACS [25,26].

Risk of complications of the ischemic event

Complications of ACS that are associated with increased risk are outlined in **Box 3**.

Left ventricular dysfunction

Evidence of LV dysfunction (Killip class ≥2, gallop rhythm, hypotension, tachycardia, or pulmonary rales) is highly predictive of a poor outcome in patients with ACS. Indeed, the presence of cardiogenic shock in patients with ACS is associated with mortality rates in excess of 50%, irrespective of whether ST-segment elevation is present on the admission ECG [42,43].

More recently, brain (B-type) natriuretic peptide and its N-terminal fragment have been shown to be powerful predictors of mortality,

---

Box 3. Complications of acute coronary syndromes associated with increased risk.

Evidence of left ventricular dysfunction:

- clinical examination
- echocardiography
- radiological or angiographic
- brain natriuretic peptide
- N-terminal brain natriuretic peptide

Ventricular arrhythmias

---

heart failure, and recurrent infarction in patients with ACS [44–46]. Moreover, in patients with MI, the predictive value of brain natriuretic peptide appears to be independent of prognostic information obtained from estimation of LV ejection fraction [47].

Ventricular arrhythmias

Ventricular arrhythmias are common in the setting of ACS. Although the predictive value of ventricular ectopy and nonsustained ventricular arrhythmias in all forms of ACS is limited, sustained ventricular arrhythmias (both early [within 24 hours] and late) or cardiac arrest are associated with a higher in-hospital and longer term mortality [7,48,49]. In addition, evidence of high-degree heart block is also associated with a worse outcome.

Risk-scoring systems

Individual clinical and biochemical variables can be used to stratify patient populations on the basis of cardiac risk in the setting of ACS. However combining these variables to allow accurate and reproducible risk prediction at an individual level is more complex and has led to the development of a number of risk-scoring systems, for patients with both STEMI [6,50,51] and non-ST elevation MI (NSTEMI) (see **Table 2**) [5,7,52].

For risk assessment to be effective, the algorithms employed need to be easy to use, accurate, and available at the bedside. One commonly used scoring system that fulfills these criteria is the TIMI risk score for use in patients presenting with ACS without ST elevation [7]. Developed from the TIMI 11B trial comparing enoxaparin with unfractionated heparin in the treatment of unstable angina and NSTEMI, the TIMI system assigns a binary score to seven independent risk factors with similar predictive value (see **Table 2**) [7]. The risk of death or recurrent ischemia rises from 4.7% with a TIMI score of 0 to a staggering 40.9%

Authors	Origin	Outcome	Component variables
Morrow et al. [6] (TIMI-STEMI)	InTIME II trial (STEMI)	Mortality	Age ≥65 years, systolic BP <100 mm Hg, heart rate >100 bpm, Killip class II–IV, anterior ST elevation or LBBB, diabetes/hypertension/angina, weight <67 kg, time to treatment >4 hours
Morrow et al. [50]	InTIME II trial (STEMI)	Mortality, recurrent infarction, or recurrent ischemia requiring revascularization	Age, heart rate, systolic BP
Califf et al. [75]	GUSTO-I (STEMI)	Mortality	Age, previous infarction, presence of heart failure, (ejection fraction), (heart rate)
Krumholz et al. [51]	Medicare database (Cooperative Cardiovascular Project database of patients >65 years with confirmed acute myocardial infarction)	Mortality	Age, cardiac arrest, territory of infarction, systolic BP, white blood cell count, serum creatinine, presence of heart failure
Antman et al. [7] (TIMI-NSTEMI/UA)	TIMI 11B (ACS without persistent ST elevation)	Mortality	Age ≥65 years, ≥3 risk factors for CAD, coronary artery stenosis >50%, ST deviation, severe prodromal angina, recent aspirin use (<7 days), elevated cardiac markers
Boersma et al. [5]	PURSUIT trial (ACS without persistent ST elevation)	Mortality	Age, gender, recent angina severity, heart rate, systolic BP, presence of heart failure, ST depression
Cohen et al. [52]	ESSENCE trial (ACS without persistent ST elevation)	Mortality, reinfarction, recurrent angina	Elevated cardiac markers, ST depression, country of enrollment, age ≥75 years, severity of prior angina, presence of pulmonary rales
Granger et al. [57]	GRACE registry (entire spectrum of ACS)	Mortality	Age, diabetes/hypertension, heart rate, systolic BP, Killip class, cardiac arrest, cardiac enzymes, serum creatinine, electrocardiographic changes

Table 2. Comparison of selected combined risk assessment models for use in patients with acute coronary syndromes (ACS). BP: blood pressure; CAD: coronary artery disease; LBBB: left bundle branch block; NSTEMI: non-ST-segment elevation myocardial infarction; STEMI: ST-segment elevation myocardial infarction; UA: unstable angina.

with a TIMI score of 6 or more [7]. Interestingly, the TIMI risk score makes no use of continuous variables such as blood pressure (BP) and heart rate, nor the presence of heart failure (all strong predictors of mortality in their own right) [42,50]. This probably reflects the need for simplicity and the relatively low incidence of heart failure in the original, highly selected, TIMI 11B population [53].

Although the TIMI risk score has been validated in both clinical trials [7,54] and unselected patient populations from registries of ACS [55], its use thus far has been limited to ACS without ST-segment elevation. A similar prognostic scoring system has been developed from clinical trials of patients presenting with STEMI [6]. This model includes an assessment of hemodynamic variables as well as the presence of heart failure and has been validated in an unselected population presenting with the entire spectrum of ACS [56].

Additional models often necessitate more complicated algorithms and include continuous variables in an effort to increase both predictive power and reliability. One such scoring system has recently been developed from GRACE, a large-scale registry of patients admitted with ACS, with or without ST-segment elevation, to 94 hospitals across 14 countries [57]. Using multivariate logistic regression, the GRACE model identified prognostically significant variables (age, diabetes/hypertension, heart rate, systolic BP, Killip class, cardiac arrest, elevated cardiac enzymes, serum creatinine, and ECG changes [see **Table 2**]) and used these to generate a nomogram of patient risk. The high predictive power of the GRACE model is due, in part, to the inclusion of two novel variables not previously incorporated in large-scale models of risk in ACS: serum creatinine and resuscitated cardiac arrest. Moreover, the advantages of this model include the absence of the selection bias normally associated with stringent trial entry criteria and its ability to accurately predict in-hospital mortality across the entire spectrum of ACS [57].

One potential drawback to the practical application of multivariate risk models that incorporate continuous variables is their complexity. It is anticipated, however, that the increasing availability of hand-held computers should facilitate the use of more complicated risk assessment protocols at the patient's bedside.

Risk prediction and response to therapy

There is now substantial evidence that risk assessment may be used to target specific therapies within the setting of ACS. The reduction in cardiac events associated with the use of LMWH and intravenous glycoprotein (GP)IIb/IIIa inhibitors in ACS appears to be largely restricted to patients with elevated troponin levels [27,58–60]. In addition, troponin-positive patients would appear to benefit most from an early invasive strategy when compared with those who are troponin negative [61–63]. In the recent TACTICS-TIMI 18 trial, there was an absolute risk reduction of 9.6% in the primary endpoint of death, MI, or readmission in troponin-positive patients with ACS who were randomized to an early invasive strategy compared with conventional conservative management [62]. This benefit was not seen in troponin-negative patients [62]. Similarly, ECG evidence of ST-segment deviation may be used to identify high-risk patients who may benefit from specific antithrombotic treatment or an early invasive strategy [18,63,64].

The ability of the TIMI risk score to predict which patients benefit from specific therapeutic strategies in ACS has also been assessed retrospectively in a number of studies. As with troponin estimation, the treatment benefits associated with LMWH [54], GPIIb/IIIa inhibitors [65], or an invasive strategy [66,67] were greater in patients with higher TIMI risk scores. In contrast, the CURE study demonstrated that the treatment benefit associated with the use of the platelet ADP receptor antagonist, clopidogrel, in combination with aspirin therapy, was similar in all patients with ACS, irrespective of their TIMI risk score

[68]. These data agree with the findings of the earlier CAPRIE study, a secondary prevention trial comparing long-term aspirin with clopidogrel in high-risk patients, and imply that platelet inhibition is advantageous in all patients with ACS [69,70].

Despite a substantial body of evidence, the use of risk stratification to target specific therapies within the spectrum of ACS has not been evaluated in prospective clinical trials. However, current European and US guidelines on the management of patients with ACS (without ST-segment elevation) recommend the integration of clinical findings, ECG data, and cardiac markers to identify high-risk patients who may benefit from specific antithrombotic therapy and an early invasive strategy [25,26].

Chest pain assessment units

Chest pain assessment units first arose from the need to administer timely and life-saving reperfusion therapy to patients presenting with acute STEMI [71,72]. Subsequent work has demonstrated that, in combination with appropriate risk-scoring algorithms, chest pain assessment units provide a safe and effective means of triaging and managing patients presenting with chest pain [73,74]. Patients identified as being at high risk are admitted to coronary care units for specific anti-ischemic therapy, whilst low-risk patients may be reassured and safely discharged with appropriate outpatient follow-up. Clinical trials have not only confirmed the efficacy of chest pain assessment units, but have demonstrated that the improvements in patient care are mirrored by significant reductions in service expenditure and resource use [73].

Professional guidelines for risk stratification

The importance of professional guidelines in the current era of clinical governance is clear. In 2000, the European Society of Cardiology and the American College of Cardiology/American Heart Association published their respective recommendations on the management of patients with ACS [25,26]. Not surprisingly, these consensus documents reach similar conclusions. Risk stratification should be performed early in the management of patients presenting with ACS, repeated throughout their management, and used both to determine the most appropriate management setting for an individual and to identify high-risk groups who might benefit from specific antithrombotic treatment or an early invasive strategy. Estimation of risk should be based on clinical presentation and examination, gender, age, historical features, ECG findings, and laboratory estimation of markers of myocardial damage, namely troponins. A single estimation of troponin is insufficient and repeat testing is recommended, either at 8–12 hours following the onset of symptoms or 6–12 hours after admission.

One important difference between the guidelines is the distinction in the European recommendations between short- and long-term risk [26]. Short-term risk is based on the acute thrombotic potential and highlights the importance of prognostic markers, such as the presence of intracoronary thrombus at angiography. Long-term risk is largely determined by the presence and extent of underlying vascular disease and its assessment should include the measurement of C-reactive protein. Both reports stress the need to continually revise risk estimation as additional information becomes available. Where appropriate, this may include echocardiographic, angiographic, or radionuclear evidence of LV dysfunction, the extent and distribution of coronary disease at angiography, and the results of noninvasive testing for myocardial ischemia.

Future developments

Our current understanding of risk stratification in ACS is based largely on information obtained retrospectively or *post hoc* from clinical trials and patient registries. Expanding this evidence base to include large-scale prospective studies will help to determine the extent to which specific biomarkers improve the prognostic accuracy of thrombotic and vascular risk assessment and confirm the clinical efficacy of risk-scoring algorithms in the management of patients with ACS.

The identification of specific genetic polymorphisms, or clusters of polymorphisms, associated with increased risk in ACS may provide more robust prognostic information than is currently available from the family history. Whether this information will simply aid risk prediction at a population level or will be applicable to the individual is unclear. One promising area within this field is the use of pharmacogenetics to identify patients in whom specific therapies may be more, or potentially less, effective, thus allowing the physician to modify risk more effectively.

Conclusions

Risk stratification has become a cornerstone in the management of patients presenting with suspected or confirmed ACS. The integration of readily available clinical and laboratory data as part of a practical risk-scoring algorithm, combined with the development of chest pain assessment units, allows physicians to target high-risk patients with appropriate therapy whilst safely discharging those identified as being at low risk for future cardiac events. Equally important in our current economic climate is the evidence that these clinical improvements are associated with significant improvements in resource use and health care expenditure.

References

1. Newby LK, Califf RM, Guerci A, et al. Early discharge in the thrombolytic era: an analysis of criteria for uncomplicated infarction from the Global Utilization of Streptokinase and t-PA for Occluded Coronary Arteries (GUSTO) trial. *J Am Coll Cardiol* 1996;27:625–32.
2. Lindahl B, Toss H, Siegbahn A, et al. Markers of myocardial damage and inflammation in relation to long-term mortality in unstable coronary artery disease. FRISC Study Group. Fragmin during Instability in Coronary Artery Disease. *N Engl J Med* 2000;343:1139–47.
3. Lee KL, Woodlief LH, Topol EJ, et al. Predictors of 30-day mortality in the era of reperfusion for acute myocardial infarction. Results from an international trial of 41,021 patients. GUSTO-I Investigators. *Circulation* 1995;91:1659–68.
4. Mueller HS, Cohen LS, Braunwald E, et al. Predictors of early morbidity and mortality after thrombolytic therapy of acute myocardial infarction. Analyses of patient subgroups in the Thrombolysis in Myocardial Infarction (TIMI) trial, phase II. *Circulation* 1992;85:1254–64.
5. Boersma E, Pieper KS, Steyerberg EW, et al. Predictors of outcome in patients with acute coronary syndromes without persistent ST-segment elevation. Results from an international trial of 9461 patients. The PURSUIT Investigators. *Circulation* 2000;101:2557–67.
6. Morrow DA, Antman EM, Charlesworth A, et al. TIMI risk score for ST-elevation myocardial infarction: A convenient, bedside, clinical score for risk assessment at presentation: An intravenous nPA for treatment of infarcting myocardium early II trial substudy. *Circulation* 2000;102:2031–7.
7. Antman EM, Cohen M, Bernink PJ, et al. The TIMI risk score for unstable angina/non-ST elevation MI: A method for prognostication and therapeutic decision making. *JAMA* 2000;284:835–42.
8. Brieger DB, Mak KH, White HD, et al. Benefit of early sustained reperfusion in patients with prior myocardial infarction (the GUSTO-I trial). Global Utilization of Streptokinase and TPA for occluded arteries. *Am J Cardiol* 1998;81:282–7.
9. Ginsberg HN. Treatment for patients with the metabolic syndrome. *Am J Cardiol* 2003;91:29E–39E.
10. Wison S, Foo K, Cunningham J, et al. Renal function and risk stratification in acute coronary syndromes. *Am J Cardiol* 2003;91:1051–4.
11. Scirica BM, Moliterno DJ, Every NR, et al. Differences between men and women in the management of unstable angina pectoris (The GUARANTEE Registry). The GUARANTEE Investigators. *Am J Cardiol* 1999;84:1145–50.
12. Hochman JS, McCabe CH, Stone PH, et al. Outcome and profile of women and men presenting with acute coronary syndromes: a report from TIMI IIIB. TIMI Investigators. Thrombolysis in Myocardial Infarction. *J Am Coll Cardiol* 1997;30:141–8.
13. Barbash GI, White HD, Modan M, et al. Significance of smoking in patients receiving thrombolytic therapy for acute myocardial infarction. Experience gleaned from the International Tissue Plasminogen Activator/Streptokinase Mortality Trial. *Circulation* 1993;87:53–8.
14. Zahger D, Cercek B, Cannon CP, et al. How do smokers differ from nonsmokers in their response to thrombolysis? (the TIMI-4 trial). *Am J Cardiol* 1995;75:232–6.
15. Braunwald E. Unstable angina. A classification. *Circulation* 1989;80:410–4.

16. Bugiardini R, Borghi A, Pozzati A, et al. Relation of severity of symptoms to transient myocardial ischemia and prognosis in unstable angina. *J Am Coll Cardiol* 1995;25:597–604.

17. Savonitto S, Ardissino D, Granger CB, et al. Prognostic value of the admission electrocardiogram in acute coronary syndromes. *JAMA* 1999;281:707–13.

18. Holmvang L, Clemmensen P, Lindahl B, et al. Quantitative analysis of the admission electrocardiogram identifies patients with unstable coronary artery disease who benefit the most from early invasive treatment. *J Am Coll Cardiol* 2003;41:905–15.

19. Johanson P, Jernberg T, Gunnarsson G, et al. Prognostic value of ST-segment resolution-when and what to measure. *Eur Heart J* 2003;24:337–45.

20. Schroder R, Wegscheider K, Schroder K, et al. Extent of early ST segment elevation resolution: a strong predictor of outcome in patients with acute myocardial infarction and a sensitive measure to compare thrombolytic regimens. A substudy of the International Joint Efficacy Comparison of Thrombolytics (INJECT) trial. *J Am Coll Cardiol* 1995;26:1657–64.

21. Patel DJ, Holdright DR, Knight CJ, et al. Early continuous ST segment monitoring in unstable angina: prognostic value additional to the clinical characteristics and the admission electrocardiogram. *Heart* 1996;75:222–8.

22. Langer A, Krucoff MW, Klootwijk P, et al. Prognostic significance of ST segment shift early after resolution of ST elevation in patients with myocardial infarction treated with thrombolytic therapy: the GUSTO-I ST Segment Monitoring Substudy. *J Am Coll Cardiol* 1998;31:783–9.

23. Cannon CP, McCabe CH, Stone PH, et al. The electrocardiogram predicts one-year outcome of patients with unstable angina and non-Q wave myocardial infarction: results of the TIMI III Registry ECG Ancillary Study. Thrombolysis in Myocardial Ischemia. *J Am Coll Cardiol* 1997;30:133–40.

24. Lev EI, Battler A, Behar S, et al. Frequency, characteristics, and outcome of patients hospitalized with acute coronary syndromes with undetermined electrocardiographic patterns. *Am J Cardiol* 2003;91:224–7.

25. Braunwald E, Antman EM, Beasley JW, et al. ACC/AHA guidelines for the management of patients with unstable angina and nonST-segment elevation myocardial infarction: executive summary and recommendations. A report of the American College of Cardiology/American Heart Association task force on practice guidelines (committee on the management of patients with unstable angina). *Circulation* 2000;102:1193–209.

26. Bertrand ME, Simoons ML, Fox KA, et al. Management of acute coronary syndromes in patients presenting without persistent ST-segment elevation. *Eur Heart J* 2002;23:1809–40.

27. Hamm CW, Heeschen C, Goldmann B, et al. Benefit of abciximab in patients with refractory unstable angina in relation to serum troponin T levels. c7E3 Fab Antiplatelet Therapy in Unstable Refractory Angina (CAPTURE) Study Investigators. *N Engl J Med* 1999;340:1623–9. Erratum in: *N Engl J Med* 1999;341:548.

28. Antman EM, Tanasijevic MJ, Thompson B, et al. Cardiac-specific troponin I levels to predict the risk of mortality in patients with acute coronary syndromes. *N Engl J Med* 1996;335:1342–9.

29. Kaul P, Newby LK, Fu Y, et al. Troponin T and quantitative ST-segment depression offer complementary prognostic information in the risk stratification of acute coronary syndrome patients. *J Am Coll Cardiol* 2003;41:371–80.

30. Freda BJ, Tang WH, Van Lente F, et al. Cardiac troponins in renal insufficiency: review and clinical implications. *J Am Coll Cardiol* 2002;40:2065–71.

31. Aviles RJ, Askari AT, Lindahl B, et al. Troponin T levels in patients with acute coronary syndromes, with or without renal dysfunction. *N Engl J Med* 2002;346:2047–52.

32. Ross R. Atherosclerosis-an inflammatory disease. *N Engl J Med* 1999;340:115–26.
33. Liuzzo G, Biasucci LM, Gallimore JR, et al. The prognostic value of C-reactive protein and serum amyloid a protein in severe unstable angina. *N Engl J Med* 1994;331:417–24.
34. Morrow DA, Rifai N, Antman EM, et al. C-reactive protein is a potent predictor of mortality independently of and in combination with troponin T in acute coronary syndromes: a TIMI 11A substudy. Thrombolysis in Myocardial Infarction. *J Am Coll Cardiol* 1998;31:1460–65.
35. Heeschen C, Hamm CW, Bruemmer J, et al. Predictive value of C-reactive protein and troponin T in patients with unstable angina: a comparative analysis. CAPTURE Investigators. Chimeric c7E3 AntiPlatelet Therapy in Unstable angina REfractory to standard treatment trial. *J Am Coll Cardiol* 2000;35:1535–42.
36. Pietila K, Harmoinen A, Teppo AM. Acute phase reaction, infarct size and in-hospital morbidity in myocardial infarction patients treated with streptokinase or recombinant tissue type plasminogen activator. *Ann Med* 1991;23:529–35.
37. Ridker PM, Rifai N, Stampfer MJ, et al. Plasma concentration of interleukin-6 and the risk of future myocardial infarction among apparently healthy men. *Circulation* 2000;101:1767–72.
38. Ridker PM, Rifai N, Pfeffer M, et al. Elevation of tumor necrosis factor-alpha and increased risk of recurrent coronary events after myocardial infarction. *Circulation* 2000;101:2149–53.
39. Lindmark E, Diderholm E, Wallentin L, et al. Relationship between interleukin 6 and mortality in patients with unstable coronary artery disease: effects of an early invasive or noninvasive strategy. *JAMA* 2001;286:2107–13.
40. Morrow DA, Rifai N, Antman EM, et al. Serum amyloid A predicts early mortality in acute coronary syndromes: A TIMI 11A substudy. *J Am Coll Cardiol* 2000;35:358–62.
41. Heeschen C, Dimmeler S, Hamm CW, et al. Soluble CD40 ligand in acute coronary syndromes. *N Engl J Med* 2003;348:1104–11.
42. Hochman JS, Sleeper LA, Webb JG, et al. Early revascularization in acute myocardial infarction complicated by cardiogenic shock. SHOCK Investigators. Should We Emergently Revascularize Occluded Coronaries for Cardiogenic Shock. *N Engl J Med.* 1999;341:625–34.
43. Holmes DR Jr, Berger PB, Hochman JS, et al. Cardiogenic shock in patients with acute ischemic syndromes with and without ST-segment elevation. *Circulation* 1999;100:2067–73.
44. Omland T, Persson A, Ng L, et al. N-terminal pro-B-type natriuretic peptide and long-term mortality in acute coronary syndromes. *Circulation* 2002;106:2913–8.
45. Omland T, Aakvaag A, Bonarjee VV, et al. Plasma brain natriuretic peptide as an indicator of left ventricular systolic function and long-term survival after acute myocardial infarction. Comparison with plasma atrial natriuretic peptide and N-terminal proatrial natriuretic peptide. *Circulation* 1996;93:1963–9.
46. de Lemos JA, Morrow DA, Bentley JH, et al. The prognostic value of B-type natriuretic peptide in patients with acute coronary syndromes. *N Engl J Med* 2001;345:1014–21.
47. Richards AM, Nicholls MG, Espiner EA, et al. B-type natriuretic peptides and ejection fraction for prognosis after myocardial infarction. *Circulation* 2003;107:2786–92.
48. Newby KH, Thompson T, Stebbins A, et al. Sustained ventricular arrhythmias in patients receiving thrombolytic therapy: incidence and outcomes. The GUSTO Investigators. *Circulation* 1998;98:2567–73.
49. Al Khatib SM, Granger CB, Huang Y, et al. Sustained ventricular arrhythmias among patients with acute coronary syndromes with no ST-segment elevation: incidence, predictors, and outcomes. *Circulation* 2002;106:309–12.

50. Morrow DA, Antman EM, Giugliano RP, et al. A simple risk index for rapid initial triage of patients with ST-elevation myocardial infarction: an InTIME II substudy. *Lancet* 2001;358:1571–5.

51. Krumholz HM, Chen J, Wang Y, et al. Comparing AMI mortality among hospitals in patients 65 years of age and older: evaluating methods of risk adjustment. *Circulation* 1999;99:2986–92.

52. Cohen M, Stinnett SS, Weatherley BD, et al. Predictors of recurrent ischemic events and death in unstable coronary artery disease after treatment with combination antithrombotic therapy. *Am Heart J* 2000;139:962–70.

53. Ohman EM, Granger CB, Harrington RA, et al. Risk stratification and therapeutic decision making in acute coronary syndromes. *JAMA* 2000;284:876–8.

54. Sabatine MS, McCabe CH, Morrow DA, et al. Identification of patients at high risk for death and cardiac ischemic events after hospital discharge. *Am Heart J* 2002;143:966–70.

55. Scirica BM, Cannon CP, Antman EM, et al. Validation of the thrombolysis in myocardial infarction (TIMI) risk score for unstable angina pectoris and nonST-elevation myocardial infarction in the TIMI III registry. *Am J Cardiol* 2002;90:303–5.

56. Ilkhanoff L, O'Donnell CJ, Camargo CA, et al. The TIMI Risk Index Predicts In-hospital and Long-term Mortality in Unselected Patients with Myocardial Infarction. *Acad Emerg Med* 2003;10:429–30.

57. Granger CB, Goldberg RJ, Dabbous O, et al. Predictors of hospital mortality in the Global Registry of Acute Coronary Events. *Arch Intern Med* 2003;163:2345–53.

58. Lindahl B, Venge P, Wallentin L. Troponin T identifies patients with unstable coronary artery disease who benefit from long-term antithrombotic protection. Fragmin in Unstable Coronary Artery Disease (FRISC) Study Group. *J Am Coll Cardiol* 1997;29:43–8.

59. Morrow DA, Antman EM, Tanasijevic M, et al. Cardiac troponin I for stratification of early outcomes and the efficacy of enoxaparin in unstable angina: a TIMI-11B substudy. *J Am Coll Cardiol* 2000;36:1812–7.

60. Heeschen C, Hamm CW, Goldmann B, et al. Troponin concentrations for stratification of patients with acute coronary syndromes in relation to therapeutic efficacy of tirofiban. PRISM Study Investigators. Platelet Receptor Inhibition in Ischemic Syndrome Management. *Lancet* 1999;354:1757–62.

61. Morrow DA, Cannon CP, Rifai N, et al. Ability of minor elevations of troponins I and T to predict benefit from an early invasive strategy in patients with unstable angina and nonST elevation myocardial infarction: results from a randomized trial. *JAMA* 2001;286:2405–12.

62. Cannon CP, Weintraub WS, Demopoulos LA, et al. Comparison of early invasive and conservative strategies in patients with unstable coronary syndromes treated with the glycoprotein IIb/IIIa inhibitor tirofiban. *N Engl J Med* 2001;344:1879–87.

63. Diderholm E, Andren B, Frostfeldt G, et al. The prognostic and therapeutic implications of increased troponin T levels and ST depression in unstable coronary artery disease: the FRISC II invasive troponin T electrocardiogram substudy. *Am Heart J* 2002;143:760–7.

64. Cohen M, Antman EM, Gurfinkel EP, et al. Enoxaparin in unstable angina/non-ST-segment elevation myocardial infarction: treatment benefits in prespecified subgroups. *J Thromb Thrombolysis* 2001;12:199-206.

65. Morrow DA, Antman EM, Snapinn SM, et al. An integrated clinical approach to predicting the benefit of tirofiban innonST elevation acute coronary syndromes. Application of the TIMI Risk Score for UA/NSTEMI in PRISM-PLUS. *Eur Heart J* 2002;23:223–9.

66. Cannon CP. Small molecule glycoprotein IIb/IIIa receptor inhibitors as upstream therapy in acute coronary syndromes. Insights from the TACTICS TIMI-18 trial. *J Am Coll Cardiol* 2003;41:43S–48S.

67. Samaha FF, Kimmel SE, Kizer JR, et al. Usefulness of the TIMI risk score in predicting both short- and long-term outcomes in the Veterans Affairs nonQ-Wave Myocardial Infarction Strategies In-Hospital (VANQWISH) Trial. *Am J Cardiol* 2002;90:922–6.

68. Budaj A, Yusuf S, Mehta SR, et al. Benefit of clopidogrel in patients with acute coronary syndromes without ST-segment elevation in various risk groups. *Circulation* 2002;106:1622–6.

69. Cannon CP. Evidence-based risk stratification to target therapies in acute coronary syndromes. *Circulation* 2002;106:1588–91.

70. Cannon CP; CAPRIE Investigators. Effectiveness of clopidogrel versus aspirin in preventing acute myocardial infarction in patients with symptomatic atherothrombosis (CAPRIE trial). *Am J Cardiol* 2002;90:760–2.

71. Bahr RD. Chest pain centers: moving toward proactive acute coronary care. *Int J Cardiol* 2000;72:101–10.

72. Newby LK, Mark DB. The chest-pain unit-ready for prime time? *N Engl J Med* 1998;339:1930–2.

73. Farkouh ME, Smars PA, Reeder GS, et al. A clinical trial of a chest-pain observation unit for patients with unstable angina. Chest Pain Evaluation in the Emergency Room (CHEER) Investigators. *N Engl J Med* 1998;339:1882–8.

74. Gibler WB, Runyon JP, Levy RC, et al. A rapid diagnostic and treatment center for patients with chest pain in the emergency department. *Ann Emerg Med* 1995;25:1–8.

75. Califf RM, Pieper KS, Lee KL, et al. Prediction of 1-year survival after thrombolysis for acute myocardial infarction in the global utilization of streptokinase and TPA for occluded coronary arteries trial. *Circulation* 2000;101:2231–8.

4
Antiplatelet agents

Anil K Taneja, Umair Mallick, & Marcus D Flather

Introduction

Acute coronary syndromes (ACS) are usually caused by plaque rupture, platelet activation, and thrombus formation leading to partial or total occlusion of a coronary artery. The main triggers of platelet activation are thromboxane A_2, epinephrine, collagen, thrombin, and ADP. Platelets, therefore, play a key role in the pathogenesis of ACS [1].

In this chapter, we discuss the role of three categories of antiplatelet agents commonly used in the early management of ACS: aspirin, thienopyridines (ticlopidine and clopidogrel), and platelet glycoprotein (GP)IIb/IIIa surface receptor antagonists (abciximab, eptifibatide, and tirofiban). Other antiplatelets such as dipyridamole are not discussed, as their efficacy in the treatment of ACS has not been established.

This chapter covers the mechanism of action, clinical trial evidence, guidelines, and clinical use of antiplatelet agents in ACS, and gives a short summary of platelet function and physiology. Each antiplatelet agent is presented in the context of ACS with and without persistent ST-segment elevation on the presenting electrocardiograph (ECG).

The Antithrombotic Therapy Trialists' (ATT) collaboration identified all randomized trials of antiplatelet therapy up to 1997 [2]. A total of 287 studies, involving 135,000 patients, compared antiplatelet therapies with placebo; in 77,000 of the patients, one agent was compared with

Figure 1. Main findings of the Antithrombotic Therapy Trialists' collaboration. A circle represents the meta-analysis of results for all trials (and 95% confidence intervals [CIs]), showing the effects of antiplatelet therapy on vascular events (stroke, myocardial infarction, or vascular death) in five high-risk categories. Squares represent the groups; horizontal lines represent the 99% CI. Adjusted control totals have been calculated after converting any unevenly randomized trials to even ones, by counting control groups more than once; other statistical calculations are based on actual numbers from individual trials. Adapted from *Br Med J* 2002;324:71–86.

another. The main findings of the ATT collaboration are summarized in **Figure 1**. Antiplatelet therapy was associated with a proportional reduction of 22% ($P = 0.0001$) in the composite outcome of vascular death, nonfatal stroke, or nonfatal myocardial infarction (MI).

Platelet function and physiology

Platelets are small cells (2–4 μm in diameter) produced as fragments of a large precursor cell (the megakaryocyte) by budding in the bone marrow. Platelets provide the initial hemostatic plug at sites of vascular injury. They also contribute to mechanisms that lead to atherosclerosis and thrombosis.

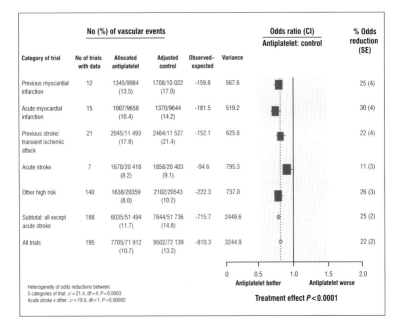

The normal human platelet count is 150,000–300,000/mm³ and normal platelets survive in the circulation for 8–12 days unless activated in response to vessel injury. Old or abnormal platelets are mostly removed by macrophages in the spleen. Platelets are involved in primary hemostasis by interacting with the vascular endothelium to stop bleeding following vessel injury. Hemostasis occurs in three main steps:

- vascular spasm (vasoconstriction at injured site)
- platelet plug formation
- coagulation

The steps involved in the mechanism of platelet action are summarized in **Figure 2**.

Figure 2. Platelet action.

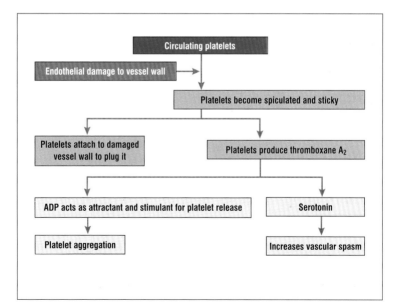

Platelet plug formation is a more complex process than vascular spasm and takes place in three consecutive steps: platelet adhesion, the release reaction, and platelet aggregation. Two types of chemical granules are held within the cytoplasm of platelets: alpha granules (which contain clotting factors, growth factors, and fibroblasts) and dense granules (which contain ADP, ATP, calcium ions, and serotonin). Nearby platelets are activated by the release of ADP and thromboxane A_2 (a prostaglandin found within platelets); this is the release reaction. Thromboxane A_2 and serotonin act to cause vasoconstriction. Platelet aggregation involves ADP acting to make the nearby platelets sticky and adhere to the other recruited platelets. When the collection is large enough, it creates a platelet plug to stop blood loss.

Aspirin

In about the 5th century BC, the Greeks discovered a substance (now called salicin) from the bark of the willow tree that could relieve pain. The first recorded use of aspirin, derived originally from salicin, was in 1828 when Johann Buchner, Professor of Pharmacy at the University of Munich, isolated salicin as a tiny amount of bitter-tasting, yellow, needle-like crystals. Two Italians, Brugnatelli and Fontana, had in fact already obtained salicin in 1826, but in a highly impure form. Because of its anti-inflammatory, analgesic, and antiplatelet properties, aspirin has been used to treat a number of indications [3].

Mechanism of action

Figures 3 and **4** illustrate aspirin's mechanism of action. It is readily absorbed from the stomach and upper intestine. It is then hydrolyzed, releasing acetyl groups that inactivate the enzyme cyclo-oxygenase (COX) in platelets. COX catalyses the conversion of arachidonic acid to prostaglandin G_2 and thromboxane A_2. The latter is a potent mediator of platelet aggregation and vasoconstriction. Inhibition of COX is irreversible and thus the effects of aspirin last until new platelets are formed [4]. Bleeding times generally return to normal within 48 hours of stopping aspirin.

However, platelet aggregation and thrombosis can occur in spite of treatment with aspirin, as ADP, collagen, and thrombin may also lead to platelet aggregation. The antiplatelet effects of aspirin may be observed within 30 minutes of oral administration (and with doses as low as 20 mg, although conventional therapeutic doses range from 75 mg to 325 mg daily). Low doses are associated with fewer side effects (see **Table 1**), but these include active peptic ulcers; hemorrhagic conditions and allergy are absolute contraindications.

Use of aspirin in patients with ST-segment elevation: clinical trials

The main evidence for the role of aspirin in ACS with ST-segment elevation comes from the ISIS-2 study, which enrolled 17,187 patients with suspected MI [5]. In a placebo-controlled design, patients were

Figure 3. Diagrammatic representation of the mode of action of different antiplatelet agents. COX: cyclo-oxygenase; TXA_2: thromboxane A_2. Adapted from *Am J Med* 1996;101:199–209.

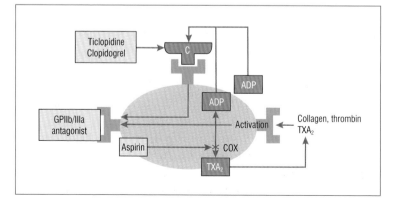

randomized to one of four groups: intravenous streptokinase (SK), oral aspirin, both, or neither.

The primary outcome was all-cause mortality, evaluated at 35 days. Aspirin (162.5 mg daily) was given within the first 24 hours (median 5 hours) after the onset of symptoms. The mortality rate in the aspirin group was 9.4% compared with 11.8% in the placebo group, a proportional reduction of 22% (95% confidence interval [CI] 0.71–0.85; $P<0.0001$). There were 8.0% vascular deaths with SK plus aspirin compared with 13.2% with placebo, indicating that aspirin has a greater benefit when combined with a thrombolytic agent.

Figure 4. Diagrammatic summary of the antiplatelet action of aspirin.

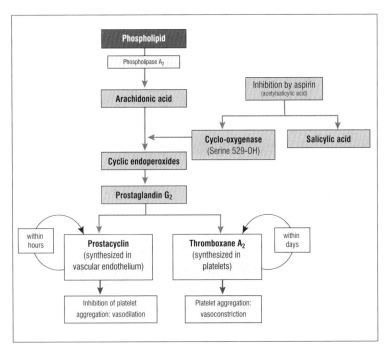

| | Aspirin | Clopidogrel | Ticlopidine | GPIIb/IIIa inhibitors | | |
				Abciximab	Tirofiban	Eptifibatide
Route of administration	Oral	Oral	Oral	Intravenous infusion for 24–72 hours	Intravenous infusion for 24–72 hours	Intravenous infusion for 24–72 hours
Recommended dose	Load: 300 mg Maintenance: 75–150 mg daily	Load: 300 mg Maintenance: 75 mg daily	250 mg twice daily	Bolus: 0.25 mg/kg Infusion: 0.10–0.15 µg/kg/min	Bolus: 0.4–0.6 µg/kg Infusion: 0.10–0.15 µg/kg/min	Bolus: 180 µg/kg with maintenance of 2 µg/kg/min
Main mechanism of action	Cyclo-oxygenase inhibited irreversibly	ADP receptor	ADP receptor	Inhibits fibrinogen and vWF binding	Inhibits fibrinogen and vWF binding	Inhibits fibrinogen and vWF binding
Pathways affected	Collagen, ADP and thromboxane A_2	ADP	ADP	ADP	Collagen, thrombin, ADP, epinephrine, serotonin, and thromboxane A_2	
Potential adverse effects	GI bleed (occurs in 1–2 patients per 1,000 per year) Intracranial bleed (occurs in 1 patient per 1,000 per 3 years) GI toxicity Hypersensitivity	Diarrhea Skin rash	Thrombocytopenia Neutropenia Diarrhea Skin rash Raised lipid levels Liver dysfunction	Thrombocytopenia Bleeding Nausea Fever Headache Rash	Thrombocytopenia Bleeding Nausea Fever Headache Rash	Thrombocytopenia Bleeding Nausea Fever Headache Rash
Contraindications	NSAID hypersensitivity Active peptic ulcer Severe hepatic/ renal disease Hemorrhagic diathesis Rare allergy	Severe hepatic disease Pregnancy Lactation	Severe hepatic disease Pregnancy Lactation	Active bleeding Concurrent warfarin use History of intracranial bleed Previous thrombocytopenia with GPIIb/IIIa antagonists Within 30 days of bleeding, major surgery, or stroke	Active bleeding Concurrent warfarin use History of intracranial bleed Previous thrombocytopenia with GPIIb/IIIa antagonists Within 30 days of bleeding, major surgery, or stroke	Active bleeding Concurrent warfarin use History of intracranial bleed Previous thrombocytopenia with GPIIb/IIIa antagonists Within 30 days of bleeding, major surgery, or stroke
Half life	20 mins	8 hours	24–36 hours	30 mins	1.2–1.6 hours	1–2 hours

Table 1. Important characteristics of antiplatelet agents used in the treatment of acute coronary syndromes, including pharmacological properties. ADP: adenosine diphosphate; GI: gastrointestinal; GP: glycoprotein; NSAID: nonsteroidal anti-inflammatory drug; vWF: von Willebrand factor.

Aspirin significantly reduced nonfatal reinfarction (1% vs 2% in the placebo group) and nonfatal stroke (0.3% vs 0.6%).

Several other smaller randomized studies have evaluated the role of aspirin in suspected acute MI, but they have not materially altered the conclusions based on the results of ISIS-2. There are no randomized studies of the use of aspirin in ST-segment elevation ACS treated with primary percutaneous coronary intervention (PCI), but it is assumed that aspirin is an effective treatment in this context because of the wealth of evidence from related coronary conditions.

Use of aspirin in patients with non-ST-segment elevation

The efficacy and safety of aspirin in ACS without ST-segment elevation have been studied in 12 trials involving about 5,000 patients with ACS. Aspirin (75–1,300 mg/day, given for a period varying from 5 days to 1 year) reduced vascular deaths or major nonfatal vascular events by about 46% ($P<0.0001$) [2]. Since the mortality risk in non-ST-segment elevation ACS is generally lower than in ST-segment elevation ACS, most of these trials have used a primary composite outcome of death and MI.

The RISC study evaluated the effects of aspirin 75 mg daily in 796 men with ACS without ST-segment elevation [6]. It used a 2×2 factorial design to compare:

- aspirin 75 mg/day versus placebo
- intravenous heparin 5,000 U bolus every 6 hours for
  5 days versus placebo

The combined endpoint of death or MI was reduced by aspirin (compared with placebo) at 5 days (2.5% vs 5.8%; $P = 0.03$) and at 90 days (6.5% vs 17.0%; $P < 0.0001$). Heparin had no significant effect on outcome, although the group treated with aspirin and heparin had the lowest number of events during the initial 5 days. Severe angina necessitating referral for coronary angiography was less common during aspirin therapy. Other studies have shown similar results [7].

Guidelines on the use of aspirin and revascularization procedures

The American Heart Association (AHA)/American College of Cardiology (ACC) and the European Society of Cardiology (ECS) guidelines [8–11] state unequivocally that aspirin should be given to all patients with ACS (with and without ST-segment elevation) as soon as possible and continued indefinitely (see **Table 2**). The ESC guidelines give aspirin a class Ia recommendation and the US guidelines give it a class I recommendation. Aspirin should be continued for percutaneous revascularization procedures and should not be a contraindication for patients proceeding to urgent coronary artery surgery.

Recommended formulations of aspirin

Aspirin formulations and doses vary from region to region. In the US, aspirin is available in doses of 81 mg, 162.5 mg, and 325 mg, while in Europe doses of 75 mg, 150 mg, and 300 mg are used. A loading dose of at least 300 mg is recommended in ACS, but a maintenance dose of 75–80 mg appears to have similar efficacy to higher doses. Some studies have administered aspirin intravenously, but this approach is not widely used as it does not seem to offer an efficacy advantage over oral aspirin.

Thienopyridines: ticlopidine and clopidogrel

Mechanisms of action

The thienopyridines ticlopidine and clopidogrel are structurally related inhibitors of ADP-dependent platelet activation (see **Figure 3** and **Table 3**). Ticlopidine became available for clinical use in 1978, and has been demonstrated to have clinical efficacy in ACS and stroke [12–15].

Ticlopidine has a number of unwanted side effects, including neutropenia and skin rashes. Severe neutropenia, which is usually

Table 2. Summary of recommendations based on European Society of Cardiology and American Heart Association/ American College of Cardiology guidelines for antiplatelet therapy for non-ST-segment elevation acute coronary syndromes (ACS) and in patients having revascularization. CABG: coronary artery bypass graft; GP: glycoprotein; PCI: percutaneous coronary intervention.

Treatment	Recommendations
Aspirin	Treatment with aspirin in all patients with suspected ACS without contraindications Acutely, with a loading dose and thereafter long-term maintenance with a low dose (level of evidence 1A).
Clopidogrel	Clopidogrel should be administered to patients intolerant to aspirin who have no contraindications to clopidogrel (level of evidence 2B). Clopidogrel for acute treatment in addition to aspirin as loading dose and in the maintenance dose thereafter for at least 1 month (level of evidence: class 1A) and up to 9–12 months (level of evidence: class 1B).
GPIIb/IIIa receptor inhibitors	GPIIb/IIIa receptor inhibitors should be administered to all patients with ACS who may undergo PCI. The infusion needs to be continued for 12 hours for abciximab and 24 hours for eptifibatide or tirofiban after the procedure (level of evidence: class 1A).
PCI	For patients undergoing PCI, GPIIb/IIIa receptor blockers along with aspirin and weight-adjusted low-dose heparin should be administered to all patients with ACS and positive troponin levels who are scheduled for early revascularization (level of evidence: class 1A). GPIIb/IIIa receptor blockers should be administered to patients (who are already on heparin, clopidogrel, and aspirin) in whom PCI is planned (level of evidence 2A). Clopidogrel administration should be continued for 9–12 months after PCI in patients not at high risk of bleeding (level of evidence: class 1B). Clopidogrel should be given to patients receiving a stent (level of evidence: class 1B).
CABG	For patients undergoing CABG GPIIb/IIIa receptor blockers should be discontinued 4 hours before (or at the time of) cardiac surgery. Eptifibatide and tirofiban have shorter half-lives, but as for patients on abciximab fresh platelet transfusion can be given postsurgery, if need be (level of evidence: class 1A). With respect to clopidogrel, pretreatment with aggressive antiplatelets for an emergency surgery is a relative contraindication to early CABG, and may require special surgical procedures and platelet transfusion to minimize bleeding. For elective CABG, clopidogrel should be stopped 5 days prior to surgery (level of evidence: class 1B).

Treatment	ST-segment elevation ACS	Non-ST-segment elevation ACS	PCI procedure (coronary angioplasty and stent)		
			Before	During	After
Aspirin	Load + maintenance dose for long-term	Load + maintenance dose for long-term	Aspirin 160–325 mg daily >2 hours prior	–	75–150 mg daily: long-term
Clopidogrel	Could be used in place of aspirin	Load + maintenance dose for 1 year (add to aspirin)	+ Clopidogrel 300 mg load at least 6 hours prior	–	75 mg daily for 12 months
GPIIb/IIIa inhibitors (dose of heparin to be reduced when given together)	Use in primary PCI No clear indication with thrombolysis	+ If high risk*	+ If high risk*	+ If high risk*	+ For 12 hours for abciximab and 24 hours for tirofiban and eptifibatide, if high risk*

Table 3. Recommended clinical indications for the use of antiplatelet agents in patients with acute coronary syndromes (ACS). GP: glycoprotein; PCI: percutaneous coronary intervention.
*High risk includes: recurrent or persistent chest pains + associated electrocardiogram changes (ST-segment depression or transient ST-segment elevation) despite anti-ischemic treatment; elevated troponin concentrations; diabetes; age >65 years; cardiac failure; major arrhythmias.

reversible, can occur in up to 1%–2% of patients taking ticlopidine, but is very rare with clopidogrel. For these reasons ticlopidine has been almost completely replaced by clopidogrel.

The white cell count should be frequently checked with continued ticlopidine administration, but this is not required with clopidogrel. Ticlopidine has also been reported to cause thrombocytopenia.

Both ticlopidine and clopidogrel are metabolized in the liver to their active forms. These covalently bind to the ADP receptor on platelets, thus inhibiting ADP-dependent platelet activation [16,17]. These effects start within 30 minutes of drug absorption and last for 4–8 days after discontinuation, reflecting the circulating lifetime of platelets.

The CAPRIE study compared clopidogrel with aspirin in 19,185 patients with a prior history of stroke, MI, and peripheral arterial disease with a mean follow-up of 1.91 years [18–21]. There was a proportional reduction of 8.7% in the risk of vascular death, MI, and stroke (95% CI 0.3–16.5; $P = 0.043$).

These findings show that clopidogrel is slightly superior to aspirin alone for the treatment of patients with chronic vascular disease. However, because clopidogrel is more expensive than aspirin, this effect is not sufficiently large for clopidogrel to become the antiplatelet of choice. Most studies of clopidogrel after CAPRIE have therefore compared its effectiveness in combination with aspirin with that of aspirin alone.

Clopidogrel in patients with ST-segment elevation

As yet there is no clear evidence for the use of clopidogrel in the treatment of ST-segment elevation ACS, but clopidogrel may be used in place of aspirin in patients intolerant to aspirin (as shown by the results of the CAPRIE study). Further ongoing clinical trials, including the CLARITY and CCS-2 (COMMIT) studies, are evaluating the use of clopidogrel plus aspirin in ST-segment elevation MI.

Indirect inference from the CURE study would suggest a beneficial role for clopidogrel in addition to aspirin for ST-segment elevation ACS [22], but the efficacy and safety of clopidogrel in combination with thrombolytic therapy need to be established. For ST-segment elevation ACS patients undergoing primary PCI, clopidogrel is recommended for routine use in addition to aspirin and, in many cases, GPIIb/IIIa receptor antagonists.

Clopidogrel in patients with non-ST-segment elevation

The CURE trial randomized 12,562 patients within 24 hours of the onset of non-ST-segment elevation ACS to aspirin alone (75–325 mg) or aspirin plus clopidogrel (300 mg loading dose of clopidogrel and then 75 mg daily) [19]. Patients included in the trial had acute myocardial ischemia on their ECGs and/or elevated biomarkers at randomization, and treatment continued for up to 12 months (mean 9 months) [22,23].

The primary composite outcome of cardiovascular death, nonfatal MI, or stroke occurred in 11.4% of patients in the aspirin-alone group compared with 9.3% in the aspirin plus clopidogrel group (relative risk ratio [RRR] 0.80; 95% CI 0.72–0.90; $P<0.001$). The main reduction was observed in the rate of MI (including Q-wave MI), and beneficial effects were observed in the first 24 hours.

About 36% of all patients had a revascularization procedure during the follow-up period of the study, with 7.2% of all patients having these procedures within 5 days of randomization. GPIIb/IIIa receptor blockers were only used in 6% of patients. Major bleeding occurred in 2.7% of patients in the aspirin-alone group, as compared with 3.7% in the combination group (RRR 1.38; 95% CI 1.13–1.67; $P = 0.001$). The risk of bleeding was associated with higher doses of concomitant aspirin.

A subgroup of 2,658 patients from the CURE study underwent PCI (PCI-CURE) [24]. The rate of the primary outcome (cardiovascular death, MI, or urgent revascularization by 30 days after PCI) was 7.2% in the aspirin-alone group and 4.2% in the aspirin plus clopidogrel group (relative risk 0.58; 95% CI 0.40–0.85; $P = 0.005$), indicating that there is a benefit from clopidogrel and aspirin compared to aspirin alone in patients undergoing PCI in non–ST-segment elevation ACS [24,25]. The relative risk of cardiovascular death or MI in patients who had PCI and were on clopidogrel until the end of follow up was 0.72 (95% CI 0.53–0.96; $P = 0.03$]. These data therefore support the use of clopidogrel for 9–12 months following PCI for the treatment of ACS patients.

Guidelines for use of thienopyridines

There is no clear evidence for the routine use of clopidogrel in the early phase of ST-segment elevation ACS as yet. Indirect evidence from the CURE study may support the use of longer-term clopidogrel and aspirin, starting a few days after ST-segment elevation ACS and continuing for about a year, but this is not strictly evidence based.

In patients with non–ST-segment elevation ACS, clopidogrel should be started early with a loading dose of 300 mg and continued at a dose of 75 mg for at least 9–12 months (level of evidence: 1B). Treatment beyond a year will depend on the risk status of the patient and the judgment of the responsible physician.

Clopidogrel should be given to ACS patients scheduled for angiography unless there is a likelihood that the patient will proceed to urgent surgery (within 5 days). Clopidogrel may also be recommended for immediate and long-term therapy in patients who do not tolerate aspirin [19], and is recommended in patients receiving a stent (level of evidence: 1B) [25]. *Post hoc* analysis from the CURE study suggests that the bleeding risk of the combination of aspirin and clopidogrel is lower if the maintenance dose of aspirin is kept to 100 mg or below.

Glycoprotein IIb/IIIa inhibitors

Mechanisms of action

The surfaces of platelets are covered with GPIIb/IIIa receptors, which bind to fibrinogen. Activated platelets aggregate with other platelets through cross-linked fibrinogen, which binds to the GPIIb/IIIa receptors forming a platelet thrombus (see **Figure 4** and **Figure 5**). This is the "final common pathway" for platelet activation and aggregation. GPIIb/IIIa inhibitors competitively bind to the surface receptors, preventing fibrinogen from forming the cross-linked bridges and thereby reducing platelet aggregation. Three intravenous GPIIb/IIIa inhibitors are licensed for use in ACS: abciximab (ReoPro), eptifibatide (Integrilin), and tirofiban (Aggrastat).

Abciximab (ReoPro)

Abciximab (c7E3) is a recombinant, chimeric mouse–human monoclonal antibody directed against the GPIIb/IIIa receptor. Its pharmacological half-life is only 10 minutes, but its physiological half-life is about 12–24 hours.

Figure 5. Mechanism of platelet aggregation and its inhibition by glycoprotein (GP)IIb/IIIa receptor blockers. Adapted from *N Engl J Med* 1995;332:1553–9.

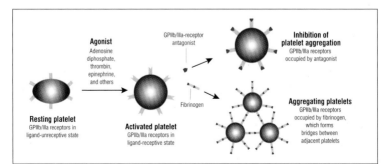

Maximum receptor blockade and inhibition of aggregation occur about 2 hours after bolus injection. The antiplatelet effect of abciximab is prolonged by redistribution from the originally bound platelet to newly produced platelets.

Abciximab inhibits the GPIIb/IIIa receptor itself, rather than direct binding to the RGD (arginine–glycine–aspartate) binding site of the receptor. It also inhibits the vitronectin receptor, which mediates platelet coagulation and endothelial and vascular smooth muscle cell proliferation. The clinical significance of this vitronectin-receptor blockade is currently being evaluated.

Eptifibatide (Integrilin)
Eptifibatide is a cyclic peptide that selectively inhibits the GPIIb/IIIa receptor. It has a short half-life and platelet function recovers 2–4 hours after cessation of treatment.

Tirofiban (Aggrastat)
Tirofiban is a small nonpeptide (derivative of tyrosine) antagonist that mimics the tripeptide sequence of fibrinogen. Onset of action is rapid, selective, and reversible within 4–6 hours.

Lamifiban, orbofiban, sibrafiban, and lefradafiban
Lamifiban is a synthetic, nonpeptide selective receptor blocker with a half-life of approximately 4 hours. Several oral GPIIb/IIIa receptor blockers have also been studied, including orbofiban, sibrafiban, and lefradafiban; none of these has been found to have a beneficial clinical profile [27].

GPIIb/IIIa inhibitors in patients with ST-segment elevation

In ACS with ST-segment elevation, two potential strategies have emerged for GPIIb/IIIa inhibitors:

- combination therapy (with modified dose regimens of fibrinolytics and GPIIb/IIIa receptor blockers)
- adjunctive GPIIb/IIIa blockade during primary angioplasty

Combination therapy

Several trials have reported improvements in infarct-related artery patency when conventional thrombolytic regimes have been compared with reduced-dose fibrinolysis in combination with a GPIIb/IIIa receptor blocker (see **Table 4**) [28–32]. Two large trials (GUSTO-V and ASSENT-3) have tested the clinical benefit and safety of these combinations [33,34].

In GUSTO-V, 16,588 patients were randomly assigned to receive a standard dose of the thrombolytic agent reteplase (two 10-U boluses, 30 minutes apart) or the combination of a standard dose of abciximab and a half dose of reteplase (two 5-U boluses, 30 minutes apart). All-cause mortality at 1 year occurred in 8.4% of patients in both groups (hazard ratio 1.00; 95% CI 0.90–1.11).

ASSENT-3 was a multinational, randomized, open-label comparison of three treatment regimens in 6,095 patients with ST-segment elevation MI (STEMI) of less than 6 hours' duration [34]:

- standard, full-dose, weight-based tenecteplase plus enoxaparin
- half-dose, weight-based tenecteplase plus abciximab plus low-dose unfractionated heparin (UFH)
- full-dose tenecteplase plus UFH

Study	Sample size	Study drug	Duration of treatment	Presentation at the time of enrolment	Primary endpoint	Comments	Period of enrolment
ASSENT-3 (open label)	6,095	Enoxaparin + tenecteplase	Enoxaparin for 12 hours to 7 days	ST-segment elevation/LBBB ACS <6 hours	Composite of 30-day mortality, in-hospital reinfarction, or refractory ischemia occurred less in enoxaparin (11.4% vs 15.4; $P = 0.0002$) and abciximab groups (11.1% vs 15.4%; $P<0.0001$) versus UFH group.	Total stroke and ICH rates were similar in the three groups. In the abciximab group, compared to the UFH group, more noncerebral bleeding complications ($P = 0.0002$), more transfusions ($P = 0.001$), and a higher rate of thrombocytopenia ($P = 0.0001$) were seen.	2000–2001
		Abciximab + tenecteplase + heparin	Abciximab for 12 hours				
		Heparin + tenecteplase	UFH for 48 hours				
TIMI-14	888	Abciximab + reteplase (5 U + 5 U)	Abciximab for 12 hours	ST-segment elevation ACS	The primary endpoint, TIMI grade 3 flow, occurred more in the tPA plus abciximab group than in the tPA alone group at 60 minutes (72% vs 43%; $P = 0.0009$) and at 90 minutes (77% vs 62%; $P = 0.02$).	The rates of major hemorrhage were 6% in tPA-alone group, 3% with abciximab alone, 10% with streptokinase + abciximab, and 1% with tPA + abciximab + low-dose heparin. Efficacy and safety were optimal for a tPA dose that was one-half the standard dose.	1997–1998
		Abciximab + reteplase (5 U + 10 U)	Heparin for 12 hours				
		Reteplase + heparin					
IMPACT-AMI	180	Eptifibatide + alteplase	24 hours	STEMI	The primary outcome was TIMI 3 flow at 90 minutes. TIMI 3 flow occurred in 66% of the high-dose eptifibatide group and in 39% of the placebo group ($P = 0.006$).	Complications were similar for the two groups.	1993–1995
		Placebo + alteplase					

Study	Sample size	Study drug	Duration of treatment	Presentation at the time of enrolment	Primary endpoint	Comments	Period of enrolment
GUSTO-V	16,588	Reteplase Abciximab + half-dose reteplase	12 hours	STEMI/ new LBBB	The primary endpoint, 30-day mortality, occurred in 5.9% of the reteplase-alone group and in 5.6% of the reteplase/ abciximab group (*P* = NS). The 30-day composite of death or reinfarction was 8.8% in the reteplase group and 7.4% in the reteplase/ abciximab group (*P* = 0.0011).	Severe or moderate bleeding occurred in 4.6% of the reteplase/ abciximab group and in 2.3% of the reteplase group (*P*<0.0001). However, hemorrhagic and nonhemorrhagic stroke rates were comparable between groups (~1.0%).	1999–2001
SPEED (GUSTO-IV Pilot)	530	Abciximab alone or with reteplase	12 hours In phase A, abciximab plus one of six reteplase dosing strategies (none, 5 U, 7.5 U, 10 U, 5 U + 2.5 U, or 5 U + 5 U) In phase B, the best combination from phase A (abciximab plus reteplase 5 U + 5 U) was compared with reteplase alone (10 U + 10 U)	STEMI/ new LBBB	Primary endpoint was TIMI 3 flow at 60–90 minutes. In phase A, TIMI 3 flow occurred in 62% of the abciximab/ reteplase (5 + 5) group and in 27% of the abciximab-only group (*P* = 0.001). In phase B, TIMI 3 flow occurred in 54% of the abciximab–reteplase (5 U + 5 U) group and in 47% of the reteplase (10 U + 10 U) only patients (*P* = 0.32).	Major bleeding in phase B occurred in 9.8% of the abciximab/reteplase (5 U +5 U) group and in 3.7% of the reteplase alone group (*P* = NS).	

Table 4 continues on page 76

75

Study	Sample size	Study drug	Duration of treatment	Presentation at the time of enrolment	Primary endpoint	Comments	Period of enrolment
INTRO-AMI	649	Eptifibatide + tPA	48 hours	STEMI	The incidences of death, reinfarction or revascularization at 30 days were similar among the treatment groups.	Lower dose tPA (groups 1 and 2) was not associated with less major bleeding.	1998–2000
RAPPORT	483	Abciximab or placebo	12 hours	Acute MI	Incidence of death, reinfarction, or revascularization at 6 months was similar (28.1% in placebo vs 28.2% in abciximab groups [$P = 0.97$]). At 30 days, urgent target-vessel revascularization rate was 1.8% for abciximab and 5.6% for placebo groups ($P = 0.03$).	The need for stenting was reduced by abciximab ($P = 0.057$). Need for unplanned stenting was reduced by 42% in abciximab group (20.4% vs 11.9%; $P = 0.008$).	1995–1997
ADMIRAL	300	Abciximab vs placebo	12 hours	STEMI	Scheduled for primary PCI and stent.	Primary endpoint- composite of death or reinfarction or any revascularization at 6 months was 6% for abciximab vs 14.6% for placebo ($P = 0.01$).	1997–1998

Table 4. Summary of randomized trials of glycoprotein (GP)IIb/IIIa receptor blockers in ST-segment elevation acute coronary syndromes (ACS). ICH: intracranial hemorrhage; LBBB: left bundle branch block; MI: myocardial infarction; NS: nonsignificant; PCI: percutaneous coronary intervention; STEMI: ST-segment elevation myocardial infarction; tPA: tissue plasminogen activator; UFH: unfractionated heparin.

The primary outcome measures were:

- a composite of 30-day mortality, in-hospital reinfarction, or in-hospital refractory ischemia (efficacy endpoint)

- a composite of 30-day mortality, in-hospital reinfarction, or in-hospital refractory ischemia plus in-hospital intracranial hemorrhage or in-hospital major bleeding complications (efficacy plus safety endpoint)

The composite efficacy endpoint occurred significantly less in the enoxaparin and abciximab groups than in the UFH group (11.4% vs 15.4% for enoxaparin [P = 0.0002] and 11.1% vs 15.4% for abciximab [$P<0.0001$]) as did the efficacy plus safety composite endpoint (13.7% vs 17.0% for enoxaparin [P = 0.0037] and 14.2% vs 17.0% for abciximab [P = 0.01416]); 30-day mortality was equal among groups.

Total stroke and intracranial hemorrhage rates were similar in the three groups. More noncerebral bleeding complications (P = 0.0002), more transfusions (P = 0.001), and a higher rate of thrombocytopenia (P = 0.0001) were seen in the abciximab group compared with the UFH group.

These data suggest that abciximab added to tenecteplase offers no advantage compared with enoxaparin and is associated with an increased bleeding rate.

Adjunctive GPIIb/IIIa blockade and primary angioplasty

The CADILLAC trial randomized 2,082 patients in an open-label, 2×2 factorial design of primary stenting versus angioplasty and abciximab treatment (n = 1,052) versus no abciximab treatment (n = 1,030) [35]. Abciximab treatment was associated with a significant reduction in the composite endpoint of death, MI, ischemia-driven target-vessel revascularization (TVR), or disabling stroke at 30 days (4.6% vs 7.0%;

relative risk 0.65; 95% CI 0.46–0.93; P = 0.01). At 12 months, however, rates of the composite endpoint did not differ significantly (18.4% for controls vs 16.9% for abciximab-treated patients; relative risk 0.92; 95% CI 0.76–1.10; P = 0.29).

There was no significant interaction between stenting and abciximab treatment. Adjunctive abciximab treatment during primary PCI significantly enhanced 30-day event-free survival, predominantly by reducing ischemia-driven TVR.

In ADMIRAL, 300 patients with acute MI were randomized in a double-blind fashion, before they underwent coronary angiography, to either abciximab plus stenting (n = 149) or placebo plus stenting (n = 151) [36].

At 30 days, the primary outcome of a composite of death, reinfarction, or urgent TVR had occurred in 6.0% of the patients in the abciximab group compared with 14.6% of those in the placebo group (P = 0.01). At 6 months, the corresponding figures were 7.4% and 15.9% (P = 0.02). The better clinical outcomes in the abciximab group were mainly related to improved TIMI flow rate.

Thus abciximab, particularly when given prior to primary PCI, markedly reduces ischemic events. At the present time, there is no clear evidence for the use of GPIIb/IIIa receptor blockers with a thrombolytic agent for ST-segment elevation ACS, although further studies are in progress.

GPIIb/IIIa receptor inhibitors in patients with non-ST-segment elevation

Several randomized trials have evaluated the efficacy and safety of intravenous GPIIb/IIIa inhibitors in non–ST-segment elevation ACS [37–43] and the results have been pooled in a meta-analysis (see **Table 3**, **Table 5**, and **Figure 6**). Most studies have compared the combination of a GPIIb/IIIa blocker plus UFH with UFH alone.

Table 5 summarizes the patient characteristics, design, and results of these trials. Overall the use of GPIIb/IIIa blockers is associated with a modest, but significant, reduction in death or MI at 30 days in patients with non-ST-segment elevation ACS.

Abciximab

The CAPTURE trial enrolled 1,265 patients with refractory ACS scheduled for PCI. Abciximab was administered from some time during the day before intervention until 1 hour afterwards [37]. In contrast, GUSTO-IV ACS studied the effect of abciximab in patients with non-ST-segment elevation ACS not scheduled for early revascularization [42].

This latter study was one of the few large trials that has not show any benefit of a GPIIb/IIIa inhibitor in non-ST-segment elevation ACS. Several explanations for this finding have been proposed, including the enrolment of low-risk patients who may not benefit from the treatment and the possibility that the dose and timing of abciximab were not optimal for patients who are not likely to have a PCI.

Tirofiban

The PRISM study enrolled 3,232 patients and compared tirofiban with UFH [38]. PRISM-PLUS enrolled patients at somewhat higher risk (those with unstable angina and ECG changes indicative of ischemia) and compared three groups: tirofiban plus UFH, tirofiban alone, and UFH alone [39]. The tirofiban-alone arm was discontinued early because, in an interim analysis, there appeared to be an elevated risk of death.

Eptifibatide

PURSUIT, the largest trial of a GPIIb/IIIa blocker in non-ST-segment elevation ACS, randomized 10,948 patients with ECG evidence of ischemia or elevated cardiac enzymes to a bolus of eptifibatide followed by an infusion for up to 72 hours, or to a placebo bolus and infusion [40].

Study	Sample size	Study drug	Duration of treatment	Presentation at the time of enrolment	Angiography and revascularization	PCI	Death or MI at 30 days	Period of enrolment
CAPTURE	1,265	Abciximab vs placebo	19–25 hours	Non-ST-segment elevation ACS	PCI planned in all subjects	98%	9.0% vs 4.8%; RR= 0.53 (P = 0.003)	1993–1995
PRISM	3,232	Tirofiban vs heparin	48 hours	Non-ST-segment elevation ACS	Mostly after 48 hours	21%	5.8% vs 7.1%; RR= 0.80 (P = 0.11)	1994–1996
PRISM-PLUS	1,915	Tirofiban vs tirofiban + heparin vs heparin	48–96 hours	Non-ST-segment elevation ACS	48–96 hours	31%	8.7% vs 11.9%; RR= 0.7 (P = 0.006)	1994–1996
PURSUIT	10,948	Eptifibatide vs placebo	Up to 96 hours	Non-ST-segment elevation ACS	At physician's discretion	24%	14.2% vs 15.7%; RR= 0.90 (P = 0.04)	1995–1997
PARAGON A	2,282	Low dose lamifiban + heparin vs high dose lamifiban + heparin vs placebo	72–120 hours	Non-ST-segment elevation ACS	Mostly after 48 hours	14%	11.3% vs 11.7%; RR= 0.96 (P = 0.80)	1995–1996
PARAGON B	5,225	Lamifiban vs placebo	72–120 hours	Non-ST-segment elevation ACS	At physician's discretion	27%	10.6% vs 11.55; RR= 0.92 (P = 0.32)	1998–1999
GUSTO-IV-ACS	7,800	Abciximab shorter duration vs abciximab longer duration vs placebo	24 hours in shorter duration and 48 hours in the longer duration arms	Non-ST-segment elevation ACS	Mostly after 60 hours	19%	8.2% vs 9.1% vs 8.0% (P = 0.19)	1998–2000
EPIC	2,099	Abciximab bolus vs abciximab bolus + infusion vs placebo	12 hours	Acute or recent MI, unstable angina or complex target lesion Angiographic morphology in association with advanced age, female gender, or diabetes mellitus	PCI-angioplasty or atherectomy	100%	11.1% vs 5% vs 0.6% (P<0.001)	1991–1992
TARGET	4,809	Abciximab vs tirofiban	12 hours abciximab and 18–24 hours tirofiban	Patients undergoing nonemergency PCI with stent placement STEMI patients were excluded	Nonemergent PCI	95%	Composite of death, MI, or urgent target vessel revascularization at 30 days: 6.0% abciximab group and 7.6% tirofiban group (P = 0.037)	1999–2000

Table 5. Main clinical trials of glycoprotein (GPIIb/IIIa) receptor blockers in non-ST-elevation acute coronary syndromes (ACS). MI: myocardial infarction; PCI: percutaneous coronary intervention; RR: risk ratio; STEMI: ST-segment elevation myocardial infarction.

Lamifiban

PARAGON-A studied low dose (300 µg bolus, 1.0 µg/min infusion) and high dose (750 µg bolus, 5.0 µg/min infusion) lamifiban. PARAGON-B used a 500 µg bolus and infusions of 1.0, 1.5, and 2.0 µg/min.

Treatment in diabetics

Diabetics with non-ST-segment elevation ACS appear to derive particular benefit from GPIIb/IIIa receptor blockers [53]. Among 6,458 diabetics, treatment was associated with a significant mortality reduction at 30 days from 6.2% to 4.6% (RRR 0.74; 95% CI 0.59–0.92; $P = 0.007$).

Figure 6. Forest plot showing odds ratio with 95% confidence interval (CI) and corresponding *P*-values for treatment effect on death or myocardial infarction (MI) at 30 days. Adapted from *Eur Heart J* 2002;23:1441–8.

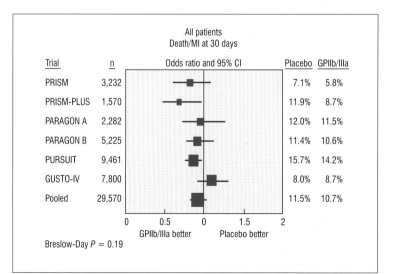

GPIIb/IIIa receptor blockers for revascularization in patients without ST-segment elevation

Patients undergoing PCI have received a clear benefit from GPIIb/IIIa receptor blocker administration in a number of clinical trials that included patients selected for PCI (EPIC, CAPTURE, EPILOG, EPISTENT, RESTORE, IMPACT-II, ESPRIT) by reducing the combined endpoint of death, MI, and TVR [37,44–49]. Abciximab showed modest superiority over tirofiban in the TARGET study of PCI, particularly in ACS patients [50].

Patients who underwent PCI in CAPTURE [37], and similar subgroups from PURSUIT [36] and PRISM-PLUS [35], showed a reduction in procedure-related events from 8.0% to 4.9% ($P = 0.001$) at up to 30-days follow-up. In the larger placebo-controlled trials, the treatment benefit of GPIIb/IIIa in ACS patients appears greater in those in whom early revascularization has been performed [37,39,40].

Subgroup analysis from the meta-analysis by Boersma and colleagues showed little benefit in patients who received GPIIb/IIIa without any intervention, compared with a 3% absolute reduction in death or MI both at 5 and 30 days in patients who had PCI or coronary artery bypass grafting (RRR 0.79; 95% CI 0.68–0.91) [51]. The comparison at 30 days showed a 1.7% absolute risk reduction (RRR 0.89; 95% CI 0.80–0.98). Since PCI is a postrandomization variable, these analyses may have over-estimated the benefits of GPIIb/IIIa blockers.

Oral GPIIb/IIIa receptor blockers

Four trials addressed prolonged treatment with oral GPIIb/IIIa inhibitors in patients with ACS or those who have undergone coronary intervention. Such prolonged treatments have shown no evidence of benefit (OPUS-TIMI-14-EXCITE, SYMPHONY 1, SYMPHONY 2). In fact, a modest but significant increase in mortality was apparent in a meta-analysis of patients receiving oral GPIIb/IIIa inhibitors [27].

Management and avoidance of bleeding complications

The bleeding risk of GPIIb/IIIa inhibitors is clearly related to the dose of adjunctive heparin and specific reduced-heparin dosing schedules are recommended. In the setting of PCI, it is recommended to reduce the dose of heparin to 70 IU/kg with a target activated clotting time of 200 seconds. When local complications occur, such as an important hematoma or continuous bleeding at the puncture site, surgical intervention may be required.

Thrombocytopenia may occur in a small percentage of patients during administration of parenteral GPIIb/IIIa receptor inhibitors. A decrease in platelet counts to <50,000/mm^3 occurred in <1% of patients in PRISM-PLUS or GUSTO-IV-ACS (24 hours). Stopping treatment usually results in a return to normal platelet levels [39,42].

GPIIb/IIIa inhibitors should ideally be discontinued at least 4 hours prior to cardiac surgery. Eptifibatide and tirofiban have a short half-life, and some recovery of platelet function should occur towards the end of the procedure when hemostasis is necessary. Abciximab has a longer effective half-life and, if excessive bleeding occurs, fresh platelet transfusions may be administered.

Finally, re-administration might be an issue for abciximab, because of its inherent immunogenicity. In practice, the re-administration registry shows similar safety and efficacy for repeat administration as compared with first time administration [50,52].

Conclusions

Antiplatelet therapy is a fundamental part of the optimum management of ST-segment and non-ST-segment elevation ACS. Aspirin should be routine for all patients, unless there are clear contraindications (when clopidogrel can be substituted), and life-long treatment is the accepted practice.

The approach of adding clopidogrel or GPIIb/IIIa inhibitors to aspirin in ST-segment elevation ACS treated with fibrinolysis has not been established, although studies are ongoing. For many patients with non-ST-segment elevation ACS, especially those with elevated biomarkers or ischemia on the ECG, adding clopidogrel to aspirin and continuing the combination for about a year reduces the risk of death, MI, and stroke.

Clopidogrel and aspirin are indicated in the context of PCI for ST-segment and non-ST-segment elevation ACS with clopidogrel continued for 9–12 months. GPIIb/IIIa inhibitors are indicated for PCI with ACS (either primary angioplasty or following non-ST-segment elevation ACS), and are also indicated for stabilization of higher risk non-ST-segment elevation patients prior to a potential PCI.

The benefits of GPIIb/IIIa inhibitors appear greater in patients with non-ST-segment elevation ACS who are treated with a more invasive approach. Taking all the data together, there is a clear role for GPIIb/IIIa inhibitors in the management of non-ST-segment elevation ACS. However, it seems that greater benefits are derived in higher risk patients (eg, those with elevated troponin levels and diabetics) and those undergoing concomitant PCI.

References

1. Falk E, Thuesen L. Pathology of coronary microembolisation and no reflow. *Heart* 2003; 89:983–5.
2. Antithrombotic Trialists Collaboration. Collaborative meta-analysis of randomised trials of antiplatelet therapy for prevention of death, myocardial infarction, and stroke in high risk patient. *Br Med J* 2002;324:71–86.
3. Wilson CO, Grisvold O, Dorge RF, editors. *Textbook of Organic Medicinal and Pharmaceutical Chemistry*. 7th ed. Philadelphia: JB Lippincott Company;1977.
4. Weksler BB, Pett SB, Alonso D, et al. Differential inhibition by aspirin of vascular and platelet prostaglandin synthesis in atherosclerotic patients. *N Eng J Med* 1983;308:800–6.
5. ISIS-2 (Second International Study of Infarct Survival) Collaborative Group. Randomised trial of intravenous streptokinase, oral aspirin, both, or neither among 17,187 cases of suspected acute myocardial infarction: ISIS-2. *Lancet* 1988;2:349–60.

6. The RISC Group. Risk of myocardial infarction and death during treatment with low dose aspirin and intravenous heparin in men with unstable coronary artery disease. *Lancet* 1990; 336:827–30.

7. Theroux P, Ouimet H, McCans J, et al. Aspirin, heparin, or both to treat acute unstable angina. *N Engl J Med* 1988;319:1105–11.

8. Van de Werf F, Chair F, Ardissino D, et al. Management of acute myocardial infarction in patients presenting with ST segment elevation. The Task Force on the Management of Acute Myocardial Infarction of the European Society of Cardiology. *Eur Heart J* 2003; 24:28–66.

9. Braunwald E, Antman EM, Beasley JW, et al. ACC/AHA guideline update for the management of patients with unstable angina and non-ST-segment elevation myocardial infarction–2002: summary article: a report of the American College of Cardiology/American Heart Association Task Force on Practice Guidelines (Committee on the Management of Patients With Unstable Angina). *Circulation* 2002;106:1893–900.

10. Ryan TJ, Antman EM, Brooks NH, et al. 1999 update: ACC/AHA Guidelines for the Management of Patients With Acute Myocardial Infarction: Executive Summary and Recommendations: A report of the American College of Cardiology/American Heart Association Task Force on Practice Guidelines (Committee on Management of Acute Myocardial Infarction). *Circulation* 1999;100:1016–30.

11. Bertrand ME, Simoons ML, Fox KA, et al; Task Force on the Management of Acute Coronary Syndromes of the European Society of Cardiology. Management of acute coronary syndromes in patients presenting without persistent ST-segment elevation. *Eur Heart J* 2002;23:1809–4. Erratum in: *Eur Heart J* 2003;24:1174–5. *Eur Heart J* 2003;24:485.

12. Panak E, Maffrand JP, Picard-Fraire C, et al. Ticlopidine: a promise for the prevention and treatment of thrombosis and its complications. *Haemostasis* 1983;13(Suppl 1):1–54.

13. Gent M, Blakely JA, Easton JD, et al; CATS Group. The Canadian American Ticlopidine Study (CATS) in thromboembolic stroke *Lancet* 1989;1:1215–20.

14. Gent M. A systematic overview of randomised trials of antiplatelet agents for the prevention of stroke, myocardial infarction and vascular death. In: Hass WK, Easton JD, editors. *Ticlopidine, Platelets and Vascular Disease*. Springer Verlag: New York, 1993:99.

15. Bhatt DL, Bertrand ME, Berger PB, et al. Meta-Analysis of randomized and registry comparisons of ticlopidine with clopidogrel after tenting. *J Am Coll Cardiol* 2002;39:9–14.

16. Meyers KM, Holmsen H, Seachord CL. Comparative study of platelet dense granules constituents. *Am J Physiol* 1982;243:R454–R461.

17. Gardner A, Jonsen J, Laland S, et al. Adenosine diphosphate in red blood cells as a factor in the adhesiveness of human blood platelets. *Nature* 1961;192:531–2.

18. Cannon CP; CAPRIE Investigators. Effectiveness of clopidogrel versus aspirin in preventing acute myocardial infarction in patients with symptomatic atherothrombosis (CAPRIE trial). *Am J Cardiol* 2002;90:760–2.

19. CAPRIE Steering Committee. A randomised, blinded, trial of clopidogrel versus aspirin in patients at risk of ischaemic events (CAPRIE). *Lancet* 1996;348:1329–39.

20. Bhatt DL, Chew DP, Hirsch AT, et al. Superiority of clopidogrel versus aspirin in patients with prior cardiac surgery. *Circulation* 2001;103:363–8.

21. Bhatt DL, Marso SP, Hirsch AT, et al. Amplified benefit of clopidogrel versus aspirin in patients with diabetes mellitus. *Am J Cardiol* 2002;90:625–8.

22. The Clopidogrel in Unstable Angina to Prevent Recurrent Events (CURE) Trial Investigators. Effects of clopidogrel in addition to aspirin in patients with acute coronary syndromes without ST-segment elevation. *N Engl J Med* 2001;345:494–502.

23. Yusuf S, Mehta SR, Zhao F, et al. Early and late effects of clopidogrel in patients with acute coronary syndromes. *Circulation* 2003;107:966–72.

24. Mehta SR, Yusuf S, Peters RJ, et al. Effects of pretreatment with clopidogrel and aspirin followed by long-term therapy in patients undergoing percutaneous coronary intervention: the PCI-CURE study. *Lancet* 2001;358:527–33.

25. Bertrand ME, Rupprecht HJ, Urban P, et al. Double-blind study of the safety of clopidogrel with and without a loading dose in combination with aspirin compared with ticlopidine in combination with aspirin after coronary stenting: the clopidogrel aspirin stent international cooperative study (CLASSICS). *Circulation* 2000;102:624–9.

26. Bhatt DL, Topol EJ. Current role of platelet glycoprotein IIb/IIIa inhibitors in acute coronary syndromes. *JAMA* 2000;284:1549–58.

27. Chew DP, Bhatt DL, Sapp S, et al. Increased mortality with oral platelet glycoprotein IIb/IIIa antagonists: a meta-analysis of the phase III multicenter randomized trials. *Circulation* 2001;103:201–6.

28. Antman EM, Giugliano CM, Gibson CM, et al. Abciximab facilitates the rate and extent of thrombolysis. Results of Thrombolysis in Myocardial Infarction (TIMI) 14 trial. The TIMI 14 Investigators. *Circulation* 1999;99:2720–32.

29. Strategies for Patency Enhancement in the Emergency Department (SPEED) Group. Trial of abciximab with and without low-dose reteplase for acute myocardial infarction. *Circulation* 2000;101:2788–94.

30. Brener SJ, Zeymer U, Adgey AA, et al. Eptifibatide and low-dose tissue plasminogen activator in acute myocardial infarction: the integrilin and low-dose thrombolysis in acute myocardial infarction (INTRO AMI) trial. *J Am Coll Cardiol* 2002;39:377–86.

31. Antman EM, Louwerenburg HW, Baars HF, et al. Enoxaparin as adjunctive antithrombin therapy for ST-elevation myocardial infarction: results of the ENTIRE-Thrombolysis in Myocardial Infarction (TIMI) 23 Trial. *Circulation* 2002;105:1642–9. Erratum in: *Circulation* 2002;105:2799.

32. Ohman M. The FASTER Study, presented at the TCT congress in Washington DC, September 2002.

33. Topol EJ; GUSTO V investigators. Reperfusion therapy for acute myocardial infarction with fibrinolytic therapy or combination reduced fibrinolytic therapy and platelet glycoprotein IIb/IIIa inhibition: the GUSTO V randomized trial. *Lancet* 2001;357:1905–14.

34. The Assessment of the Safety and Efficacy of a New Thrombolytic Regimen (ASSENT)-3 Investigators. Efficacy and safety of tenecteplase in combination with enoxaparin, abciximab, or unfractionated heparin: *Lancet* 2001;358:605–13.

35. Tcheng JE, Kandzari DE, Grines CL, et al; CADILLAC Investigators. Benefits and risks of abciximab use in primary angioplasty for acute myocardial infarction: the Controlled Abciximab and Device Investigation to Lower Late Angioplasty Complications (CADILLAC) trial. *Circulation* 2003;108:1316–23.

36. Montalescot G, Barragan P, Wittenberg O, et al; ADMIRAL Investigators. Abciximab before Direct Angioplasty and Stenting in Myocardial Infarction Regarding Acute and Long-Term Follow-up. Platelet glycoprotein IIb/IIIa inhibition with coronary stenting for acute myocardial infarction *N Engl J Med* 2001;344:1895–903.

37. Randomised placebo-controlled trial of abciximab before and during coronary intervention in refractory unstable angina: the CAPTURE Study. *Lancet* 1997;349:1429–35.

38. Platelet Receptor Inhibition in Ischemic Syndrome Management (PRISM) Study Investigators. A comparison of aspirin plus tirofiban with aspirin plus heparin for unstable angina. *N Engl J Med* 1998;338:1498–505.

39. PRISM–PLUS. Inhibition of the platelet glycoprotein IIb/ IIIa receptor with tirofiban in unstable angina and non-Q-wave myocardial infarction. Platelet Receptor Inhibition in Ischemic Syndrome Management in Patients Limited by Unstable Signs and Symptoms (PRISM-PLUS) Study Investigators. *N Engl J Med* 1998;338:1488–97.

40. PURSUIT Investigators. Inhibition of platelet glycoprotein IIb/IIIa with eptifibatide in patients with acute coronary syndromes. The PURSUIT Trial Investigators. Platelet Glycoprotein IIb/IIIa in Unstable Angina: Receptor Suppression Using Integrilin Therapy. *N Engl J Med* 1998;339:436–43.

41. PARAGON Investigators. International, randomized, controlled trial of lamifiban (a platelet glycoprotein IIb/IIIa inhibitor), heparin, or both in unstable angina. The PARAGON Investigators. Platelet IIb/IIIa Antagonism for the Reduction of Acute coronary syndrome events in a Global Organization Network. *Circulation* 1998;97:2386–95.

42. Simoons ML; GUSTO IV-ACS Investigators. Effect of glycoprotein IIb/IIIa receptor blocker abciximab on outcome in patients with acute coronary syndromes without early coronary revascularisation: the GUSTO IV-ACS randomised trial. *Lancet* 2001;357:1915–24.

43. PARAGON-B investigators. Randomized, placebocontrolled trial of titrated IV Lamifiban for acute coronary syndrome. *Circulation* 2002;105:316–21.

44. EPIC Investigators. Use of a monoclonal antibody directed against the platelet glycoprotein IIb/IIIa receptor in high-risk angioplasty. *N Engl J Med* 1994;330:956–61.

45. EPILOG investigators. Platelet glycoprotein IIb/IIIa receptor blockade and low-dose heparin during percutaneous coronary revascularization. The EPILOG Investigators. *N Engl J Med* 1997;336:1689–96.

46. EPISTENT Investigators. Randomised placebo-controlled and balloon-angioplasty-controlled trial to assess safety of coronary stenting with use of platelet glycoprotein-IIb/IIIa blockade. The EPISTENT Investigators. Evaluation of Platelet IIb/IIIa Inhibitor for Stenting. *Lancet* 1998;352:87–92.

47. RESTORE Investigators. Effects of platelet glycoprotein IIb/IIIa blockade with tirofiban on adverse cardiac events in patients with unstable angina or acute myocardial infarction undergoing coronary angioplasty. The RESTORE Investigators. Randomized Efficacy Study of Tirofiban for Outcomes and Restenosis. *Circulation* 1997;96:1445–53.

48. IMPACT–II Investigators. Randomised placebo-controlled trial of effect of eptifibatide on complications of percutaneous coronary intervention: IMPACT-II. Integrilin to Minimise Platelet Aggregation and Coronary Thrombosis-II. *Lancet* 1997;349:1422–8.

49. ESPRIT Investigators. Novel dosing regimen of eptifibatide in planned coronary stent implantation (ESPRIT): a randomised, placebo-controlled trial. *Lancet* 2000;356:2037–44.

50. Stone GW, Moliterno DJ, Bertrand M, et al. Impact of clinical syndrome activity on the differential response to 2 glycoprotein IIb/IIIa inhibitors in patients undergoing coronary stenting: the TARGET trial. *Circulation* 2002;105:2347–54.

51. Boersma E, Harrington R, Moliterno D, et al. Platelet glycoprotein IIb/IIIa inhibitors in acute coronary syndromes: A meta-analysis of all-major randomised clinical trials. *Lancet* 2002;359:189–98.

52. Leebeek FWG, Boersma E, Cannon CP, et al. Oral glycoprotein IIb/IIIa receptor inhibitors in patients with cardiovascular disease: why were the results so unfavourable? *Eur Heart J* 2002;23:444–57.

53. Roffi M, Moliterno DJ, Meier B, et al; TARGET Investigators. Impact of different platelet glycoprotein IIb/IIIa receptor inhibitors among diabetic patients undergoing percutaneous coronary intervention: Do Tirofiban and ReoPro Give Similar Efficacy Outcomes Trial (TARGET) 1-year follow-up. *Circulation* 2002;105:2730–6.

5

Anticoagulants

Jonas Oldgren & Lars Wallentin

Introduction

The exposure of the thrombogenic contents of an atherosclerotic plaque triggers activation of both platelets and the coagulation system. These two fundamental mechanisms of thrombogenesis are closely linked *in vivo*, as thrombin is a potent platelet activator and activated platelets augment the coagulation process. Both anticoagulants and platelet inhibitors, or a combination of the two, are therefore beneficial in the treatment of acute coronary syndromes (ACS).

Coagulation

The coagulation system is a series of reactions involving procoagulant and anticoagulant proteins circulating in the plasma as proenzymes or pro-cofactors.

The lipid-rich core of the disrupted atherosclerotic plaque has a high content of tissue factor (TF), a small glycoprotein (GP) expressed on stimulated monocytes, macrophages, endothelial cells, and smooth muscle cells.

TF initiates activation of the extrinsic coagulation cascade (see **Figure 1**). Factor VII binds TF on the cell surface and the factor VIIa/TF complex then activates factors IX and X. Factor Xa assembles on the surface of activated platelets as part of the prothrombinase complex, consisting of factors Xa, Va, and calcium, and converts prothrombin to thrombin.

Thrombin has multiple effects and plays a central role in the process of thrombus formation; it converts fibrinogen to fibrin and is also a strong platelet activator. Fibrin is stabilized by factor XIIIa (which is also activated by thrombin). It forms a fibrin network, thus stabilizing the platelet–rich clot. The presence of a persistent prothrombotic state after the acute phase of ACS has passed is supported by the finding of high levels of molecular markers of coagulation activity up to 6 months after the index event.

Figure 1. The coagulation cascade. F: factor; TFPI: tissue factor pathway inhibitor.

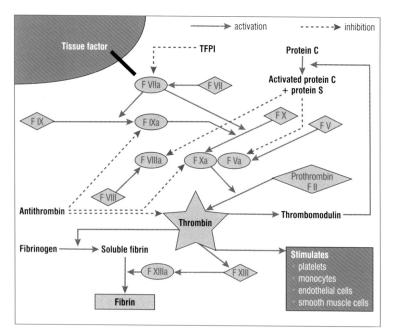

Anticoagulants

There are several physiological anticoagulant pathways. Antithrombin forms inactive complexes with coagulation factors Xa, IIa (thrombin), IXa, and XIa, which are then removed by the liver. Another important anticoagulant is TF pathway inhibitor (TFPI), an endothelium-bound protein that inactivates factors VIIa and Xa. Thrombin bound to thrombomodulin furthermore activates protein C, which, in the presence of protein S, degrades factors Va and VIIIa on platelet surfaces, thereby slowing blood clotting.

Unfractionated heparin

The inhibition of coagulation by antithrombin is markedly increased in the presence of heparin. Treatment with unfractionated heparin (UFH) has several limitations, including the need for intravenous infusion, nonlinear dose–response, high interindividual variability of anticoagulant response, requirement for endogenous cofactors, and nonspecific binding to plasma proteins and cells.

UFH treatment should be closely monitored since activated partial thromboplastin times (aPTT) >70 seconds are associated with an increased risk of bleeding and mortality. However, the relationship between anticoagulant efficacy and aPTT is less clear. Activated clotting time (ACT) is used to monitor the higher doses of heparin that are administered during percutaneous coronary intervention (PCI).

Low molecular weight heparin

Compared with UFH, the low molecular weight heparins (LMWHs) exhibit an increased inhibition of factor Xa, increased bioavailability (following subcutaneous administration), less plasma protein binding, and a 2- to 4-fold longer half-life. They are therefore easier to administer (as twice-daily subcutaneous weight-adjusted injections) and do not require monitoring.

Direct thrombin inhibitors

Direct thrombin inhibitors (DTIs) work independently of antithrombin and heparin cofactor II and are not inactivated by heparinases. Like heparins, DTIs inhibit free thrombin, but they also inhibit fibrin-bound thrombin and might thereby more effectively inhibit thrombin activity in ACS.

Hirudin, a 65- or 66-amino acid polypeptide originally found in the saliva of the medicinal leech, is now available through recombinant DNA technology. Bivalirudin is a synthetic 20-amino acid polypeptide with a shorter plasma half-life than hirudin. Hirudin is approved for the treatment of heparin-induced thrombocytopenia, whereas bivalirudin is approved as a heparin substitute in patients undergoing PCI.

Oral anticoagulants

The oral anticoagulant warfarin, a coumarin derivate, induces hepatic production of partially decarboxylated coagulation factors II, VII, IX, and X by inhibiting the vitamin K conversion cycle, resulting in reduced coagulant activity. The onset of anticoagulation is slow and careful monitoring is required during treatment to maintain the international normalized ratio (INR) within the therapeutic range while avoiding bleeding complications, which is especially important when warfarin is used in combination with antiplatelet agents.

ST-segment elevation MI

Unfractionated heparin

Randomized clinical trials performed before the reperfusion era reported a reduction in mortality and reinfarction with UFH treatment. However, patients in the control groups were not treated with aspirin, so the results are not applicable to current practice [1].

UFH, administered as a 24–48 hour infusion, is routinely used as an adjunct to aspirin and tissue plasminogen activator (tPA)-based fibrinolytics [2,3], although no placebo-controlled trials have proven its efficacy [4]. Two small studies have shown that UFH improves the surrogate endpoint of coronary patency up to 2 days after tPA-based fibrinolysis, but these results have been questioned by other studies. No difference in patency has been shown with the addition of UFH to streptokinase [1]. **Box 1** provides dosing guidance for UFH in ST-segment elevation myocardial infarction (STEMI).

Low molecular weight heparin

Treatment with LMWH as an adjunct to fibrinolytics might provide a bridge to late revascularization after successful primary lysis. Two recent large-scale trials comparing fibrinolytic treatment in combination with either LMWH or UFH have revealed both increased antithrombotic efficacy and increased risk of major hemorrhages with

Box 1. Anticoagulant dose regimens in ST-segment elevation myocardial infarction. ACT: activated clotting time; aPTT: activated partial thromboplastin time; GP: glycoprotein; IV: intravenous; LMWH: low molecular weight heparin; PCI: percutaneous coronary intervention; SC: subcutaneous; tPA: tissue plasminogen activator; UFH: unfractionated heparin.

Unfractionated heparin

A. In conjunction with tPA-based fibrinolytics [2,36]:
- IV bolus 60 U/kg body weight, maximum 4,000 U followed by
- IV infusion 12 U/kg/h, maximum 1,000 U/h, 24–48 hours
- aPTT at 3, 6, 12, and 24 hours after treatment onset, aiming at aPTT 50–70 seconds

B. During direct PCI without GPIIb/IIIa receptor inhibitor [1]:
- IV bolus 100–175 U/kg aiming at ACT 300–350 seconds
- IV bolus 10–15 U/kg/h

C. During direct PCI with GPIIb/IIIa receptor inhibitor [1]:
- IV bolus 50–70 U/kg aiming at ACT >200 seconds
- repeated bolus doses only if complicated, prolonged procedure

LMWH administration [5,6]. Further studies are required to determine the appropriate dose of LMWH before it can routinely be used in this setting (see **Table 1**).

Direct thrombin inhibitors

Hirudin has not shown any clear benefit over UFH in Phase III trials of STEMI patients treated with tPA-derived fibrinolytics (see **Table 2**) [7,8]. The recent HERO-2 study of STEMI patients treated with streptokinase and randomized to 48-hour infusion with bivalirudin or UFH showed no reduction in the primary endpoint of mortality at 30 days with bivalirudin, but did find a significantly reduced rate of in-hospital reinfarctions (median stay 14 and 13 days, respectively) (see **Table 2**) [9].

Oral anticoagulants

Oral anticoagulants are not indicated in the acute phase of STEMI because of their slow onset of anticoagulation, with antithrombotic efficacy only developing after 3–4 days of treatment. Patients

Table 1. Low molecular weight heparin versus placebo (in addition to aspirin and tenecteplase) in ST-segment elevation myocardial infarction (STEMI) patients. Randomized studies with more than 500 patients in each treatment group. AMI: acute myocardial infarction; IV: intravenous; NS: nonsignificant.

Study (number of patients)	Study treatment and duration	Control and duration	Study vs control (P value)		
			Death + AMI in-hospital	Death + AMI + refractory angina at 30 d	Major bleeding
ASSENT-III (4,078) [5]	Enoxaparin IV bolus 30 mg + 1 mg/kg bid, max. 7 days	UFH infusion, 48 hours	6.8% vs 9.1% ($P = 0.02$)	11.4% vs 15.4% 15.4% ($P<0.001$)	3.0% vs 2.2% (NS)
ASSENT-III PLUS (1,639) [6]	Enoxaparin IV bolus 30 mg + 1 mg/kg bid, max. 7 days	UFH infusion, 48 hours	3.5% vs 5.8% ($P = 0.03$) Only AMI	14.2% vs 17.4% ($P = 0.08$)	4.0% vs 2.8% (NS)

already on oral anticoagulants have an increased bleeding risk if fibrinolytics are administered, although lytic treatment is not absolutely contraindicated.

Several attempts have been made to combine low intensity oral anticoagulants (INR <2.0) and aspirin, though the results have been discouraging. Three recent trials of long-term treatment with moderate-to-high intensity oral anticoagulants (INR >2.0) plus aspirin, as compared with aspirin alone in post-myocardial infarction (MI) patients, demonstrated fewer reocclusions after successful lysis and, in the group receiving oral anticoagulants, a reduced rate of death, reinfarction, and stroke (see **Table 3**) [10]. However, this benefit was at the cost of an increase in major nonfatal bleeding complications, despite the careful monitoring of anticoagulation.

Table 2. Direct thrombin inhibitors versus unfractionated heparin (UFH) (in addition to fibrinolysis and aspirin) in ST-segment elevation myocardial infarction (STEMI) patients. Randomized studies with more than 500 patients in each treatment group. AMI: acute myocardial infarction; NS: nonsignificant. *Data for the total GUSTO-IIB cohort (STEMI + NSTEMI), see also **Table 7**. †Includes heart failure and cardiogenic shock.

Study (number of patients)	Study treatment and duration	Control and duration	Study vs control (P value)		
			Death + AMI in-hospital	Death + AMI at 30 d	Major bleeding
GUSTO-IIb (4,131) [7]	Hirudin bolus + infusion 0.1 mg/kg/h, 3–5 days	UFH bolus + infusion, 3–5 days	2.3% vs 3.1% (P = 0.001) at 48 hours*	9.9% vs 11.3% (P = 0.12)	1.1% vs 1.5% (NS)
TIMI-9B (3,002) [8]	Hirudin bolus + infusion 0.1 mg/kg/h, 96 hours	UFH bolus + infusion, 96 hours	7.7% vs 8.1% (NS)	12.9% vs 11.9%† (NS)	4.6% vs 5.3% (NS)
HERO-2 (17,073) [9]	Bivalirudin bolus + infusion 0.5 mg/kg/h, 12 hours + 0.25 mg/kg/h, 36 hours	UFH bolus + infusion, 48 hours	2.8% vs 3.6% (P = 0.005) Only AMI	12.6% vs 13.6% (P = 0.07)	0.7% vs 0.5% (P = 0.07)

The balance between risk and benefit of oral anticoagulants in the real-life setting is difficult to evaluate. Thus, routine use of aspirin plus oral anticoagulation is not generally recommended. Oral anticoagulation alone is the best alternative in patients hypersensitive to aspirin [11], and might furthermore be the best treatment option after MI in patients with atrial fibrillation.

Non-ST-segment elevation MI/ unstable angina

Unfractionated heparin

A combination of UFH infusion and aspirin has been the standard therapy in many clinical guidelines [12], although there is no solid evidence of long-term benefits. A meta-analysis of six randomized trials has shown a nonsignificant 2.4% absolute risk reduction in death or MI during treatment with UFH plus aspirin in comparison with aspirin alone [13]. After cessation of treatment, there are signs of

Table 3. Oral anticoagulation (moderate to high intensity) plus aspirin versus aspirin alone in postmyocardial infarction patients. Randomized studies with more than 100 patients in each treatment group. AMI: acute myocardial infarction; INR: international normalized ratio; NS: nonsignificant; OAC: oral anticoagulant. *Total bleeding.

Study (number of patients)	Study treatment (reached INR) and duration	Control and duration	Study vs control (P value)		
			Reocclusion	Death + AMI + stroke	Major bleeding
APRICOT-II (308) [47]	OAC (INR 2.6) + aspirin 80 mg, 3 months	Aspirin 80 mg, 3 months	18% vs 30% ($P = 0.02$)	–	5% vs 3% (NS)*
ASPECT-II (668) [48]	OAC (INR 2.4) + aspirin 80 mg, median 12 months	Aspirin 160 mg, median 12 months	–	5.1% vs 9.0% ($P<0.05$)	2% vs 1% per year (NS)
WARIS-2 (2,414) [49]	OAC (INR 2.2) + aspirin 80 mg, mean 48 months	Aspirin 160 mg, mean 48 months	–	15% vs 20% ($P<0.01$)	0.57% vs 0.17% per year ($P<0.001$)

reactivation of coagulation activity, as manifested both biochemically and by new clinical events [14,15]. **Box 2** provides dosing guidance for non-ST-segment elevation MI (NSTEMI)/unstable angina.

Low molecular weight heparin

LMWH plus aspirin is the current standard of care in the acute phase of NSTEMI/unstable angina [16]. There is consistent evidence that LMWH is superior to placebo [17] and at least as effective as UFH (see **Table 4**). LMWH has a safety profile similar to that of UFH when used in combination with GPIIb/IIIa receptor antagonists (see **Table 5**) [18].

Box 2. Anticoagulant dose regimens in non-ST-segment elevation myocardial infarction (NSTEMI)/ unstable angina. ACT: activated clotting time; aPTT: activated partial thromboplastin time; GP: glycoprotein; IV: intravenous; LMWH: low molecular weight heparin; PCI: percutaneous coronary intervention; SC: subcutaneous; UFH: unfractionated heparin.

UFH	LMWH
A. UFH might be administered in the cardiac care unit although LMWH is preferred [12,36] • IV bolus 60–70 U/kg (maximum 5,000 U) followed by • IV infusion 12–15 U/kg/h to aPTT at 50–70 seconds	A. In the cardiac care unit and continued for 2–8 days or until revascularization • enoxaparin 1 mg/kg body weight SC bid [40] • dalteparin 120 IU/kg body weight SC bid (maximum 10,000 IU bid) [38]

B. During early PCI without GPIIb/IIIa receptor inhibitor [23,24]
 	
• IV bolus 70–100 U/kg aiming at
 	
• ACT 300–350 seconds (Hemachron) or 250–300 seconds (Hematec)
 	
• additional IV bolus 2,500–5,000 U might be administered
	B. During early PCI with or without GPIIb/IIIa receptor inhibitor [18,26]
	
	• no extra heparin if <8 hours since last dose of LMWH
	
	• if 8–12 hours since last dose of SC enoxaparin:
	
	   – IV bolus enoxaparin 0.3 mg/kg or
	
	   – IV bolus UFH
	
	• if >8 hours since last dose of SC dalteparin:
	
	   – IV bolus UFH

C. During early PCI with GPIIb/IIIa receptor inhibitor [16,23] • IV bolus 70 U/kg aiming at ACT 200–250 seconds • repeated bolus doses only if complicated prolonged procedure	

Although initial intense anticoagulation improves clinical outcomes in ACS patients, an increased risk of new thrombotic events persists for several weeks, providing the rationale for prolonged LMWH treatment. A meta-analysis of four randomized placebo-controlled trials showed only a modest, nonsignificant reduction in ischemic events with LMWH (see **Table 6**) [19]. Nevertheless, full-dose LMWH may be beneficial in the first 4–6 weeks of treatment in patients awaiting revascularization [20].

Direct thrombin inhibitors

A meta-analysis of several large-scale NSTEMI/unstable angina studies has revealed a significant but modest reduction in death or MI at 30 days, from 8.1% in heparin-treated patients to 7.3% in patients treated with DTIs [21] – mainly as a result of

Table 4. Low molecular weight heparin versus unfractionated heparin (UFH) (in addition to aspirin) in patients with unstable angina. Randomized studies with more than 500 patients in each treatment group. AMI: acute myocardial infarction; NS: nonsignificant; SC: subcutaneous.

Study (number of patients)	Study treatment and duration	Control and duration	Study vs control (P value)			
			Death + AMI at 1–5 d	Death + AMI at 30 d	Death + AMI + refr. angina at 30–45 d	Major bleeding
FRIC (1,482) [37]	Dalteparin bid, 5–7 days	UFH infusion, 2–3 days UFH SC 2 days	3.9% vs 3.6% (NS)	4.3% vs 4.7% (NS), day 6–45	12.3% vs 12.3%, day 6–45 (NS)	1.6% vs 1.4% (NS)
ESSENCE (3,171) [40]	Enoxaparin bid, 2.6 days	UFH infusion, 2.6 days	1.1% vs 1.3% (NS)	6.1% vs 7.7% (NS)	19.8% vs 23.3% (P = 0.02)	7.0% vs 6.5 % (NS)
TIMI 11B (3,910) [39]	Enoxaparin bid, 4.6 days + long-term enoxaparin	UFH infusion, 3 days + placebo	4.1% vs 5.3% (NS), after 8 days	5.7% vs 6.8% (NS), after 14 days	17.3% vs 19.6% (P<0.05)	1.5% vs 1.0% (NS), in hospital
FRAX.I.S (2,317) [41]	Nadroparin bid, 6 ± 3 days	UFH infusion, 6 ± 3 days	3.1% vs 3.1% (NS), after 6 days	8.6% vs 7.9% (NS), after 3 months	22% vs 22% (NS), after 3 months	1% vs 1% (NS), in hospital

decreases in myocardial (re-)infarctions (see **Table 7**). No DTI has yet been approved for the acute treatment of NSTEMI/unstable angina, though the on-going ACUITY trial is examining bivalirudin in this setting.

Oral anticoagulants

The use of oral anticoagulants has been addressed in only one large-scale NSTEMI/unstable angina study, in which 3,712 patients were randomized to receive either oral anticoagulation therapy in addition to aspirin for 5 months or standard aspirin therapy. The trial demonstrated no significant reduction in cardiovascular death, MI, or stroke [22]. However, the ASPECT-2 study (in which more than 50% of patients had NSTEMI/unstable angina) and the WARIS-2 study (in which approximately 40% of patients had a non-Q-wave MI) found an advantage of combination therapy at the cost of increased bleeding risk (see **Table 3**).

Table 5. Low molecular weight heparin versus unfractionated heparin (UFH) during glycoprotein IIb/IIIa receptor inhibition (in addition to aspirin) in non-ST-segment elevation myocardial infarction/unstable angina patients. Randomized studies with more than 200 patients in each treatment group. AMI: acute myocardial infarction; NS: nonsignificant.

Study (number of patients)	Study treatment and duration	Control and duration	Study vs control (P value)		
			Death + AMI at 7 d	Death + AMI at 30 d	Major bleeding
ACUTE-II (525) [42]	Enoxaparin bid + tirofiban 24–96 hours	UFH bolus + infusion + tirofiban 24–96 hours	–	9.2% vs 9.0% (NS)	0.3% vs 1.0% (NS)
GUSTO-IV dalteparin substudy (5,202) [43]	Dalteparin bid 5 days + abciximab 24–48 hours (n = 646)	UFH bolus + infusion 48 hours + abciximab 24–48 hours (n = 4,556)	4.8% vs 3.9% (NS)	9.6% vs 8.5% (NS)	1.2% vs 0.7% (NS)
INTERACT (746) [44]	Enoxaparin bid + eptifibatide 48 hours	UFH bolus + infusion + eptifibatide 48 hours	–	5% vs 9% (P = 0.03)	1.8% vs 4.6% (P = 0.03)

Percutaneous coronary intervention

Unfractionated heparin

Despite dosing uncertainties and unpredictable therapeutic response, UFH is the standard anticoagulant treatment during direct PCI for STEMI [23] and in early PCI for NSTEMI/unstable angina [16]. ACT should be monitored during treatment. The dose should be reduced when UFH is used in combination with GPIIb/IIIa receptor inhibitors. Infusion of UFH after the intervention gives no clinical benefit, but increases bleeding risk [24].

Low molecular weight heparin

There is growing evidence from both randomized trials and observational studies [25] that early coronary intervention in NSTEMI/unstable angina

Table 6. Prolonged low molecular weight heparin versus placebo (in addition to aspirin) in non-ST-elevation myocardial infarction unstable angina – randomized studies with more than 500 patients in each treatment group. AMI: acute myocardial infarction; NS: nonsignificant. *Events during the initial phase with active treatment in both arms are not included in the FRIC results.

Study (number of patients)	Study treatment and duration	Control and duration	Study vs control* (P value)		
			Death + AMI at 30–45 d	Death + AMI + refr. angina at 30–45 d	Major bleeding
FRISC I (1,498) [17]	Dalteparin bid, 45 days	Placebo	8.0% vs 10.7% (P = 0.07)	18.0% vs 23.7% (P = 0.005)	1.2% vs 0.8%
FRIC ([1,123] long-term) [37]	UFH infusion or dalteparin bid 5–7 days + dalteparin od 45 days	UFH infusion or dalteparin bid 5–7 days + placebo	4.3% vs 4.7% (NS)*	12.3% vs 12.3% (NS)*	0.5% vs 0.4% (during long-term treatment)
FRISC II (2,250) [38]	Dalteparin bid, 90 days	Dalteparin bid 5–7 days + placebo	6.2% vs 8.4% (P = 0.048)	19.5% vs 25.7% (P = 0.001)	3.3% vs 1.5% (during long-term treatment)
TIMI 11B (3,910) [39]	Enoxaparin bid, 42 days	UFH infusion 3 days + placebo	5.7% vs 6.8% (14 days, NS)	17.3% vs 19.6% (P = 0.048)	2.9% vs 1.5% (during long-term treatment)

can be both effectively and safely performed with LMWH treatment, both with and without concomitant treatment with GPIIb/IIIa receptor inhibitors (see **Table 5**) [18,26]. Large-scale randomized trials, such as the ongoing SYNERGY study [27], will generate further information on this topic.

Direct thrombin inhibitors

Only two randomized studies have directly compared DTIs with UFH in ACS patients undergoing PCI (see **Table 8**), although a meta-analysis of 8,497 ACS patients undergoing PCI during treatment with DTIs or UFH showed a significant 32% relative risk reduction in death or MI at the end of DTI treatment [28]. The benefit was most pronounced with bivalirudin as compared with UFH [29], where the combined endpoint of death, MI, or repeat revascularization was significantly reduced at 90 days. Bleeding was also significantly reduced.

Bivalirudin is therefore considered as an alternative to UFH in patients undergoing PCI, although no studies

Table 7. Direct thrombin inhibitors versus unfractionated heparin (UFH) (in addition to aspirin) in non-ST-elevation myocardial infarction/ unstable angina patients. Randomized studies with more than 500 patients in each treatment group. *Data for the total GUSTO-IIb cohort (STEMI + NSTEMI), see also Table 2.

Study (number of patients)	Study treatment and duration	Control and duration	Study vs control (P value)		
			Death + AMI in-hospital	Death + AMI at 30–35 d	Major bleeding
GUSTO-IIb (8,011) [7]	Hirudin bolus + infusion 0.1 mg/kg/h, 3–5 days	UFH bolus + infusion, 3–5 days	2.3% vs 3.1% at 48 hours* (P = 0.001)	8.3% vs 9.1% (NS)	1.3% vs 0.9% (P = 0.06)
OASIS-2 (10,141) [45]	Hirudin bolus + infusion 0.15 mg/kg/h, 72 hours	Heparin bolus + infusion, 72 hours	3.6% vs 4.2% (P = 0.08)	6.8% vs 7.7% (P = 0.06)	1.2% vs 0.7 % (P = 0.01)

in high-risk ACS patients have been performed in the era of stents and GPIIb/IIIa receptor antagonists [30].

Oral anticoagulants

Oral anticoagulants were previously used to prevent thrombosis after coronary stenting. However, ADP-receptor blockers in combination with aspirin are more effective in reducing the risk of thrombotic events as well as bleeding complications when compared with oral anticoagulants [31].

Bleeding complications

Severe bleeding complications in ACS are unusual, despite modern aggressive antithrombotic treatment of ACS, including various combinations of antiplatelets and anticoagulants. Minor bleeding is usually treated by local measures to stop bleeding and/or discontinuation of treatment, although the long half-life of oral anticoagulants needs to be taken into account.

Table 8. Direct thrombin inhibitors versus unfractionated heparin (UFH) during percutaneous coronary intervention (in addition to aspirin) in non-ST-segment elevation myocardial infarction/unstable angina patients. Randomized studies with more than 300 patients in each treatment group. AMI: acute myocardial infarction; NS: nonsignificant; SC: subcutaneous. *Includes coronary bypass surgery, bailout procedure, and second angioplasty.

Study (number of patients)	Study treatment and duration	Control and duration	Study vs control* (P value) Death + AMI at 4–7 d	Death + AMI + revascularization at >90 d	Major bleeding
HELVETICA (1,141) [4,6]	Hirudin bolus + infusion 24 hours + hirudin/placebo SC bid, 3 days	UFH bolus + infusion 24 hours + placebo SC bid 3 days	6.7%* vs 11%* (P = 0.02)	34% vs 33% (NS) 30 weeks	6.6% vs 6.2% (NS)
Bivalirudin Angioplasty Study (4,312) [29]	Bivalirudin bolus + infusion 2.5 mg/kg/h, 4 hours + 0.2 mg/kg/h, 20 hours	UFH bolus + infusion, 24 hours	6.2% vs 7.9% (P = 0.04)	15.7% vs 18.5% (P = 0.01) 90 days	3.5% vs 9.3% (P<0.001)

Major bleeding, such as intracranial hemorrhages, hematemesis, or melena, is unusual except in combination with fibrinolytics, but may require supportive measures such as transfusions of erythrocytes, freshly frozen plasma, and/or platelets.

UFH is fully reversed by protamine sulfate, which neutralizes the anti-factor IIa activity, but only partially reverses the anti-factor Xa activity of LMWHs. The anticoagulant effect of coumarin derivates is slowly reversed by vitamin K administration and immediately reversed by administration of prothrombin complex concentrate. There are no antidotes to DTIs, but recombinant factor VIIa might be useful in the event of life-threatening bleeding.

Novel anticoagulants

Factor Xa inhibitors

A new class of selective antithrombin-dependent factor Xa inhibitors has been developed. Fondaparinux is a synthetic pentasaccharide with nearly complete bioavailability after subcutaneous injection. Four Phase III studies have demonstrated that fondaparinux (compared with LMWH) reduces the incidence of asymptomatic venous thromboembolism in orthopedic surgery by approximately 50% [32], although this is at the cost of an increased bleeding risk. Fondaparinux is furthermore as effective and safe as LMWH and UFH in the treatment of deep venous thrombosis and pulmonary embolism, respectively [33].

Phase II studies with once-daily subcutaneous injections of fondaparinux in ACS (STEMI and NSTEMI/unstable angina) have demonstrated similar efficacy and safety to UFH and LMWH, although no clear dose–effect relationship has been established [33]. Phase III studies are ongoing.

An interesting future approach will be the development of pentasaccharides with longer half-life, allowing once weekly injections. This might be feasible for long-term treatment.

Oral direct thrombin inhibitors

Orally available DTIs are under investigation and might be advantageous in prolonged anticoagulant treatment. Ximelagatran has no food or drug interactions and predictable pharmacokinetics, and therefore does not require laboratory monitoring of its antithrombotic effect. Fixed-dose ximelagatran has been evaluated in comparison with LMWH in Phase III trials for elective hip or knee arthroplasty [34]; with LMWH–warfarin and placebo in the treatment and prophylaxis of venous thromboembolism; and with warfarin in the prophylaxis of arterial thromboembolism in atrial fibrillation. The balance between efficacy and bleeding risk generally favors ximelagatran.

Promising results have recently been presented from a Phase II study (ESTEEM) of 6 months' treatment with ximelagatran and aspirin, versus aspirin alone, in 1,883 patients with a recent MI. The primary endpoint of death, MI, and severe recurrent ischemia at 6 months was significantly reduced from 16.3% in the aspirin group to 12.7% in the group treated with ximelagatran plus aspirin [35]. As with fondaparinux, there appeared to be no dose–response relationship and no increase in major bleeding. In the future, long-term oral treatment with ximelagatran might be an alternative to warfarin as a complement to platelet inhibition in ACS.

References

1. Hirsh J, Anand SS, Halperin JL, et al. AHA Scientific Statement: Guide to anticoagulant therapy: heparin: a statement for healthcare professionals from the American Heart Association. *Arterioscler Thromb Vasc Biol* 2001;21:e9–e33.
2. Ryan TJ, Antman EM, Brooks NH, et al. 1999 update: ACC/AHA Guidelines for the Management of Patients With Acute Myocardial Infarction: Executive Summary and Recommendations: A report of the American College of Cardiology/American Heart Association Task Force on Practice Guidelines (Committee on Management of Acute Myocardial Infarction). *Circulation* 1999;100:1016–30.

3. Van de Werf F, Ardissino D, Betriu A, et al. Management of acute myocardial infarction in patients presenting with ST-segment elevation. The Task Force on the Management of Acute Myocardial Infarction of the European Society of Cardiology. *Eur Heart J* 2003;24:28–66.

4. Collins R, MacMahon S, Flather M, et al. Clinical effects of anticoagulant therapy in suspected acute myocardial infarction: systematic overview of randomized trials. *Br Med J* 1996;313:652–9.

5. ASSENT-3 Investigators. Efficacy and safety of tenecteplase in combination with enoxaparin, abciximab, or unfractionated heparin: the ASSENT-3 randomized trial in acute myocardial infarction. *Lancet* 2001;358:605–13.

6. Wallentin L, Goldstein P, Armstrong PW, et al. Efficacy and safety of tenecteplase in combination with the low-molecular-weight heparin enoxaparin or unfractionated heparin in the prehospital setting: the Assessment of the Safety and Efficacy of a New Thrombolytic Regimen (ASSENT)-3 PLUS randomized trial in acute myocardial infarction. *Circulation* 2003;108:135–42.

7. GUSTO-2B. A comparison of recombinant hirudin with heparin for the treatment of acute coronary syndromes. The Global Use of Strategies to Open Occluded Coronary Arteries (GUSTO) IIb investigators. *N Engl J Med* 1996;335:775–82.

8. Antman EM. Hirudin in acute myocardial infarction. Thrombolysis and Thrombin Inhibition in Myocardial Infarction (TIMI) 9B trial. *Circulation* 1996;94:911–21.

9. White H. Thrombin-specific anticoagulation with bivalirudin versus heparin in patients receiving fibrinolytic therapy for acute myocardial infarction: the HERO-2 randomized trial. *Lancet* 2001;358:1855–63.

10. Hirsh J, Fuster V, Ansell J, et al. American Heart Association/American College of Cardiology Foundation guide to warfarin therapy. *J Am Coll Cardiol* 2003;41:1633–52.

11. Brouwer MA, Verheugt FW. Oral anticoagulation for acute coronary syndromes. *Circulation* 2002;105:1270–4.

12. Braunwald E, Antman EM, Beasley JW, et al. ACC/AHA guidelines for the management of patients with unstable angina and non-ST-segment elevation myocardial infarction: executive summary and recommendations. A report of the American College of Cardiology/American Heart Association task force on practice guidelines (committee on the management of patients with unstable angina). *Circulation* 2000;102:1193–209.

13. Oler A, Whooley MA, Oler J, et al. Adding heparin to aspirin reduces the incidence of myocardial infarction and death in patients with unstable angina. A meta-analysis. *JAMA* 1996;276:811–5.

14. Theroux P, Ouimet H, McCans J, et al. Aspirin, heparin, or both to treat acute unstable angina. *N Engl J Med* 1988;319:1105–11.

15. RISC. Risk of myocardial infarction and death during treatment with low dose aspirin and intravenous heparin in men with unstable coronary artery disease. The RISC Group. *Lancet* 1990;336:827–30.

16. Bertrand ME, Simoons ML, Fox KA, et al. Management of acute coronary syndromes in patients presenting without persistent ST-segment elevation. *Eur Heart J* 2002;23:1809–40.

17. FRISC. Low-molecular-weight heparin during instability in coronary artery disease. *Lancet* 1996;347:561–8.

18. Wong GC, Giugliano RP, Antman EM. Use of low-molecular-weight heparins in the management of acute coronary artery syndromes and percutaneous coronary intervention. *JAMA* 2003;289:331–42.

19. Bahit MC, Granger CB, Wallentin L. Persistence of the prothrombotic state after acute coronary syndromes: implications for treatment. *Am Heart J* 2002;143:205–16.

20. Husted SE, Wallentin L, Lagerqvist B, et al. Benefits of extended treatment with dalteparin in patients with unstable coronary artery disease eligible for revascularization. *Eur Heart J* 2002;23:1213–8.
21. Eikelboom J, White H, Yusuf S. The evolving role of direct thrombin inhibitors in acute coronary syndromes. *J Am Coll Cardiol* 2003;41:70S–78S.
22. OASIS-2. Effects of long-term, moderate-intensity oral anticoagulation in addition to aspirin in unstable angina. The Organization to Assess Strategies for Ischemic Syndromes (OASIS) Investigators. *J Am Coll Cardiol* 2001;37:475–84.
23. Smith SC Jr, Dove JT, Jacobs AK, et al. ACC/AHA guidelines of percutaneous coronary interventions (revision of the 1993 PTCA guidelines) – executive summary. A report of the American College of Cardiology/American Heart Association Task Force on Practice Guidelines (committee to revise the 1993 guidelines for percutaneous transluminal coronary angioplasty). *J Am Coll Cardiol* 2001;37:2215–39.
24. Popma JJ, Prpic R, Lansky AJ, et al. Heparin dosing in patients undergoing coronary intervention. *Am J Cardiol* 1998;82:19P–24P.
25. Collet JP, Montalescot G, Lison L, et al. Percutaneous coronary intervention after subcutaneous enoxaparin pretreatment in patients with unstable angina pectoris. *Circulation* 2001;103:658–63.
26. Kereiakes DJ, Montalescot G, Antman EM, et al. Low-molecular-weight heparin therapy for non-ST-elevation acute coronary syndromes and during percutaneous coronary intervention: an expert consensus. *Am Heart J* 2002;144:615–24.
27. SYNERGY. The SYNERGY trial: study design and rationale. *Am Heart J* 2002;143:952–60.
28. DTI trialists collaborative group. Direct thrombin inhibitors in acute coronary syndromes: principal results of a meta-analysis based on individual patients' data. *Lancet* 2002;359:294–302.
29. Bittl JA, Chaitman BR, Feit F, et al. Bivalirudin versus heparin during coronary angioplasty for unstable or postinfarction angina: Final report reanalysis of the Bivalirudin Angioplasty Study. *Am Heart J* 2001;142:952–9.
30. Lincoff AM, Bittl JA, Harrington RA, et al. Bivalirudin and provisional glycoprotein IIb/IIIa blockade compared with heparin and planned glycoprotein IIb/IIIa blockade during percutaneous coronary intervention: REPLACE-2 randomized trial. *JAMA* 2003;289:853–63.
31. Steinhubl S, Berger P. What is the role for improved long-term antiplatelet therapy after percutaneous coronary intervention? *Am Heart J* 2003;145:971–8.
32. Turpie AG, Bauer KA, Eriksson BI, et al. Fondaparinux vs enoxaparin for the prevention of venous thromboembolism in major orthopedic surgery: a meta-analysis of 4 randomized double-blind studies. *Arch Intern Med* 2002;162:1833–40.
33. Samama MM, Gerotziafas GT. Evaluation of the pharmacological properties and clinical results of the synthetic pentasaccharide (fondaparinux). *Thromb Res* 2003;109:1–11.
34. Eriksson BI. Clinical experience of melagatran/ximelagatran in major orthopaedic surgery. *Thromb Res* 2003;109(Suppl. 1):S23–S9.
35. Wallentin L, Wilcox RG, Weaver WD, et al. Oral ximelagatran for secondary prophylaxis after myocardial infarction: the ESTEEM randomized controlled trial. *Lancet* 2003;362:789–97.
36. Menon V, Berkowitz SD, Antman EM, et al. New heparin dosing recommendations for patients with acute coronary syndromes. *Am J Med* 2001;110:641–50.

37. Klein W, Buchwald A, Hillis SE, et al. Comparison of low-molecular-weight heparin with unfractionated heparin acutely and with placebo for 6 weeks in the management of unstable coronary artery disease. Fragmin in unstable coronary artery disease study (FRIC). *Circulation* 1997;96:61–8.

38. FRISC-II. Long-term low-molecular-mass heparin in unstable coronary-artery disease: FRISC II prospective randomized multicentre study. *Lancet* 1999;354:701–7.

39. Antman EM, McCabe CH, Gurfinkel EP, et al. Enoxaparin Prevents Death and Cardiac Ischemic Events in Unstable Angina/Non-Q-Wave Myocardial Infarction: Results of the Thrombolysis In Myocardial Infarction (TIMI) 11B Trial. *Circulation* 1999;100:1593–601.

40. Cohen M, Demers C, Gurfinkel EP, et al. A comparison of low-molecular-weight heparin with unfractionated heparin for unstable coronary artery disease. Efficacy and Safety of Subcutaneous Enoxaparin in Non-Q-Wave Coronary Events Study Group. *N Engl J Med* 1997;337:447–52.

41. FRAX.I.S. Comparison of two treatment durations (6 days and 14 days) of a low molecular weight heparin with a 6-day treatment of unfractionated heparin in the initial management of unstable angina or non-Q wave myocardial infarction: FRAX.I.S. (FRAxiparine in Ischaemic Syndrome). *Eur Heart J* 1999;20:1553–62.

42. Cohen M, Theroux P, Borzak S, et al. Randomized double-blind safety study of enoxaparin versus unfractionated heparin in patients with non-ST-segment elevation acute coronary syndromes treated with tirofiban and aspirin: the ACUTE II study. The Antithrombotic Combination Using Tirofiban and Enoxaparin. *Am Heart J* 2002;144:470–7.

43. James S, Armstrong P, Califf R, et al. Safety and efficacy of abciximab combined with dalteparin in treatment of acute coronary syndromes. *Eur Heart J* 2002;23:1538–45.

44. Goodman SG, Fitchett D, Armstrong PW, et al. Randomized evaluation of the safety and efficacy of enoxaparin versus unfractionated heparin in high-risk patients with non-ST-segment elevation acute coronary syndromes receiving the glycoprotein IIb/IIIa inhibitor eptifibatide. *Circulation* 2003;107:238–44.

45. OASIS-2. Effects of recombinant hirudin (lepirudin) compared with heparin on death, myocardial infarction, refractory angina, and revascularisation procedures in patients with acute myocardial ischaemia without ST elevation: a randomized trial. Organisation to Assess Strategies for Ischemic Syndromes (OASIS-2) Investigators. *Lancet* 1999;353:429–38.

46. Serruys PW, Herrman JP, Simon R, et al. A comparison of hirudin with heparin in the prevention of restenosis after coronary angioplasty. Helvetica Investigators. *N Engl J Med* 1995;333:757–63.

47. Brouwer MA, van den Bergh PJ, Aengevaeren WR, et al. Aspirin plus coumarin versus aspirin alone in the prevention of reocclusion after fibrinolysis for acute myocardial infarction: results of the Antithrombotics in the Prevention of Reocclusion In Coronary Thrombolysis (APRICOT)-2 Trial. *Circulation* 2002;106:659–65.

48. van Es RF, Jonker JJ, Verheugt FW, et al. Aspirin and coumadin after acute coronary syndromes (the ASPECT-2 study): a randomized controlled trial. *Lancet* 2002;360:109–13.

49. Hurlen M, Abdelnoor M, Smith P, et al. Warfarin, aspirin, or both after myocardial infarction. *N Engl J Med* 2002;347:969–74.

6

Fibrinolysis

Peter Sinnaeve & Frans Van de Werf

Introduction

Since its first use in the 1950s, fibrinolytic therapy has become the cornerstone of contemporary treatment of acute myocardial infarction (MI). Improvement in therapy has led to the consistent achievement of early, complete, and sustained infarct-related artery patency, resulting in a reduction in average 30-day mortality from 18% in the prefibrinolytic era, to less than 6% in the context of contemporary clinical trials [1].

Infarct-related coronary artery patency can be achieved by administration of fibrinolytic agents or by primary percutaneous coronary intervention (PCI). While primary angioplasty achieves higher patency rates and carries a lower risk of intracranial bleeding complications, pharmacologic reperfusion can be given earlier, is less costly, and is more widely available. Recent guidelines recommend using primary PCI if the procedure can be performed by an experienced team within 90 minutes of initial medical contact. Nevertheless, fibrinolytic therapy is still used for acute MI in the majority of centers worldwide. Data from the GRACE registry indicate that, while only 7 out of 10 patients eligible for reperfusion therapy actually receive treatment, 43% of these patients receive lytic therapy whilst 17% undergo mechanical intervention [2].

Fibrinolytic agents

Rationale and mechanism

Acute MI is generally caused by rupture of an atherosclerotic plaque, triggering the formation of an occlusive coronary thrombus [3]. When the occlusion persists, typical ST-segment elevations appear on the electrocardiogram (ECG). To rescue myocardial muscle at risk of undergoing necrosis, rapid restoration of coronary blood flow is essential. Clot lysis can be achieved by activating the endogenous fibrinolytic system using plasminogen activating agents. These agents convert plasminogen to plasmin which then degrades fibrin, a major constituent of clots (see **Figure 1**).

Fibrinolytic drugs are divided into two groups: fibrin-specific agents and non-fibrin-specific agents

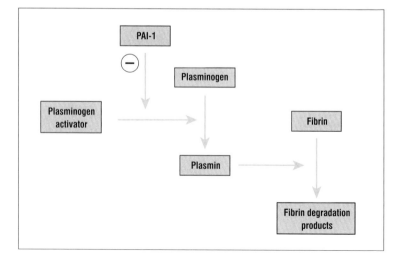

Figure 1. The conversion of plasminogen to plasmin and its degradation to fibrin. PAI-1: plasminogen activator inhibitor-1.

(see **Table 1**). Fibrin-specific drugs are more efficient at dissolving thrombi and they do not deplete systemic coagulation factors, in contrast to non-fibrin-specific agents. However, this potential asset can increase the risk of reocclusion: the reocclusion rate is twice as high (13%) with the fibrin-specific drug alteplase than with non-fibrin-specific drugs [4]. As a consequence, concomitant treatment with heparin is advised in patients receiving fibrin-specific fibrinolytics. **Table 2** provides a summary of the appropriate dosing for frequently used fibrinolytic agents.

Although contemporary pharmacologic reperfusion strategies focus on antithrombotic co-therapies and improvements in, for example, prehospital treatment, the search for the ideal fibrinolytic agent continues. Indeed, standard fibrinolytic regimens suffer from several well-known limitations.

- Fibrinolytics need on average 30–45 minutes to recanalize the infarct-related artery, and complete patency is only achieved in 60%–80% of patients.

- Reocclusion due to prothrombotic effects is common, occurring in 5%–15% of successfully recanalized arteries [5].

Table 1. Fibrin-specific and non-fibrin-specific fibrinolytic agents.

Fibrin-specific agents		Non-fibrin-specific agents
Alteplase	Amediplase	Streptokinase
Reteplase	Monteplase	Urokinase
Tenecteplase	Pametiplase	Anistreplase
Lanoteplase	Staphylokinase	

- Even when blood flow to the infarct-related artery is restored, microcirculatory reperfusion can still be absent ("no-reflow" phenomenon) [6].

- Bleeding complications, especially intracranial hemorrhage (ICH), continue to be a concern.

- Pre-existing antibodies or an immune response to streptokinase or anistreplase may reduce their fibrinolytic capacity or rule out readministration.

Non-fibrin-specific fibrinolytic agents
Streptokinase

Streptokinase is a non-fibrin-specific fibrinolytic agent that indirectly activates plasminogen. Due to its lack of fibrin specificity, streptokinase induces a systemic lytic state. No benefit of concomitantly administered heparin has been convincingly

Table 2. Frequently used fibrinolytic agents: dosing.

Streptokinase	1.5 million IU/hour
Alteplase	15-mg bolus
	90-minute infusion (total dose not to exceed 100 mg):
	• 0.75 mg/kg over 30 minutes (max 50 mg)
	• 0.50 mg/kg over next hour (max 35 mg)
Reteplase	Initial 10 U bolus, followed by second 10 U bolus 30 minutes later
Tenecteplase	Weight-adjusted single bolus:
	• 30 mg if <60 kg
	• 35 mg if 60–69 kg
	• 40 mg if 70–79 kg
	• 45 mg if 80–89 kg
	• 50 mg if ≥90 kg

demonstrated in clinical trials, and the use of heparin is thus at the discretion of the treating physician.

Pre-existing antistreptokinase antibodies impede reperfusion after treatment with streptokinase in patients with acute MI [7]. Administration of streptokinase also invariably induces formation of antistreptokinase antibodies, thus precluding readministration [8]. Although new fibrin-specific fibrinolytics have theoretical advantages, streptokinase remains widely used, in part because of its low cost.

Anistreplase

Anisoylated plasminogen streptokinase activator complex (APSAC, or anistreplase) is a combination of streptokinase and lys-plasminogen. Its active site is protected by an acyl group, thus increasing its half-life. In the ISIS-3 study, anistreplase failed to improve outcomes compared with streptokinase, but was associated with more bleeding complications [9].

Fibrin-specific fibrinolytic agents

Alteplase

Recombinant tissue-type plasminogen activator (rt-PA or alteplase) is a single-chain tissue-type plasminogen activator molecule. Despite its fibrin-specificity, alteplase nevertheless induces mild systemic fibrinogen depletion. Due to its short half-life, alteplase requires a continuous infusion.

Reteplase

The development of reteplase, a second-generation thrombolytic agent, was an attempt to improve on the shortcomings of alteplase (see **Table 3**). It is a mutant of alteplase in which the finger domain (kringle-1) and the epidermal growth factor domain are removed. This results in a decreased plasma clearance, allowing double-bolus administration. However, the removal of the finger domain diminishes fibrin specificity [10]. Like alteplase, reteplase has no resistance to plasminogen activator inhibitor-1 (PAI-1) inactivation.

Tenecteplase

Tenecteplase (TNK-t-PA) is derived from alteplase. It has mutations at three sites (**T**103, **N**117, **K**HRR296–299), which increase the plasma half-life, fibrin binding, fibrin specificity, and resistance to PAI-1. Its slower clearance allows convenient single-bolus administration. Administration of tenecteplase leads to faster recanalization compared with alteplase [11], and it has higher thrombolytic potency on platelet-rich clots than its parent molecule [12].

Lanoteplase

In the InTIME-II trial, lanoteplase (another alteplase variant) was shown to be associated with an increased incidence of ICH and major bleeding [13]. Further development has ceased [13].

Table 3. Properties of selected fibrinolytic agents. PAI-1: plasminogen activator inhibitor 1.

Agent	Fibrin specificity	Half-life (min)	PAI-1 resistance
Streptokinase	–	18–23	–
Anistreplase	–	40–90	–
Alteplase	↑	3–4	–
Reteplase	↓	15–18	–
Tenecteplase	↑↑	20–24	↑
Lanoteplase	↓	30–45	↑
Pametiplase	↑	30–47	–
Monteplase	↑	23	↑
Staphylokinase	↑↑↑	13	–

fibrin specificity [10]. Like alteplase, reteplase has no resistance to plasminogen activator inhibitor-1 (PAI-1) inactivation.

Tenecteplase

Tenecteplase (TNK-t-PA) is derived from alteplase. It has mutations at three sites (**T**103, **N**117, **K**HRR296–299), which increase the plasma half-life, fibrin binding, fibrin specificity, and resistance to PAI-1. Its slower clearance allows convenient single-bolus administration. Administration of tenecteplase leads to faster recanalization compared with alteplase [11], and it has higher thrombolytic potency on platelet-rich clots than its parent molecule [12].

Lanoteplase

In the InTIME-II trial, lanoteplase (another alteplase variant) was shown to be associated with an increased incidence of ICH and major bleeding [13]. Further development has ceased [13].

Table 3. Properties of selected fibrinolytic agents. PAI-1: plasminogen activator inhibitor 1.

Agent	Fibrin specificity	Half-life (min)	PAI-1 resistance
Streptokinase	–	18–23	–
Anistreplase	–	40–90	–
Alteplase	↑	3–4	–
Reteplase	↓	15–18	–
Tenecteplase	↑↑	20–24	↑
Lanoteplase	↓	30–45	↑
Pametiplase	↑	30–47	–
Monteplase	↑	23	↑
Staphylokinase	↑↑↑	13	–

Other fibrinolytics in the pipeline

Staphylokinase

Staphylokinase (STAR) is a fibrin-specific profibrinolytic agent of bacterial origin [14]. In addition to having high fibrinolytic potency and high fibrin specificity, staphylokinase is very effective at dissolving platelet-rich thrombi. Polyethylene glycol-derived mutant variants with reduced immunogenicity and increased half-lives are currently being studied in clinical trials; these permit single-bolus administration [15].

Amediplase

Amediplase is a chimeric fusion protein consisting of the kringle-2 domain of tissue plasminogen activator (t-PA) and the catalytic domain of urokinase-PA. It is fibrin-specific and nonimmunogenic, and can be given as a single bolus. In two angiographic studies (2k2 and 3k2) [16,17], 50% of patients receiving ≈ 1 mg/kg amediplase achieved TIMI 3 flow, and administration was shown to be safe. Phase III trials are in the planning phase.

BB-10153

BB-10153 represents a completely new approach to pharmacologic reperfusion. BB-10153 is not a plasminogen activator; rather, it is a recombinant variant of human plasminogen, modified so that it can be activated by thrombin, a key enzyme involved in thrombus formation. Because thrombin activity is localized at the site of thrombus formation, administration of BB-10153 triggers site-selective production of plasmin. As a result, thrombus dissolution may be achieved without systemic lytic side-effects. BB-10153 will be investigated by the TIMI group.

Indications and contraindications for the use of fibrinolytic therapy

Indications

ST-segment elevation

Administration of fibrinolytic drugs should be considered in patients with typical chest pain and/or other infarct-related symptoms, and patients who present with typical ECG changes (see **Box 1**). Treatment has to be initiated as soon as possible, preferably within 6 hours of symptom onset, although patients can benefit from fibrinolytics up to 12 hours after symptom onset. Although some controversy surrounds the use of pharmacologic reperfusion in patients over 75 years of age, current guidelines advocate the use of fibrinolytics in this age group when primary angioplasty is not available.

Non-ST-segment elevation

Fibrinolytic therapy is not recommended for non–ST-segment elevation acute coronary syndromes (ACS). Although alteplase led to a substantial reduction in thrombus formation compared with placebo in the TIMI IIIa ACS trial [18], the overview by the Fibrinolytic Therapy Trialists (FTT) showed an increased mortality in patients with ST-segment depression treated with fibrinolytics [19].

Reinfarction

Reinfarction after fibrinolysis occurs in 4% of patients and is associated with a more than 3-fold increase in 30-day mortality [20]. When timely revascularization is not available, repeat fibrinolytic therapy is a

---

Box 1. Indications for fibrinolysis.

Presentation and history suggestive of acute myocardial infarction

Persistent ST-segment elevation ≥ 0.1 mV in two or more contiguous leads

New left bundle branch block

---

valuable alternative. Results from GUSTO-I and ASSENT-2 indicated that repeat fibrinolysis significantly improves outcome: 30-day mortality was 11% for repeat fibrinolysis or urgent revascularization compared with 28% for conservative treatment [21]. Nevertheless, readministration of fibrinolytic agents should be carefully weighed against the increased risk of bleeding complications.

Contraindications

Patients at risk of major side effects, including major bleeding and ICH, should not receive fibrinolytics; other absolute and relative contraindications are listed in **Table 4**. Over the past years, an increase in the incidence of ICH has been observed in thrombolytic trials. This is probably the result of several factors: better and more frequent use of brain imaging, inclusion of more patients at high risk

Table 4. Contraindications to fibrinolytic therapy. CNS: central nervous system; CPR: cardiopulmonary resuscitation; ICH: intracranial hemorrhage; TIA: transient ischemic attack.

Absolute contraindications	Relative contraindications
Active bleeding or known bleeding disorder	Uncontrollable hypertension
Recent major surgery or trauma (2–4 weeks)	Previous exposure to streptokinase or staphylokinase
History of ICH	Use of oral anticoagulation with international normalized ratio >2.0
History of ischemic stroke or TIA within past 6 months	History of ischemic stroke or TIA
CNS malformation or tumor	Noncompressible vascular puncture
Aortic dissection	Previous surgery within past 2 weeks
	Retinopathy
	Prolonged CPR (>10 min)
	Pregnancy

(such as the elderly), and more frequent use of revascularization procedures. It is important to identify patients who are at increased risk of bleeding complications (see **Box 2**). In these patients, primary PCI should be considered.

It is not clear why women and those with low body weight have an increased risk of ICH, but it is probably a result of relative overdosing, and recent trials have incorporated weight-adjusted dosing regimens. However, in the ASSENT-2 trial more incidents of ICH were observed in patients with a lower body weight, even with weight-adjusted doses for both tenecteplase and alteplase [16,23].

Evaluation of reperfusion

Reperfusion can be assessed:

- clinically – resolution of chest pain
- angiographically – infarct-related artery patency
- electrocardiographically – ST–T segment resolution on 12-lead ECGs and continuous ST–T segment monitoring
- enzymatically – rapid rise of myoglobin

Traditionally, most clinical trials have used an endpoint of early (60 or 90 minute) angiographic patency of the infarct-related vessel on

Box 2. Patients at increased risk for intracranial hemorrhage.
Age above 75 years
Female gender
Low body weight
High blood pressure or pulse pressure on admission
Prior history of cerebrovascular disease
African descent

angiography as indicative of successful fibrinolysis. A TIMI flow grade of less than 3 in the infarct-related artery is associated with increased mortality and poor recovery of left ventricular function. Unfortunately, angiography only provides a snapshot of the dynamic process of coronary occlusion and recanalization. Myocardial tissue reperfusion correlates better with outcome than epicardial coronary artery patency [16,24], but restored epicardial blood flow does not adequately reflect reperfusion at the tissue level. Restoration of reperfusion at the tissue level can be assessed noninvasively with contrast echocardiography, magnetic resonance imaging, positron emission tomography, and continuous ST-segment monitoring. Results from ASSENT-2 and ASSENT Plus showed that continuous ST-segment monitoring during the first hour after treatment initiation effectively predicts 30-day mortality [25]. In addition, even in patients with TIMI grade 3 flow, failure to achieve early ST-segment recovery was associated with a worse 5-year outcome [16,26].

Fibrinolytic trials

Landmark outcome trials

The first large trial to show a significant reduction in mortality with a fibrinolytic agent was the GISSI-1 trial [27]. In this study, over 11,000 patients with acute MI presenting within 12 hours of symptom onset were randomized to either streptokinase or standard nonfibrinolytic therapy. In-hospital mortality was 10.7% in patients treated with intravenous streptokinase compared with 13.1% in control patients, representing 23 lives saved per 1,000 patients treated. This benefit in mortality was preserved at both 1-year and 10-year follow-up [28,29].

The ISIS-2 study confirmed the results of GISSI-1, but also showed a clear benefit of adding aspirin to the pharmacologic reperfusion regimen [30]. Treatment with aspirin (160 mg/day for 1 month) or streptokinase alone resulted in a significant reduction in mortality

(23% and 24%, respectively). Treatment with both agents combined resulted in a 43% reduction in mortality, demonstrating that this benefit was additive. Aspirin also significantly reduced nonfatal reinfarction (1.0% vs 2.0%).

In a meta-analysis of nine large randomized controlled trials, each with more than 1,000 patients and together totaling over 58,000 patients, the FTT reported a significant 18% reduction in mortality with fibrinolysis in the first 35 days after an acute MI [19]. This benefit was evident across all subgroups.

The question of which fibrinolytic drug reduces mortality most effectively was addressed in the first GUSTO trial, GUSTO-I [31]. A 3-hour infusion of alteplase had previously been shown to result in higher patency rates than streptokinase [4]. In the 40,000 patient GUSTO-I trial, however, a "front-loaded" 90-minute dosing regimen of alteplase was used, which had been shown to achieve higher patency rates than the 3-hour scheme [32]. Mortality at 30 days was significantly lower in patients receiving alteplase (6.3%) compared with those treated with streptokinase (7.4%, $P = 0.001$). Alteplase was also shown to be superior to anistreplase in the TIMI 4 trial (6-week mortality: 2.2% vs 8.8%, respectively) [33].

Trials with new fibrinolytic agents

Encouraged by higher early patency rates in the RAPID I and RAPID II trials (see **Figure 2**) [34,35], reteplase was compared with streptokinase (INJECT) and alteplase (GUSTO-III) in two outcome trials. In the INJECT trial [36], 6,010 patients with acute MI who presented within 12 hours of symptom onset were randomized to either double-bolus reteplase or streptokinase. Double-bolus reteplase (10 MU, given 30 minutes apart) was shown to be at least equivalent to streptokinase (35-day mortality: 9.0% vs 9.5%, respectively). In the GUSTO-III trial [37], which was designed as a superiority trial, 15,059 patients were randomized to double-bolus reteplase or front-loaded alteplase. Mortality at 30 days was similar in both treatment arms (7.47% vs 7.24%, respectively) (see **Figure 3**), as was the incidence of hemorrhagic stroke and other major bleeding complications. Similar mortality rates were maintained for both treatment groups at 1-year follow-up (11.2% vs 11.1%, respectively) [38]. Thus, although reteplase achieves higher early TIMI 3 flow rates, this benefit does not result in improved outcome. This might partially be explained by increased platelet activation with reteplase compared with alteplase [39].

After encouraging patency rates in the TIMI-10A and TIMI-10B trials (see **Figure 2**) [40,41], the double-blind ASSENT-2 trial randomized 16,949 patients to single-bolus tenecteplase or weight-adjusted front-loaded alteplase [42]. This study

Figure 2. Ninety-minute patency rates with alteplase (rt-PA), reteplase (r-PA), and tenecteplase (TNK-t-PA).

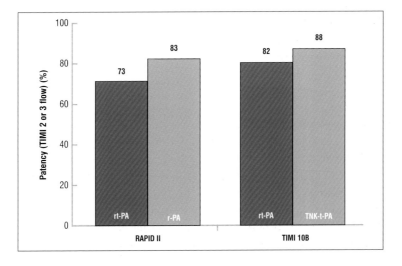

showed that 30-day mortality was similar in the tenecteplase and alteplase arms (6.18% vs 6.15%, respectively) (see **Figure 3**), although, in patients treated ≥4 hours after symptom onset, 30-day mortality was lower in the tenecteplase arm. In the total population studied the incidence of major noncerebral bleeding complications was significantly reduced in the tenecteplase arm (26.1% vs 28.4%, $P<0.0003$). In a subsequent analysis, patients at risk for bleeding complications tended to have lower rates of major bleeding or ICH after treatment with tenecteplase [23]. **Table 5** summarizes key clinical trials in fibrinolysis.

Recent trials testing combination strategies

In GUSTO-V, a noninferiority trial, 16,588 patients were randomized to either reteplase or half-dose reteplase with weight-adjusted abciximab, a

Figure 3. Thirty-day mortality with alteplase (rt-PA), reteplase (r-PA), and tenecteplase (TNK-t-PA).

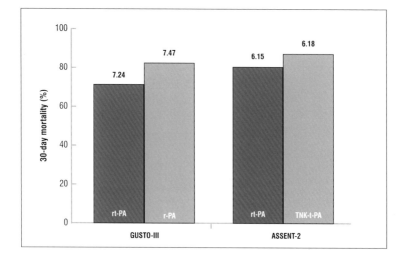

glycoprotein (GP)IIb/IIIa antagonist (see **Table 6**) [43]. In the preceding SPEED trial, patency rate had been shown to be higher with the combination of reteplase and abciximab [44]. In GUSTO-V, 30-day mortality rates were 5.9% for reteplase and 5.6% for the combined reteplase–abciximab group, fulfilling the criteria for noninferiority. Combination therapy

Table 5. Key clinical trials in fibrinolysis. ICH: intracranial hemorrhage; IV: intravenous; SC: subcutaneous. *In GISSI-1, a definite cause (hemorrhagic vs ischemic) was only determined in 27% of all patients with a stroke.

Trial	Patients	Regimen	Mortality (%)	ICH (%)
GISSI-1 [27]	11,806	Control	13.1	*
		Streptokinase	10.7	*
ISIS-2 [30]	17,186	Streptokinase	10.4	0.3
		Streptokinase + aspirin	8.0	0.3
GISSI-2 [22]	20,891	Streptokinase	8.5	0.29
		Alteplase	8.9	0.42
ISIS-3 [9]	41,299	Streptokinase	10.6	0.24
		Alteplase	10.3	0.66
		Anistreplase	10.5	0.55
GUSTO-I [31]	41,021	Streptokinase + SC heparin	7.2	0.46
		Streptokinase + IV heparin	7.4	0.57
		Alteplase + IV heparin	6.3	0.70
		Alteplase + streptokinase	7.0	0.88
GUSTO-III [37]	15,059	Alteplase	7.2	0.87
		Reteplase	7.5	0.91
ASSENT-2 [42]	16,949	Alteplase	6.2	0.94
		Tenecteplase	6.2	0.93
GUSTO-V [43]	16,588	Reteplase	5.9	0.6
		Reteplase + abciximab	5.6	0.6
ASSENT-3 [45]	6,095	Tenecteplase + heparin	6.0	0.9
		Tenecteplase + enoxaparin	5.4	0.9
		Tenecteplase + abciximab	6.6	0.9

with reteplase and abciximab resulted in a significant reduction in ischemic complications after acute MI, but this benefit was offset by an increased risk of serious bleeding complications, particularly in elderly patients.

In the ASSENT-3 study, the low molecular weight heparin (LMWH) enoxaparin, unfractionated heparin (UFH), and abciximab were compared in combination with tenecteplase (see **Table 7**) [45]. A total of 6,095 patients with acute MI received either full-dose weight-adjusted single-bolus tenecteplase with weight-adjusted enoxaparin or UFH, or half-dose tenecteplase with abciximab and weight-adjusted low-dose UFH. Primary endpoints were the composites of 30-day mortality, in-hospital reinfarction, or refractory ischemia at 30 days (primary efficacy endpoint), and the above plus in-hospital ICH or major bleeding (primary efficacy plus safety endpoint). Both enoxaparin plus full-dose tenecteplase and abciximab plus half-dose tenecteplase significantly reduced the risk of ischemic complications (reinfarction and refractory ischemia). A significant improvement in the primary efficacy plus safety endpoint was seen with tenecteplase and enoxaparin, but not with tenecteplase and abciximab,

Table 6. Dosing in GUSTO-V.

	Reteplase	Abciximab	Heparin
Standard	Two boluses of 10 U, 30 min apart		5,000 U bolus 800 (<80 kg) or 1,000 (>80 kg) U/h
Combination	Two boluses of 5 U, 30 min apart	0.25 mg/kg bolus followed by 0.125 μg/kg/min for 12 hours	60 U/kg UFH bolus 7 U/kg infusion

when compared with standard tenecteplase and UFH. ICH rates were very similar in the three treatment arms, but major and minor bleeding complications, thrombocytopenia, and transfusions were more frequent in the half-dose tenecteplase–abciximab arm. As in the GUSTO-V trial, patients in the abciximab group who were older than 75 years experienced significantly more bleeding complications.

Guidelines for fibrinolytic therapy

Current US (American College of Cardiology [ACC]/ American Heart Association [AHA]) and European (European Society of Cardiology [ESC]) guidelines emphasize the importance of prompt early revascularization [46,47]. Both advocate the use of fibrinolytic therapy in eligible patients, regardless of age, when primary PCI cannot be performed by an

Table 7. Dosing in ASSENT-3. UFH: unfractionated heparin.

	Tenecteplase	UFH	Enoxaparin	Abciximab
UFH group	Weight-adjusted single bolus (30 mg <60 kg, 35 mg 60–69 kg, 40 mg 70–79 kg, 45 mg 80–89 kg, 50 mg ≥90 kg)	60 mg/kg bolus (max 4,000 U) 12 U/kg/h infusion (max 1,000)	–	–
Enoxaparin group	Weight-adjusted single bolus (30 mg <60 kg, 35 mg 60–69 kg, 40 mg 70–79 kg, 45 mg 80–89 kg, 50 mg ≥90 kg)	–	30 mg intravenous bolus, then 1 mg/kg every 12 hours subcutaneously for 7 days	–
Abciximab group	Weight-adjusted half-dose single bolus	40 mg/kg bolus (max 3,000 U) 7 U/kg/h infusion (max 800 U/h)		0.25 mg/kg bolus followed by 0.125 µg/kg/min for 12 hours

experienced team within 90 minutes of first medical contact. In patients presenting with cardiogenic shock or contraindications to fibrinolytic therapy (see **Table 4**), primary PCI is indicated.

All patients should receive aspirin. Weight-adjusted UFH is recommended as adjunctive therapy to tenecteplase or alteplase, but is optional for patients receiving streptokinase. The choice of fibrinolytic agent is determined by balancing benefit and risk, and depends on cost and local availability. However, a more fibrin-specific fibrinolytic (such as tenecteplase or alteplase) is recommended in patients presenting more than 4 hours after symptom onset [47].

Improving pharmacologic reperfusion strategies

Time to reperfusion

Current guidelines limit the use of fibrinolytics to a maximum of 12 hours after symptom onset [46]. Overwhelming evidence exists to support administration within 6 hours, but some controversy surrounds the use of fibrinolytics after 6 hours. Nevertheless, in GISSI-1, patients treated 6–12 hours after symptom onset had improved survival with streptokinase [27]. Similarly, in the LATE trial alteplase was shown to be effective in patients presenting after 6 hours, when compared with placebo [48].

Although infarct-related artery patency is the primary goal, rapid reperfusion upon diagnosis is equally essential. Numerous studies have shown the importance of early treatment [49]. Indeed, treatment delay jeopardizes possible muscle recovery and is associated with increased mortality.

Minimizing the delay between symptom onset and treatment initiation can be targeted at multiple levels:

- patient education: symptom awareness and the importance of seeking professional help
- transport to hospital
- detection of MI patients and implementation of critical pathways
- recognition of atypical presentation
- treatment initiation: bolus administration and prehospital treatment

Fibrin specificity

Current guidelines recommend the use of fibrin-specific agents in patients presenting late [47]. After 3 hours, TIMI 3 flow rates are significantly lower with the non–fibrin-specific streptokinase than with alteplase or reteplase [50]. Similar results have been found in outcome trials. In the GUSTO-III trial, 30-day mortality was higher in patients treated 4 hours after symptom onset with reteplase (fibrin-specific) than with alteplase (more fibrin-specific) [37]. Similarly, in the ASSENT-2 trial, mortality in patients treated 4 hours after symptom onset was significantly lower after treatment with the more fibrin-specific tenecteplase [42].

Critical pathways

Comparison between the GUSTO-I and GUSTO-III trials indicates that median time to treatment did not decrease between 1995 and 2002 [51]. Nevertheless, reperfusion delays can be reduced by implementing critical pathways [52]. Data from randomized trials have shown that prompt evaluation and management of admitted patients, using fast-track algorithms, can halve door-to-drug times [53].

Prehospital treatment

Early patency is thought to be associated with improved outcomes. Indeed, mortality rates in randomized trials are consistently lower when patients are treated within 2 hours of symptom onset. Prehospital treatment is therefore an attractive approach to improve outcome after acute MI. A meta-analysis of six trials including 6,434 patients observed an ~1-hour reduction in time to thrombolysis with prehospital treatment, resulting in a 17% mortality reduction [54]. The advent of bolus fibrinolytic agents has also facilitated prehospital reperfusion protocols. The combination of single-bolus tenecteplase plus enoxaparin, which emerged as a convenient and attractive therapy in the ASSENT-3 study, has recently been investigated in the prehospital setting in the ASSENT-3 Plus trial. In this trial, 1,639 patients with acute MI received prehospital tenecteplase and were randomized to either enoxaparin or UFH: a reduction of 47 minutes was observed in time to thrombolysis, increasing the fraction of patients treated within 2 hours of symptom onset from 29% in ASSENT-3 to 52% in ASSENT-3 Plus. Early treatment (<2 hours) was associated with a lower 30-day mortality (4.4% [<2 hours] vs 6.2 [2–4 hours] and 10.4% [4–6 hours]), but no significant difference in outcome was observed between enoxaparin and heparin. Together with findings from the meta-analysis, these results underscore the critical link between early treatment and outcome.

Facilitated PCI

The next logical step towards improving treatment for acute MI is to combine the benefits of primary PCI and fibrinolysis. Much time is often lost between diagnosis and PCI either due to delays in obtaining suitable transport to another center or due to long waiting times for a catheterization laboratory or team to become available. On the other hand, primary PCI allows immediate treatment of the culprit lesion, and, in qualified high-volume centers, is associated with lower mortality rates. Facilitated PCI refers to the administration of a fibrinolytic agent before taking the patient to the catheterization lab. The rationale behind this approach is that reperfusion can be obtained sooner than with PCI alone, while PCI allows immediate recanalization if fibrinolysis fails. The addition of a GPIIb/IIIa antagonist or a direct thrombin inhibitor could help to improve tissue perfusion and hence outcome. Indeed, both classes of antithrombotic agents have been shown to improve outcome in patients with ACS undergoing early PCI [55,56]. Early observations suggest that the combination of fibrinolysis and GPIIb/IIIa antagonism facilitates PCI [57]. Results from the PACT study also show that this strategy leads to more frequent early recanalization and left ventricular function preservation [58]. Currently, both full-dose lytic therapy and combination therapy with half-dose lytic plus a GPIIb/IIIa antagonist followed by immediate PCI are being tested in the setting of facilitated PCI (in the ASSENT-4 PCI, FINESSE, CARESSE, and the prematurely terminated ADVANCE-MI studies).

Conclusions

Fibrinolytic therapy significantly improves patient outcomes after acute MI. Recently, new fibrinolytics have been developed that have several advantages over standard agents. Although they do not seem to have an impact on mortality, they are easier to administer and induce fewer side effects. Further improvement can be expected from novel antithrombotic drugs, reduction of reperfusion injury, and reduced time-to-reperfusion through facilitated PCI and prehospital treatment.

References

1. de Vreede JJ, Gorgels AP, Verstraaten GM, et al. Did prognosis after acute myocardial infarction change during the past 30 years? A meta-analysis. *J Am Coll Cardiol* 1991;18:698–706.
2. Eagle KA, Goodman SG, Avezum A, et al. Practice variation and missed opportunities for reperfusion in ST-segment-elevation myocardial infarction: findings from the Global Registry of Acute Coronary Events (GRACE). *Lancet* 2002;359:373–7.
3. Davies MJ. The pathophysiology of acute coronary syndromes. *Heart* 2000;83:361–6.
4. Granger CB, Califf RM, Topol EJ. Thrombolytic therapy for acute myocardial infarction. A review. *Drugs* 1992;44:293–325. Erratum in: *Drugs* 1993;45:894.
5. Topol EJ. Acute myocardial infarction: thrombolysis. *Heart* 2000;83:122–6.
6. Ito H, Tomooka T, Sakai N, et al. Lack of myocardial perfusion immediately after successful thrombolysis. A predictor of poor recovery of left ventricular function in anterior myocardial infarction. *Circulation* 1992;85:1699–705.
7. Juhlin P, Bostrom PA, Torp A, et al. Streptokinase antibodies inhibit reperfusion during thrombolytic therapy with streptokinase in acute myocardial infarction. *J Intern Med* 1999;245:483–8.

8.   Battershill PE, Benfield P, Goa KL. Streptokinase. A review of its pharmacology and therapeutic efficacy in acute myocardial infarction in older patients. *Drugs Aging* 1994;4:63–86.

9.   ISIS-3: a randomised comparison of streptokinase vs tissue plasminogen activator vs anistreplase and of aspirin plus heparin vs aspirin alone among 41,299 cases of suspected acute myocardial infarction. ISIS-3 (Third International Study of Infarct Survival) Collaborative Group. *Lancet* 1992;339:753–70.

10.   Hoffmeister HM, Kastner C, Szabo S, et al. Fibrin specificity and procoagulant effect related to the kallikrein-contact phase system and to plasmin generation with double-bolus reteplase and front-loaded alteplase thrombolysis in acute myocardial infarction. *Am J Cardiol* 2000;86:263–8.

11.   Binbrek A, Rao N, Absher PM, et al. The relative rapidity of recanalization induced by recombinant tissue-type plasminogen activator (r-tPA) and TNK-tPA, assessed with enzymatic methods. *Coron Artery Dis* 2000;11:429–35.

12.   Collen D, Stassen JM, Yasuda T, et al. Comparative thrombolytic properties of tissue-type plasminogen activator and of a plasminogen activator inhibitor-1-resistant glycosylation variant, in a combined arterial and venous thrombosis model in the dog. *Thromb Haemost* 1994;72:98–104.

13.   InTIME-II Investigators. Intravenous NPA for the treatment of infarcting myocardium early; InTIME-II, a double-blind comparison of single-bolus lanoteplase vs accelerated alteplase for the treatment of patients with acute myocardial infarction. *Eur Heart J* 2000;21:2005–13.

14.   Collen D, Vanderschueren S, Van de Werf FJ. Fibrin-selective thrombolytic therapy with recombinant staphylokinase. *Haemostasis* 1996;26(Suppl 4):294–300.

15.   Collen D, Sinnaeve P, Demarsin E, et al. Polyethylene glycol-derivatized cysteine-substitution variants of recombinant staphylokinase for single-bolus treatment of acute myocardial infarction. *Circulation* 2000;102:1766–72.

16.   Charbonnier B, Pluta W, De Ferrari G, et al. Evaluation of Two Weight-Adjusted Single Bolus Doses of Amediplase to Patients with Acute Myocardial Infarction: the 3k2 Trial (ABSTRACT). *Circulation* 2001;107:II–538.

17.   Vermeer F, Oldrovd K, Pohl J, et al. Safety and angiography data of Amediplase, a new fibrin specific thrombolytic agent, given as a single bolus to patients with acute myocardial infarction: the 2K2 Dose Finding Trial (ABSTRACT). *Circulation* 2001;104:II–538.

18.   Early effects of tissue-type plasminogen activator added to conventional therapy on the culprit coronary lesion in patients presenting with ischemic cardiac pain at rest. Results of the Thrombolysis in Myocardial Ischemia (TIMI IIIA) Trial. *Circulation* 1993;87:38–52.

19.   Indications for fibrinolytic therapy in suspected acute myocardial infarction: collaborative overview of early mortality and major morbidity results from all randomised trials of more than 1000 patients. Fibrinolytic Therapy Trialists' (FTT) Collaborative Group. *Lancet* 1994;343:311–22. Erratum in: *Lancet* 1994;343:742.

20.   Hudson MP, Granger CB, Topol EJ, et al. Early reinfarction after fibrinolysis: experience from the global utilization of streptokinase and tissue plasminogen activator (alteplase) for occluded coronary arteries (GUSTO I) and global use of strategies to open occluded coronary arteries (GUSTO III) trials. *Circulation* 2001;104:1229–35.

21.   Barbash GI, Birnbaum Y, Bogaerts K, et al. Treatment of reinfarction after thrombolytic therapy for acute myocardial infarction: an analysis of outcome and treatment choices in the global utilization of streptokinase and tissue plasminogen activator for occluded coronary arteries (GUSTO I) and assessment of the safety of a new thrombolytic (ASSENT 2) studies. *Circulation* 2001;103:954–60.

22. The International Study Group. In-hospital mortality and clinical course of 20,891 patients with suspected acute myocardial infarction randomised between alteplase and streptokinase with or without heparin. *Lancet* 1990;336:71–5.

23. Van de Werf FJ, Barron HV, Armstrong PW, et al. Incidence and predictors of bleeding events after fibrinolytic therapy with fibrin-specific agents: a comparison of TNK-tPA and rt-PA. *Eur Heart J* 2001;22:2253–61.

24. Ito H, Maruyama A, Iwakura K, et al. Clinical implications of the 'no reflow' phenomenon. A predictor of complications and left ventricular remodeling in reperfused anterior wall myocardial infarction. *Circulation* 1996;93:223–8.

25. Johanson P, Jernberg T, Gunnarsson G, et al. Prognostic value of ST-segment resolution–when and what to measure. *Eur Heart J* 2003;24:337–45.

26. French JK, Andrews J, Manda SO, et al. Early ST-segment recovery, infarct artery blood flow, and long-term outcome after acute myocardial infarction. *Am Heart J* 2002;143:265–71.

27. Effectiveness of intravenous thrombolytic treatment in acute myocardial infarction. Gruppo Italiano per lo Studio della Streptochinasi nell'Infarto Miocardico (GISSI). *Lancet* 1986;1:397–402.

28. Gruppo Italiano per lo Studio della Streptochi-nasi nell'Infarto Miocardico (GISSI). Long-term effects of intravenous thrombolysis in acute myocardial infarction: final report of the GISSI study. *Lancet* 1987;2:871–4.

29. Franzosi MG, Santoro E, De Vita C, et al. Ten-year follow-up of the first megatrial testing thrombolytic therapy in patients with acute myocardial infarction: results of the Gruppo Italiano per lo Studio della Sopravvivenza nell'Infarto-1 study. The GISSI Investigators. *Circulation* 1998;98:2659–65.

30. ISIS-2 (Second International Study of Infarct Survival) Collaborative Group. Randomised trial of intravenous streptokinase, oral aspirin, both, or neither among 17,187 cases of suspected acute myocardial infarction: ISIS-2. *Lancet* 1988;2:349–60.

31. The GUSTO investigators. An international randomized trial comparing four thrombolytic strategies for acute myocardial infarction. *N Engl J Med* 1993;329:673–82.

32. Neuhaus KL, Feuerer W, Jeep-Tebbe S, et al. Improved thrombolysis with a modified dose regimen of recombinant tissue-type plasminogen activator. *J Am Coll Cardiol* 1989;14:1566–9.

33. Cannon CP, McCabe CH, Diver DJ, et al. Comparison of front-loaded recombinant tissue-type plasminogen activator, anistreplase and combination thrombolytic therapy for acute myocardial infarction: results of the Thrombolysis in Myocardial Infarction (TIMI) 4 trial. *J Am Coll Cardiol* 1994;24:1602–10.

34. Bode C, Smalling RW, Berg G, et al. Randomized comparison of coronary thrombolysis achieved with double-bolus reteplase (recombinant plasminogen activator) and front-loaded, accelerated alteplase (recombinant tissue plasminogen activator) in patients with acute myocardial infarction. The RAPID II Investigators. *Circulation* 1996;94:891–8.

35. Smalling RW, Bode C, Kalbfleisch J, et al. More rapid, complete, and stable coronary thrombolysis with bolus administration of reteplase compared with alteplase infusion in acute myocardial infarction. RAPID Investigators. *Circulation* 1995;91:2725–32.

36. Randomised, double-blind comparison of reteplase double-bolus administration with streptokinase in acute myocardial infarction (INJECT): trial to investigate equivalence. International Joint Efficacy Comparison of Thrombolytics. *Lancet* 1995;346:329–36. Erratum in: *Lancet* 1995;346:980.

37. The Global Use of Strategies to Open Occluded Coronary Arteries (GUSTO III) Investigators. A comparison of reteplase with alteplase for acute myocardial infarction. *N Engl J Med* 1997;337:1118–23.

38. Topol EJ, Ohman EM, Armstrong PW, et al. Survival outcomes 1 year after reperfusion therapy with either alteplase or reteplase for acute myocardial infarction: results from the Global Utilization of Streptokinase and t-PA for Occluded Coronary Arteries (GUSTO) III Trial. *Circulation* 2000;102:1761–5.

39. Gurbel PA, Serebruany VL, Shustov AR, et al. Effects of reteplase and alteplase on platelet aggregation and major receptor expression during the first 24 hours of acute myocardial infarction treatment. GUSTO-III Investigators. Global Use of Strategies to Open Occluded Coronary Arteries. *J Am Coll Cardiol* 1998;31:1466–73.

40. Cannon CP, McCabe CH, Gibson CM, et al. TNK-tissue plasminogen activator in acute myocardial infarction. Results of the Thrombolysis in Myocardial Infarction (TIMI) 10A dose-ranging trial. *Circulation* 1997;95:351–6.

41. Cannon CP, Gibson CM, McCabe CH, et al. TNK-tissue plasminogen activator compared with front-loaded alteplase in acute myocardial infarction: results of the TIMI 10B trial. Thrombolysis in Myocardial Infarction (TIMI) 10B Investigators. *Circulation* 1998;98:2805–14.

42. Single-bolus tenecteplase compared with front-loaded alteplase in acute myocardial infarction: the ASSENT-2 double-blind randomised trial. Assessment of the Safety and Efficacy of a New Thrombolytic Investigators. *Lancet* 1999;354:716–22.

43. Topol EJ; GUSTO V Investigators. Reperfusion therapy for acute myocardial infarction with fibrinolytic therapy or combination reduced fibrinolytic therapy and platelet glycoprotein IIb/IIIa inhibition: the GUSTO V randomised trial. *Lancet* 2001;357:1905–14.

44. Trial of abciximab with and without low-dose reteplase for acute myocardial infarction. Strategies for Patency Enhancement in the Emergency Department (SPEED) Group. *Circulation* 2000;101:2788–94.

45. Assessment of the Safety and Efficacy of a New Thrombolytic Regimen (ASSENT)-3 Investigators. Efficacy and safety of tenecteplase in combination with enoxaparin, abciximab, or unfractionated heparin: the ASSENT-3 randomised trial in acute myocardial infarction. *Lancet* 2001;358:605–13.

46. Ryan TJ, Antman EM, Brooks NH, et al. 1999 update: ACC/AHA guidelines for the management of patients with acute myocardial infarction. A report of the American College of Cardiology/American Heart Association Task Force on Practice Guidelines (Committee on Management of Acute Myocardial Infarction). *J Am Coll Cardiol* 1999;34:890–911.

47. Van de Werf FJ, Ardissino D, Betriu A, et al; Task Force on the Management of Acute Myocardial Infarction of the European Society of Cardiology. Management of acute myocardial infarction in patients presenting with ST-segment elevation. *Eur Heart J* 2003;24:28–66.

48. Late Assessment of Thrombolytic Efficacy (LATE) study with alteplase 6–24 hours after onset of acute myocardial infarction. *Lancet* 1993;342:759–66.

49. Cannon CP, Antman EM, Walls R, et al. Time as an adjunctive agent to thrombolytic therapy. *J Thromb Thrombolysis* 1994;1:27–34.

50. Zeymer U, Tebbe U, Essen R, et al. Influence of time to treatment on early infarct-related artery patency after different thrombolytic regimens. ALKK-Study Group. *Am Heart J* 1999;137:34–8.

51. Gibler WB, Armstrong PW, Ohman EM, et al. Persistence of delays in presentation and treatment for patients with acute myocardial infarction: The GUSTO-I and GUSTO-III experience. *Ann Emerg Med* 2002;39:123–30.

52. Emergency department: rapid identification and treatment of patients with acute myocardial infarction. National Heart Attack Alert Program Coordinating Committee, 60 Minutes to Treatment Working Group. *Ann Emerg Med* 1994;23:311–29.

53. Cannon CP, Johnson EB, Cermignani M, et al. Emergency department thrombolysis critical pathway reduces door-to-drug times in acute myocardial infarction. *Clin Cardiol* 1999;22:17–20.

54. Morrison LJ, Verbeek PR, McDonald AC, et al. Mortality and prehospital thrombolysis for acute myocardial infarction: A meta-analysis. *JAMA* 2000;283:2686–92.

55. Boersma E, Akkerhuis KM, Theroux P, et al. Platelet glycoprotein IIb/IIIa receptor inhibition in non-ST-elevation acute coronary syndromes: early benefit during medical treatment only, with additional protection during percutaneous coronary intervention. *Circulation* 1999;100:2045–8.

56. Roe MT, Granger CB, Puma JA, et al. Comparison of benefits and complications of hirudin versus heparin for patients with acute coronary syndromes undergoing early percutaneous coronary intervention. *Am J Cardiol* 2001;88:1403–6, A6.

57. Herrmann HC, Moliterno DJ, Ohman EM, et al. Facilitation of early percutaneous coronary intervention after reteplase with or without abciximab in acute myocardial infarction: results from the SPEED (GUSTO-4 Pilot) Trial. *J Am Coll Cardiol* 2000;36:1489–96.

58. Ross AM, Coyne KS, Reiner JS, et al. A randomized trial comparing primary angioplasty with a strategy of short-acting thrombolysis and immediate planned rescue angioplasty in acute myocardial infarction: the PACT trial. PACT investigators. Plasminogen-activator Angioplasty Compatibility Trial. *J Am Coll Cardiol* 1999;34:1954–62.

7

Long-term prevention strategies

Eric Boersma, Jeroen J Bax, & Don Poldermans

Introduction

Patients presenting with ST-segment elevation acute coronary syndromes (ACS) are at serious risk of dying shortly after the acute event: a 30-day mortality rate of 6%–7% was observed among patients who participated in recently conducted clinical trials (see **Figure 1**). Trial participants with non-ST-segment elevation ACS had a better short-term prognosis, with 30-day mortality rates around 3%–4%. Interestingly, ST and non-ST-segment elevation ACS patients who survived the first month had a similar risk of dying within 1 year of the index event (3.2% and 3.7%, respectively). This illustrates the fact that the incidence of an acute coronary event is a marker of a chronic, yet dynamic, process of atherosclerosis. Episodes of unstable angina pectoris and fatal or nonfatal myocardial infarction (MI) may occur at any stage of the disease, independent of any previous acute events. It is crucial to recognize this concept when assessing treatment strategies aimed at preventing adverse cardiovascular events during long-term follow-up.

Most Phase III trials in secondary prevention of coronary artery disease (CAD) have been undertaken in patients classified according to their discharge diagnosis (such as MI and unstable angina pectoris). However, non-ST-segment elevation ACS is not a synonym for unstable angina pectoris and, although the majority of patients presenting with

ST-segment elevation ACS will develop MI, ST-segment elevation ACS and MI are not equivalent. Nevertheless, as long as we interpret ST-segment elevation ACS and non–ST-segment elevation ACS as events that may occur during one and the same disease process, the results of these trials can still provide useful information.

Figure 1. Thirty-day mortality (dark bars) and 1-year mortality (light bars) after hospital admission for ST-segment elevation (upper panel) and non-ST-segment elevation (lower panel) acute coronary syndromes in recently conducted large Phase III clinical trials [52–60]. *Six-month mortality results.

An ACS incident indicates that the patient has established coronary disease; secondary prevention measures should then be taken to reduce the risk of subsequent incidents by modifying the underlying disease. All secondary prevention guidelines emphasize the need for risk factor management (see **Box 1**) [1–3]. These long-term prevention

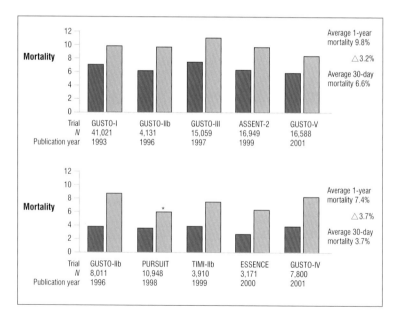

strategies include lifestyle modification, antiplatelet and anticoagulant therapy, the use of beta-blockers, angiotensin-converting enzyme (ACE) inhibitors, and angiotensin II (AT_2)-antagonists, statins, calcium antagonists, and nitrates, and glycemic control in diabetics.

Lifestyle modification

Efforts should be made to increase patient awareness of classical cardiovascular risk factors and to ensure smoking cessation and control of blood pressure, blood lipids, blood glucose, and body weight [4]. Current recommendations on lifestyle changes can be encapsulated by three statements:

- stop smoking tobacco
- make healthy food choices
- be physically active

Box 1. Secondary prevention targets.

Stop smoking tobacco

Healthy food choices
- total fat intake <30% of total energy intake
- increase intake of fresh fruits, cereals, and vegetables

Physical activity
- aerobic exercise, including walking, swimming, or cycling, for 20–30 min 4–5 times a week

Achieve ideal weight
- body mass index <25 kg/m^2
- waist circumference <94 cm (37 inches) in men, <80 cm (31 inches) in women

Blood pressure control
- target <140/90 mm Hg

Blood lipid control
- target low-density lipoprotein cholesterol <2.6 mmol/L (100 mg/dL)

Blood glucose control in diabetes
- target hemoglobin A1c <7%

Stopping smoking

In a meta-analysis of 19 randomized trials in patients with established coronary disease ($N = 13,019$), smoking cessation was associated with a 38% reduced incidence of all-cause death during long-term follow-up (17% events in quitters vs 25% in continued smokers; odds ratio [OR] 0.62; 95% confidence interval [CI] 0.57–0.68). The incidence of all-cause death or nonfatal MI was reduced by 43% (23% vs 34%; OR 0.57; 95% CI 0.53–0.62) [5]. The highest success rates are obtained in programs that are prolonged and multidisciplinary and that include a high number of face-to-face contacts [5].

Making healthy food choices

There is growing evidence that adherence to a traditional Mediterranean diet reduces cardiovascular mortality and morbidity in the general population, as well as in patients with established coronary disease [6–8]. Such a diet is characterized by a high intake of vegetables, legumes, fruit and nuts, unrefined cereals, and olive oil (but a low intake of saturated lipids), a moderately high intake of fish, a low intake of meat and poultry, and a regular but moderate intake of red wine.

Being physically active

A sedentary lifestyle is associated with an increased risk of cardiovascular disease and all-cause mortality, and even modest changes in such a lifestyle can have beneficial effects [9]. In a meta-analysis of 22 trials of rehabilitation after MI, which included an exercise program as part of a multifactorial scheme ($N = 4,554$), the rehabilitation/exercise was associated with a 20% reduction in all-cause mortality during 3 years of follow-up (OR 0.80; 95% CI 0.66–0.96), and with a 22% reduction in cardiovascular mortality (OR 0.78; 95% CI 0.63–0.96) [10]. However, no reduction was observed in the incidence of nonfatal myocardial reinfarction.

Antiplatelet and anticoagulant therapy

It is now understood that the dominant underlying mechanism of acute vascular events is thrombosis caused by a ruptured or eroded atherosclerotic plaque. Thrombi result from a complex series of events involving platelets, coagulation factors, red blood cells, and the vessel wall. Therefore, in order to prevent vascular complications in patients suspected of being at high risk, several treatment regimens that act on the platelet and coagulant cascade have been investigated.

Aspirin
The available evidence for long-term antiplatelet treatment in patients who have had ACS is mostly derived from a meta-analysis of 12 postinfarction trials (N = 20,009) of antiplatelet therapy in the secondary prevention of cardiovascular disease [11]. Long-term aspirin use was associated with a 12% reduction in all-cause death (9.2% vs 10.3%; OR 0.88; 95% CI 0.80–0.96) and a 25% reduction in fatal or nonfatal vascular events including MI and stroke (13.5% vs 17.0%; OR 0.75; 95% CI 0.70–0.82). The meta-analysis provides some evidence that aspirin doses of 75–150 mg are as effective as higher doses and cause fewer side effects. In view of these data, treatment guidelines strongly recommend long-term aspirin use in all post-ACS patients [1–3,12].

Clopidogrel
The CURE investigators compared the efficacy and safety of early and long-term use of clopidogrel (a thienopyridine) plus aspirin with that of aspirin alone in 12,562 patients presenting with non-ST-segment elevation ACS [17]. At 1-year follow-up, combination therapy was associated with a significant 20% reduction in the composite endpoint of cardiovascular death, MI, and stroke (9.3% vs 11.4% events; hazard ratio 0.80; 95% CI 0.72–0.90). The incidence of Q-wave MI was particularly reduced (1.9% vs 3.1% events; hazard ratio 0.60; 95% CI

0.48–0.76). The combination therapy was associated with an increased risk of major bleeding complications. Based on the CURE data, treatment with aspirin plus clopidogrel is recommended in non-ST-segment elevation ACS patients for at least 9 months (the average treatment duration in CURE) [2]. In ST-segment elevation patients, clopidogrel or oral anticoagulant therapy is recommended in those who do not tolerate aspirin [1]. Ongoing trials are evaluating dual antiplatelet therapy in patients with ST-segment elevation ACS.

Anticoagulant therapy

Oral anticoagulation agents could also be used in the long term, although most clinical trials with these agents were undertaken before the widespread use of aspirin [13]. Several clinical trials have shown that treatment with a combination of aspirin and low-intensity oral anticoagulant is not associated with a reduction in events [13,14]. However, in two clinical trials (ASPECT-2 and WARIS-2, together $N = 4,623$), combined aspirin and more intensive oral anticoagulation therapy (target international normalized ratio >2.0) was associated with a significant 32% reduction in the composite endpoint of all-cause death, MI, and stroke during long-term follow-up (12.8% vs 17.6% events; OR based on both trials 0.68; 95% CI 0.56–0.84), albeit at the cost of an increased risk of nonfatal bleeding complications [15,16].

Beta-blockers

Beta-blockers form a class of agents with great cardioprotective potential. Beta-blockers reduce myocardial oxygen demand (by decreasing heart rate and myocardial contractility) and reduce adrenergic activity, which results in reduced levels of free fatty acid, causing a shift in myocardial metabolism towards glucose uptake. These mechanisms may help stabilize coronary plaques that are prone to rupture.

In a meta-analysis of 31 trials (N = 24,974), long-term beta-blocker use in post-MI patients was found to be associated with a 23% reduction in the incidence of all-cause mortality (OR 0.77; 95% CI 0.70–0.84) [18]. The meta-analysis estimated the annual mortality reduction to be 12 deaths per 1,000 patients treated with beta-blockers (95% CI 6–17). The annual reduction in nonfatal MI was estimated at 9 per 1,000 treated patients (95% CI 3–16). The beneficial effect of beta-blockers was seen in patients both with and without preserved left ventricular (LV) function [19]. Based on these data, all patients with established coronary disease, without contraindications, should receive beta-blockers.

ACE inhibitors and AT_2 antagonists

The neurohormone AT_2 plays an important role in the origination of coronary atherosclerosis through a diversity of mechanisms. AT_2 affects endothelial function (it acts as a potent vasopressor), smooth muscle cell migration, and macrophage activation, and promotes platelet aggregation [20]. AT_2 is produced in the lungs from AT_1 via ACE [21]. Thus, inhibition of ACE may retard the progression of coronary atherosclerosis, and may help prevent the incidence of cardiac events in patients with established coronary disease.

ACE inhibitors

Several large randomized trials have addressed the efficacy and safety of ACE inhibitors in post-MI patients. Overview analyses of the results obtained in these trials are complicated by intertrial differences in the duration and starting point of study medication (the starting points ranged from 24 hours to a few weeks or months after the onset of symptoms) [22–26]. Thus, the heterogeneous nature of the trials needs to be taken into account when making estimates of the treatment effect on mortality and morbidity based on meta-analyses.

In a systematic overview that included three trials in post-MI patients (SAVE, AIRE, and TRACE) [22–24] and one trial in heart failure patients (SOLVD) [25,26] (together $N = 12,763$), ACE inhibitor use was associated with a significant 15% reduction in the incidence of all-cause death at 1-year follow-up, as compared with the control treatment (11.3% vs 13.0% events; OR 0.85; 95% CI 0.76–0.94), and a 20% reduction in all-cause death at 4-year follow-up (22.2% vs 26.0% events; OR 0.80; 95% CI 0.74–0.87) [27]. A 28% reduction was observed in the incidence of the composite endpoint of all-cause death, MI, and hospital admission for heart failure (33.8% vs 41.0% events; OR 0.72; 95% CI 0.67–0.78).

Similar results were observed in the HOPE study, which included 9,297 patients at suspected high risk of adverse cardiac events, including patients with diabetes mellitus, but no heart failure [28]. Patients randomized to ramipril had a 16% lower incidence of all-cause death at 4-year follow-up than patients receiving placebo (10.4% vs 12.2% events; hazard ratio 0.84; 95% CI 0.75–0.95). A 22% reduction was observed in the incidence of the primary endpoint of cardiovascular death, MI, and stroke (14.0% vs 17.8% events; hazard ratio 0.78; 95% CI 0.70–0.86). A combined analysis of the HOPE and MICRO-HOPE trials showed a significant beneficial effect of ramipril on cardiovascular events and overt nephropathy in 3,577 patients with diabetes mellitus [29]. The investigators emphasized that the beneficial effect on cardiovascular complications was greater than that attributable to the effects on blood pressure.

Based on several clinical studies, and provided that there are no major contraindications for their use, ACE inhibitors should be considered in the early phase after hemodynamic stabilization [30]. The efficacy in the early phase is probably greatest in patients who are at high risk, such as the elderly, those with Killip class II or greater, and asymptomatic patients with depressed LV function. If treatment is well tolerated, it should be continued indefinitely during long-term follow-up.

Additional support for the long-term use of ACE inhibitors after ACS was provided by the recently published EUROPA study ($N = 12,218$). Patients with established, stable coronary disease who were randomized to receive perindopril had a 20% lower incidence of the composite endpoint of cardiovascular death, MI, or cardiac arrest than patients receiving placebo (mean follow-up 4.2 years; 8.0% vs 9.9% events; hazard ratio 0.80; 95% CI 0.71–0.91) [31].

AT$_2$ antagonists

Since ACE inhibition does not affect AT$_2$ production in the heart and so will only result in partial AT$_2$ blockade [21], several groups have investigated whether a selective AT$_2$ antagonist could produce similar, or even better, results than an ACE inhibitor.

The OPTIMAAL trial studied 5,477 post-MI patients who had symptoms of heart failure during the acute phase [32]. Patients who were randomized to the AT$_2$ antagonist losartan had an apparent, though not significant, higher incidence of all-cause death during long-term follow-up (mean 2.7 years) than those receiving the ACE inhibitor captopril (18.2% vs 16.4% events; hazard ratio 1.13; 95% CI 0.99–1.28). Losartan was also associated with an increased risk of sudden cardiac death or resuscitated cardiac arrest (8.7% vs 7.4% events; hazard ratio 1.19; 95% CI 0.98–1.43).

Similar results were found in the ELITE II trial ($N = 3,152$) comparing losartan with captopril in patients with symptomatic heart failure [33]. Based on these results, losartan cannot be recommended as an alternative to captopril for long-term cardiovascular protection in post-MI patients with heart failure. Other trials comparing AT$_2$ antagonists with ACE inhibitors, including the ongoing VALIANT trial [34], may reveal the extent to which the results observed in OPTIMAAL and ELITE II are representative of the class of AT$_2$ antagonists.

Statins

There is strong evidence that elevated low-density lipoprotein (LDL) levels have an adverse effect on the risk of cardiovascular events in individuals without coronary disease, as well as in patients with established coronary disease. Lipid-lowering agents from the class of 3-hydroxy 3–methylglutaryl coenzyme A reductase inhibitors (statins), which block endogenous synthesis of cholesterol, reduce LDL levels. The clinical efficacy and safety of these agents have been demonstrated in a number of Phase III trials in a broad range of patients. In contrast to LDL, elevated levels of high-density lipoprotein (HDL) are associated with reduced cardiovascular event rates. HDL-raising strategies, which may in the future complement treatment with statins, are currently being evaluated.

The landmark 4S trial comparing simvastatin with placebo in patients with angina pectoris or previous MI and moderate hypercholesterolemia (N = 4,444) demonstrated a 30% reduction in all-cause mortality during long-term follow-up with simvastatin (8.7% vs 12.4% events; hazard ratio 0.70; 95% CI 0.58–0.85) [35]. A 42% reduction in the incidence of cardiovascular death was observed. Other benefits included a 37% reduction in myocardial revascularization procedures. These results were confirmed in the CARE and LIPID trials (together N = 13,173) of pravastatin in patients with previous MI or unstable angina, which both reported a 25% reduction in the incidence of cardiovascular death or nonfatal MI during 5- to 6-year follow-up (11.7% vs 15.0% events; hazard ratio based on both trials 0.75; 95% CI 0.67–0.83) [36,37]. On the basis of these results, treatment guidelines recommend statin use in patients with documented coronary disease if, in spite of dietary measures, elevated cholesterol levels >5 mmol/L (190 mg/dL) persist.

The recently completed Heart Protection Study investigated 20,536 high-risk individuals, including patients with coronary disease and diabetes mellitus, with total cholesterol levels >3.5 mmol/L (135 mg/dL) [38]. During long-term follow-up, patients randomized to simvastatin had a 13% lower mortality than those receiving placebo (12.9% vs 14.7% events; hazard ratio 0.87; 95% CI 0.81–0.94). The incidence of major cardiovascular events was reduced by 24% (19.8% vs 25.2% events; hazard ratio 0.76; 95% CI 0.72–0.81). These data suggest that statin treatment should be extended to patients with cholesterol levels <5 mmol/L (190 mg/dL). It should be noted that the observed beneficial effect of statins in the large Phase III trials was only reached after long-term use (5–6 years). The cost-effectiveness of treatment of patients with a limited life-expectancy is therefore questionable [39], although elderly patients do benefit from treatment with statins.

Beyond lowering lipids, statins have favorable effects on platelet adhesion, thrombosis, endothelial function, plaque stability, and inflammation [40]. Therefore, it has been postulated that early statin therapy may play a beneficial role in ACS patients. Data from the MIRACL trial (N = 3,086) support this hypothesis [41]. Between 24 and 96 hours after hospitalization, patients with unstable angina or non-Q-wave MI were randomly assigned to receive atorvastatin or placebo for 16 weeks. Fewer adverse cardiovascular events were observed in patients randomized to atorvastatin. The incidence of symptomatic ischemia was particularly reduced (6.2% vs 8.4% events; OR 0.74; 95% CI 0.57–0.95). Data from MIRACL also support the safety of early statin therapy, a point of previous contention. Observational studies in patients with non-ST-elevation ACS, as well as in patients undergoing percutaneous coronary intervention, also demonstrated lower cardiovascular event rates after early initiation of statins [40,42]. Thus, evidence from recent investigations supports the notion that the initiation of statin therapy in patients with a clear indication should not be delayed until hospital discharge.

Calcium antagonists

Calcium antagonists prevent the entry of calcium into vascular smooth muscle cells and cardiac muscle cells, and thus form another group of agents with vasculo- and cardioprotective potential. As a pharmacological class, calcium antagonists can be divided into two categories: dihydropyridine agents (which act primarily as vasodilators) and nondihydropyridine agents (which act primarily to lower the heart rate but also affect the conduction system). A number of trials have revealed discrepancies between the different classes of calcium antagonists. Several trials in post-MI and post-unstable angina patients have shown that the dihydropyridine agent nifedipine does not reduce the incidence of long-term cardiovascular events [43]. In some of these trials, nifedipine even tended to increase the risk of death. The heart rate-lowering calcium antagonists verapamil and diltiazem seem to reduce the incidence of MI, but not mortality, in post-MI patients during long-term follow-up [44–46]. It should be appreciated that the Phase III trials conducted so far have lacked the power to demonstrate clinically meaningful treatment effects. Therefore, on the basis of these studies, the routine use of calcium antagonists for secondary prevention after ACS cannot be recommended. Properly sized randomized trials in post-ACS patients are warranted to assess the clinical efficacy and safety of long-term treatment with heart rate-lowering calcium antagonists.

Nitrates

Vasodilator therapy with nitrates has been used for years to bring relief to patients suffering from angina pectoris, and it has been suggested that nitrates may have long-term cardioprotective effects. However, based on the large GISSI-3 ($N = 19,394$) and ISIS-4 ($N = 58,050$) trials in post-MI patients, there is no rationale for the use of nitrates to prevent cardiovascular events in (asymptomatic) post-ACS patients [47,48]. In

GISSI-3, patients were randomly assigned to 6 weeks of nitrates or open control. Nitrates were not associated with a mortality reduction (OR 0.94; 95% CI 0.84–1.05) or a reduction in the incidence of a composite endpoint of all-cause death and severe LV dysfunction [47]. ISIS-4 also failed to demonstrate a mortality reduction with 5 weeks of nitrate use as compared with an open control (OR 0.97; 95% CI 0.91–1.03) [48].

Glycemic control in diabetics

Approximately 20% of patients with ACS have prevalent diabetes mellitus, and are at increased risk of death during the acute phase, as well as during long-term follow-up. The unfavorable outcome in diabetic patients is related to metabolic factors causing an increased oxygen consumption of free fatty acids during acute myocardial ischemia. An association between glycemia with microvascular complications and glycemia with macrovascular complications was seen in a prospective observational study of 4,585 diabetic patients [49]. Each 1% reduction in updated hemoglobin A1c was associated with a 21% diabetes-related mortality reduction and a 14% reduction in the incidence of MI during 10-year follow-up. The DIGAMI investigators demonstrated that long-term metabolic control improves the prognosis for MI patients with previously diagnosed diabetes mellitus or an abnormal blood glucose concentration during the acute phase [50]. Patients enrolled in the DIGAMI trial (N = 620) were randomized to receive either one 24-hour insulin–glucose infusion, followed by subcutaneous insulin four times daily for at least 3 months, or control therapy (control patients were treated according to standard practice and did not receive any insulin unless clinically indicated). Long-term metabolic control was associated with a 35% reduced incidence of all-cause death during 1-year follow-up (18.6% vs 26.1% events; OR 0.65; 95% CI 0.44–0.95). One-year mortality among hospital survivors was reduced by 43%. Strict glycemic control should therefore be part of the routine management of diabetic patients after ACS [51].

Conclusions

Aspirin, beta-blockers, ACE inhibitors, clopidogrel, and statins are effective agents for the secondary prevention of coronary disease in ACS patients. Somewhat weaker evidence exists for intensive oral anticoagulation therapy. In diabetic patients, glycemic control is particularly effective. The evidence for the efficacy of prophylactic drug therapy in preventing major cardiovascular events during long-term use after ACS is summarized in **Table 1**. The goals for chronic medical therapy should be related to modification of the major cardiovascular risk factors, including smoking, obesity, physical inactivity, hypertension, hyperlipidemia, and diabetes

Table 1. Prophylactic drug therapy after acute coronary syndromes. ACE: angiotensin-converting enzyme; AT: angiotensin.

Drug	Evidence for efficacy in preventing major cardiovascular events during long-term use
Aspirin	Mortality reduction; low dosages (>75 mg) are effective
Clopidogrel	Reduction in composite endpoint of death, myocardial infarction, and stroke; increased risk of bleeding complications; alternative to aspirin in selected patients
Anticoagulation agents	Reduction in composite endpoint of death, myocardial infarction, and stroke if target international normalized ratio >2.0; increased risk of bleeding complications; alternative to aspirin in selected patients
Beta-blockers	Mortality reduction
ACE inhibitors	Mortality reduction, especially in patients with heart failure
AT_2 antagonists	Insufficient evidence for event reduction; possibly increased risk of death as compared with ACE inhibitors; ongoing trials may lead to a better understanding; alternative to ACE inhibitors in patients with cough
Statins	Mortality reduction, also in patients with moderately elevated blood lipids
Calcium antagonists	Evidence for adverse effects of (short-acting) dihydropyridine agents; insufficient evidence for event reduction with nondihydropyridine agents
Nitrates	No evidence of efficacy on major cardiovascular events
Insulin	Evidence for mortality reduction in diabetics

mellitus. One of the challenges for the clinical cardiologist is to tailor the medical regimen to the specific needs of the individual patient. The mnemonic ABCDE (antiplatelets, ACE inhibitors, and antianginals, beta-blockers and blood pressure, cholesterol and cigarettes, diet and diabetes, education and exercise) might be useful in this respect [2].

References

1. Van de Werf F, Ardissino D, Betriu A, et al. Management of acute myocardial infarction in patients presenting with ST-segment elevation. The Task Force on the Management of Acute Myocardial Infarction of the European Society of Cardiology. *Eur Heart J* 2003;24:28–66.

2. Braunwald E, Antman EM, Beasley JW, et al and the American College of Cardiology and the American Heart Association. Committee on the Management of Patients With Unstable Angina. ACC/AHA 2002 guideline update for the management of patients with unstable angina and non-ST-segment elevation myocardial infarction–summary article: a report of the American College of Cardiology/American Heart Association task force on practice guidelines (Committee on the Management of Patients With Unstable Angina). *J Am Coll Cardiol* 2002;40:1366–74.

3. Ryan TJ, Anderson JL, Antman EM, et al. ACC/AHA guidelines for the management of patients with acute myocardial infarction. A report of the American College of Cardiology/American Heart Association Task Force on Practice Guidelines (Committee on Management of Acute Myocardial Infarction). *J Am Coll Cardiol* 1996;28:1328–428.

4. Prevention of coronary heart disease in clinical practice. Recommendations of the Second Joint Task Force of European and other Societies on Coronary Prevention. *Eur Heart J* 1998;19:1434–503.

5. Van Berkel TF, Boersma H, Roos-Hesselink JW, et al. Impact of smoking cessation and smoking interventions in patients with coronary heart disease. *Eur Heart J* 1999;20:1773–82.

6. Trichopoulou A, Costacou T, Bamia C, et al. Adherence to a Mediterranean diet and survival in a Greek population. *N Engl J Med* 2003;348:2599–608.

7. Singh RB, Niaz MA, Singh R, et al. Effect of an Indo-Mediterranean diet on progression of coronary artery disease in high risk patients (Indo-Mediterranean diet heart study): a randomised single-blind trial. *Lancet* 2002;360:1455–61.

8. Barzi F, Woodward M, Marfisi RM, et al. Mediterranean diet and all-causes mortality after myocardial infarction: results from the GISSI-Prevenzione trial. *Eur J Clin Nutr* 2003;57:604–11.

9. Blair SN, Kohl HW 3rd, Barlow CE, et al. Changes in physical fitness and all-cause mortality. A prospective study of healthy and unhealthy men. *JAMA* 1995;273:1093–8.

10. O'Connor GT, Buring JE, Yusuf S, et al. An overview of randomized trials of rehabilitation with exercise after myocardial infarction. *Circulation* 1989;80:234–44.

11. Antithrombotic Trialists' Collaboration. Collaborative meta-analysis of randomised trials of antiplatelet therapy for prevention of death, myocardial infarction, and stroke in high risk patients. *Br Med J* 2002;324:71–86.

12. Bertrand ME, Simoons ML, Fox KA, et al; Task Force on the Management of Acute Coronary Syndromes of the European Society of Cardiology. Management of acute coronary syndromes in patients presenting without persistent ST-segment elevation. *Eur Heart J* 2002;23:1809–40.

13. Anand SS, Yusuf S. Oral anticoagulant therapy in patients with coronary artery disease: a meta-analysis. *JAMA* 1999;282:2058–67. Erratum in: *JAMA* 2000;284:45.

14. Coumadin Aspirin Reinfarction Study (CARS) Investigators. Randomised double-blind trial of fixed low-dose warfarin with aspirin after myocardial infarction. *Lancet* 1997;350:389–96.

15. van Es RF, Jonker JJ, Verheugt FW, et al and the Antithrombotics in the Secondary Prevention of Events in Coronary Thrombosis-2 (ASPECT-2) Research Group. Aspirin and coumadin after acute coronary syndromes (the ASPECT-2 study): a randomised controlled trial. *Lancet* 2002;360:109–13.

16. Hurlen M, Abdelnoor M, Smith P, et al. Warfarin, aspirin, or both after myocardial infarction. *N Engl J Med* 2002;347:969–74.

17. Yusuf S, Zhao F, Mehta SR, et al, for the Clopidogrel in Unstable Angina to Prevent Recurrent Events Trial Investigators. Effects of clopidogrel in addition to aspirin in patients with acute coronary syndromes without ST-segment elevation. *N Engl J Med* 2001;345:494-502. Errata in: *N Engl J Med* 2001;345:1716; *N Engl J Med* 2001;345:1506.

18. Freemantle N, Cleland J, Young P, et al. Beta blockade after myocardial infarction: systematic review and meta regression analysis. *Bt Med J* 1999;318;1730–7.

19. Freemantle N, Urdah H, Eastaugh J, et al. What is the place of beta-blockade in patients who have experienced a myocardial infarction with preserved left ventricular function? Evidence and (mis)interpretation. *Prog Cardiovasc Dis* 2002;44:243–50.

20. Dzau VJ, Pratt R, Gibbons GH. Angiotensin as local modulating factor in ventricular dysfunction and failure due to coronary artery disease. *Drugs* 1994;47 S4:1–13.

21. Boehm M, Nabel EG. Angiotensin-converting enzyme 2–a new cardiac regulator. *N Engl J Med* 2002;347:1795–7.

22. Pfeffer MA, Braunwald E, Moye LA, et al. Effect of captopril on mortality and morbidity in patients with left ventricular dysfunction after myocardial infarction. Results of the survival and ventricular enlargement trial. The SAVE Investigators. *N Engl J Med* 1992;327:669–77.

23. The Acute Infarction Ramipril Efficacy (AIRE) Study Investigators. Effect of ramipril on mortality and morbidity of survivors of acute myocardial infarction with clinical evidence of heart failure. *Lancet* 1993;342:821–8.

24. Kober L, Torp-Pedersen C, Carlsen JE, et al. A clinical trial of the angiotensin-converting-enzyme inhibitor trandolapril in patients with left ventricular dysfunction after myocardial infarction. Trandolapril Cardiac Evaluation (TRACE) Study Group. *N Engl J Med* 1995;333:1670–6.

25. The SOLVD Investigators. Effect of enalapril on survival in patients with reduced left ventricular ejection fractions and congestive heart failure. *N Engl J Med* 1991;325:293–302.

26. The SOLVD Investigators. Effect of enalapril on mortality and the development of heart failure in asymptomatic patients with reduced left ventricular ejection fractions. *N Engl J Med* 1992;327:685–91.

27. Flather MD, Yusuf S, Kober L, et al. Long-term ACE-inhibitor therapy in patients with heart failure or left-ventricular dysfunction: a systematic overview of data from individual patients. ACE-Inhibitor Myocardial Infarction Collaborative Group. *Lancet* 2000;355:1575–81.

28. Yusuf S, Sleight P, Pogue J, et al. Effects of an angiotensin-converting-enzyme inhibitor, ramipril, on cardiovascular events in high-risk patients. The Heart Outcomes Prevention Evaluation Study Investigators. *N Engl J Med* 2000;342:145–53. Errata in: 2000;342:1376; *N Engl J Med* 2000;342:748.

29. The Heart Outcomes Prevention Evaluation Study Investigators. Effects of ramipril on cardiovascular and microvascular outcomes in people with diabetes mellitus: results of the HOPE study and MICRO-HOPE substudy. *Lancet* 2000;355:253–9. Erratum in: *Lancet* 2000;356:860.

30. ACE Inhibitor Myocardial Infarction Collaborative Group. Indications for ACE inhibitors in the early treatment of acute myocardial infarction. Systematic overview of individual data from 100 000 patients in randomized trials. *Circulation* 1998;97:2202–12.

31. The EUROPA investigators. Efficacy of perindopril in reduction of cardiovascular events among patients with stable coronary artery disease: randomised double-blind, placebo-controlled, multicentre trial (the EUROPA study). *Lancet* 2003;362:782–8.

32. Dickstein K, Kjekshus J and the OPTIMAAL Steering Committee of the OPTIMAAL Study Group. Effects of losartan and captopril on mortality and morbidity in high-risk patients after acute myocardial infarction: the OPTIMAAL randomised trial. Optimal Trial in Myocardial Infarction with Angiotensin II Antagonist Losartan. *Lancet* 2002;360:752–60.

33. Pitt B, Poole-Wilson PA, Segal R, et al. Effect of losartan compared with captopril on mortality in patients with symptomatic heart failure: randomised trial–the Losartan Heart Failure Survival Study ELITE II. *Lancet* 2000;355:1582–7.

34. Pfeffer MA, McMurray J, Leizorovicz A, et al. Valsartan in acute myocardial infarction trial (VALIANT): rationale and design. *Am Heart J* 2000;140:727–50.

35. The Scandinavian Simvastatin Survival Study Group. Randomised trial of cholesterol lowering in 4444 patients with coronary heart disease: the Scandinavian Simvastatin Survival Study (4S). *Lancet* 1994;344:1383–9.

36. Sacks FM, Pfeffer MA, Moye LA, et al. The effect of pravastatin on coronary events after myocardial infarction in patients with average cholesterol levels. Cholesterol and Recurrent Events Trial investigators. *N Engl J Med* 1996;335:1001–9.

37. The Long-Term Intervention with Pravastatin in Ischaemic Disease (LIPID) Study Group. Prevention of cardiovascular events and death with pravastatin in patients with coronary heart disease and a broad range of initial cholesterol levels. *N Engl J Med* 1998;339:1349–57.

38. Heart Protection Study Collaborative Group. MRC/BHF Heart Protection Study of cholesterol lowering with simvastatin in 20,536 high-risk individuals: a randomised placebo-controlled trial. *Lancet* 2002;360:7–22.

39. Van Hout BA, Simoons ML. Cost-effectiveness of HMG coenzyme reductase inhibitors; whom to treat? *Eur Heart J* 2001;22:751–61.

40. Chan AW, Bhatt DL, Chew DP, et al. Early and sustained survival benefit associated with statin therapy at the time of percutaneous coronary intervention. *Circulation* 2002;105:691–6.

41. Schwartz GG, Olsson AG, Ezekowitz MD, et al and the Myocardial Ischemia Reduction with Aggressive Cholesterol Lowering (MIRACL) Study Investigators. Effects of atorvastatin on early recurrent ischemic events in acute coronary syndromes: the MIRACL study: a randomized controlled trial. *JAMA* 2001;285:1711–8.

42. Aronow HD, Topol EJ, Roe MT, et al. Effect of lipid-lowering therapy on early mortality after acute coronary syndromes: an observational study. *Lancet* 2001;357:1063–8.

43. Held PH, Yusuf S, Furberg CD. Calcium channel blockers in acute myocardial infarction and unstable angina: an overview. *Br Med J* 1989;299:1187–92.

44. The Danish Study Group on Verapamil in Myocardial Infarction. Effect of verapamil on mortality and major events after acute myocardial infarction (the Danish Verapamil Infarction Trial II–DAVIT II). *Am J Cardiol* 1990;66:779–85.

45. The Multicenter Diltiazem Postinfarction Trial Research Group. The effect of diltiazem on mortality and reinfarction after myocardial infarction. *N Engl J Med* 1988;319:385–92.

46. Boden WE, van Gilst WH, Scheldewaert RG, et al. Diltiazem in acute myocardial infarction treated with thrombolytic agents: a randomised placebo-controlled trial. Incomplete Infarction Trial of European Research Collaborators Evaluating Prognosis post-Thrombolysis (INTERCEPT). *Lancet* 2000;355:1751–6.

47. Gruppo Italiano per lo Studio della Sopravvivenza nell'infarto Miocardico. GISSI-3: effects of lisinopril and transdermal glyceryl trinitrate singly and together on 6-week mortality and ventricular function after acute myocardial infarction. *Lancet* 1994;343:1115–22.

48. ISIS-4 (Fourth International Study of Infarct Survival) Collaborative Group. ISIS-4: a randomised factorial trial assessing early oral captopril, oral mononitrate, and intravenous magnesium sulphate in 58,050 patients with suspected acute myocardial infarction. *Lancet* 1995;345:669–85.

49. Stratton IM, Adler AI, Neil HA, et al. Association of glycaemia with macrovascular and microvascular complications of type 2 diabetes (UKPDS 35): prospective observational study. *Br Med J* 2000;321:405–12.

50. Malmberg K, Ryden L, Efendic S, et al. Randomized trial of insulin–glucose infusion followed by subcutaneous insulin treatment in diabetic patients with acute myocardial infarction (DIGAMI study): effects on mortality at 1 year. *J Am Coll Cardiol* 1995;26:57–65.

51. Nattrass M. Managing diabetes after myocardial infarction. *Br Med J* 1997;314:1497.

52. The GUSTO investigators. An international randomized trial comparing four thrombolytic strategies for acute myocardial infarction. *N Engl J Med* 1993;329:673–82.

53. GUSTO-2b investigators. A comparison of recombinant hirudin with heparin for the treatment of acute coronary syndromes. *N Engl J Med* 1996;335:775–82.

54. The Global Use of Strategies to Open Occluded Coronary Arteries (GUSTO III) Investigators. A comparison of reteplase with alteplase for acute myocardial infarction. *N Engl J Med* 1997;337:1118–23.

55. The ASSENT-3 investigators. Efficacy and safety of tenecteplase in combination with enoxaparin, abciximab, or unfractionated heparin: the ASSENT-3 randomised trial in acute myocardial infarction. *Lancet* 2001;358:605–13.

56. Topol EJ and the GUSTO V Investigators. Reperfusion therapy for acute myocardial infarction with fibrinolytic therapy or combination reduced fibrinolytic therapy and platelet glycoprotein IIb/IIIa inhibition: the GUSTO V randomised trial. *Lancet* 2001;357:1905–14.

57. The PURSUIT Trial Investigators. Inhibition of platelet glycoprotein IIb/IIIa with eptifibatide in patients with acute coronary syndromes. *N Engl J Med* 1998;339:436–43.

58. Antman EM, McCabe CH, Gurfinkel EP, et al. Enoxaparin prevents death and cardiac ischemic events in unstable angina/non-Q-wave myocardial infarction. Results of the thrombolysis in myocardial infarction (TIMI) 11B trial. *Circulation* 1999;100:1593–601.

59. Cohen M, Demers C, Gurfinkel EP, et al. A comparison of low–molecular-weight heparin with unfractionated heparin for unstable coronary artery disease. Efficacy and Safety of Subcutaneous Enoxaparin in Non-Q-Wave Coronary Events Study Group. *N Engl J Med* 1997;337:447–52.
60. Simoons ML and the GUSTO IV-ACS Investigators. Effect of glycoprotein IIb/IIIa receptor blocker abciximab on outcome in patients with acute coronary syndromes without early coronary revascularisation: the GUSTO IV-ACS randomised trial. *Lancet* 2001;357:1915–24.

8
Interventional strategies

Michael S Chen & Deepak L Bhatt

Introduction

The management of acute coronary syndromes (ACS) depends on the presence or absence of ST-segment elevation on the electrocardiogram (ECG), although treatment of each is based on medical therapy and percutaneous coronary intervention (PCI), with a more limited role for coronary artery bypass graft (CABG) surgery. In this chapter, we compare primary PCI with thrombolytics for ST-segment elevation ACS, highlight the operational issues pertinent to primary PCI, and discuss the merits of invasive and conservative strategies in non-ST-segment elevation ACS. Finally, we review adjunctive pharmacotherapy for PCI performed during ACS [1].

ST-segment elevation ACS

PCI versus thrombolytics

The predominant treatments for ST-segment elevation ACS are thrombolytics and primary PCI. **Table 1** lists the advantages of each. In the American College of Cardiology (ACC)/American Heart Association (AHA) guidelines, primary PCI is a class I indication for ST-segment elevation ACS or new left bundle branch block if performed within 12 hours of symptom onset (see **Table 2**) [2,3]. Several randomized trials and two large meta-analyses have compared thrombolytics with primary PCI (see **Figure 1** and **Table 3**). Weaver and colleagues analyzed 10 trials involving 2,606 patients and found that percutaneous transluminal coronary angioplasty (PTCA) resulted in significantly lower 30-day mortality and stroke rates [4]. A subsequent meta-analysis incorporating more patients (7,739 patients from 23 trials) and advances in PCI (stents in 12 trials and glycoprotein [GP]IIb/IIIa inhibitors in eight trials) found lower short- and long-term individual endpoints of death, myocardial infarction (MI), and stroke with PCI [5]. In retrospective analysis, the benefits of primary PCI over thrombolytics extend to include patients over 65 years of age, with PCI resulting in improved 30-day and 1-year survival [6].

A theoretical advantage of thrombolytics over PCI is reduced time-to-therapy. The possible benefits of prehospital administration of thrombolytics were investigated in the CAPTIM trial (see **Table 3**), which compared prehospital thrombolytics with primary PCI [7]. Although neither strategy was found to be superior, the study was terminated prematurely (with only 70% of planned enrollment) and hence underpowered. Furthermore, administration

Table 1. Comparison of the advantages of thrombolytics and percutaneous coronary intervention (PCI)

Thrombolytics	PCI
Quicker time to onset of therapy	Superior efficacy in clinical trials
Wider availability, given lack of hospitals performing primary PCI	Lower risk for bleeding, including intracranial hemorrhage
Not operator-dependent	Defines coronary anatomy
	More patients eligible for PCI than thrombolytics
	Decreases length of hospital stay
	Less time-dependent (more useful with delayed patient presentation)

of prehospital thrombolytics requires close coordination between paramedics, emergency departments, and cardiologists, and is currently not an option in most areas. Overall, PCI is superior to in-hospital thrombolytics for the treatment of ST–segment elevation ACS.

PTCA versus stent

Although PTCA has been the mainstay of therapy in interventional cardiology, stenting has rapidly gained favor over the last few years. Stents are increasingly used in PCI, with over 70% of PCI procedures involving stents [2].

Figure 1. Short and long-term outcomes of primary percutaneous coronary intervention (PCI) versus thrombolytics in ST–segment elevation acute coronary syndromes (ACS). Outcomes of a quantitative review of 23 randomized trials comparing PCI with thrombolysis in ST–segment elevation ACS; both short-term and long-term outcomes are improved with PCI. *Data not available. (Reprinted with permission from *Lancet* 2003;361:13–20). PTCA: percutaneous transluminal coronary angioplasty.

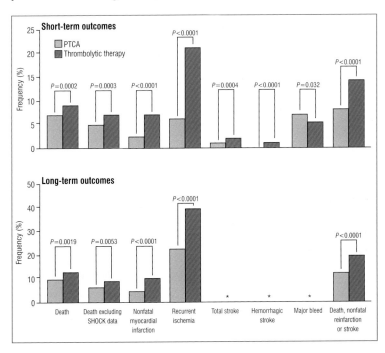

ST-segment elevation ACS – recommendations for primary PCI [3]

Class I
- As an alternative to thrombolytics in ST-elevation ACS or new LBBB, if performed within 12 hours of the onset of symptoms or >12 hours if ischemic symptoms persist
- Within 36 hours of ST-elevation ACS (or new LBBB) in patients who develop cardiogenic shock are <75 years old, and in whom revascularization can be performed within 18 hours of onset of shock

Class II
- As a reperfusion strategy in patients with contraindications to thrombolytics (IIa)
- In patients with MI without ST-elevation but with decreased flow of IRA and when PCI can be performed within 12 hours of symptom onset

Class III
- In patients who undergo elective PCI of non-IRA
- In patients >12 hours after the onset of symptoms who lack evidence for ischemia
- In patients who have received thrombolytics and have no symptoms of ischemia
- In patients who are thrombolysis candidates and are undergoing primary PCI by a low-volume operator in a facility without surgical capability

ST-segment elevation ACS patients not undergoing primary PCI – recommendations for early coronary angiography [3]

Class I
- None

Class II
- In patients with cardiogenic shock or hemodynamic instability (IIa)
- In patients with evolving large or anterior infarcts treated with thrombolytics in whom the artery is not thought to be patent and adjuvant PCI is planned (IIb)

Class III
- In patients who undergo routine angiography within 24 hours of thrombolytics

ST-segment elevation ACS – recommendations for emergency CABG [3]

Class I (assumes coronary anatomy suitable for CABG)
- In patients with failed PCI with persistent pain or hemodynamic instability
- In patients with MI with persistent or recurrent ischemia refractory to medical therapy and coronary anatomy not suitable for PCI
- Concurrent with surgical repair of VSD or mitral regurgitation

Class II (assumes coronary anatomy suitable for CABG)
- In patients with cardiogenic shock (IIa)
- After failed PCI, when small area of myocardium is at risk and the patient is hemodynamically stable (IIb)

Class III
- When surgical mortality rate exceeds medical therapy mortality rate

Non-ST-segment elevation ACS – recommendations for early invasive strategy [49]

Class I	Class II	Class III

• In patients with:
  – recurrent angina/ischemia despite medical management
  – elevated troponin
  – new ST-segment depression
  – recurrent angina/ischemia with CHF or new/worsening mitral regurgitation
  – high-risk findings on noninvasive stress test
  – hemodynamic instability or sustained ventricular tachycardia
  – PCI within 6 months or prior CABG
	• After repeated ACS presentations in patients on medical therapy and without evidence of ischemia (IIa)	• In patients with extensive comorbidities in whom risks of angiography exceed the benefits
		• In patients with acute chest pain and low likelihood of ACS
		• When the physician is unable to obtain informed consent

Non-ST-segment elevation ACS – recommendations for revascularization with PCI or CABG [49]

Class I	Class II	Class III
• CABG for significant left main CAD • CABG for three-vessel CAD • CABG for two-vessel CAD involving proximal LAD and either EF <50% or ischemia on noninvasive testing • PCI or CABG for one- or two-vessel CAD without proximal LAD involvement but with large area of viable myocardium and high-risk noninvasive stress test result • PCI for multivessel CAD with normal EF and no diabetes	• Repeat CABG for multiple SVG stenosis, especially with SVG–LAD disease (IIa) • PCI for focal SVG lesions or multiple stenosis in poor surgical candidates (IIa) • PCI or CABG for one- or two-vessel CAD (no proximal LAD involvement) and moderate area of ischemia (IIa) • PCI or CABG in one-vessel CAD involving proximal LAD (IIa) • CABG with IMA for multivessel disease in diabetics (IIa) • PCI for two-vessel or three-vessel disease with proximal LAD involvement, with either diabetes or abnormal EF (IIb)	• PCI or CABG in one- or two-vessel CAD without proximal LAD involvement and with mild symptoms in patients who have not received adequate trial of medical therapy and have no ischemia on stress testing • PCI or CABG in coronary stenosis <50% • PCI in left main CAD in CABG candidates

Table 2. ACC/AHA guidelines for revascularization in ST-segment elevation and non-ST-segment elevation acute coronary syndromes (ACS). CABG: coronary artery bypass graft; CAD: coronary artery disease; CHF: congestive heart failure; EF: ejection fraction; IMA: internal mammary artery; IRA: infarct-related artery; LAD: left anterior descending; LBBB: left bundle branch block; MI: myocardial infarction; PCI: percutaneous coronary intervention; SVG: saphenous vein graft; VSD: ventricular septal defect.

Trial	Patients	Treatment	Results	Conclusions
Quantitative review of 10 randomized controlled trials (PCI vs thrombolytics in ST-segment elevation ACS) [4]	2,606 ST-segment elevation ACS patients	Primary PTCA vs thrombolytics. Four trials used SK, three used 3–4 hour tPA infusion, and three used 90-minute "accelerated" tPA.	Primary PTCA resulted in lower rates of 30-day mortality (4.4% vs 6.5%, $P = 0.02$), death or nonfatal reinfarction (7.2% vs 11.9%, $P<0.001$), and total stroke (0.7% vs 2.0%, $P = 0.007$).	Primary PTCA results in improved outcomes over thrombolytics in ST-segment elevation ACS.
Quantitative review of 23 randomized controlled trials (PCI vs thrombolytics in ST-segment elevation ACS) [5]	7,739 ST-segment elevation ACS patients	Primary PTCA (n = 3,872) vs thrombolytics (n = 3,867). GPIIb/IIIa inhibitors were used in eight trials and stents in 12 trials.	Primary PCI resulted in lower short-term mortality (7% vs 9%, $P<0.0002$), nonfatal reinfarction (3% vs 7%, $P<0.0001$), and stroke (1% vs 2%, $P = 0.0004$). Differences persisted long-term.	Primary PCI is better than thrombolytics in ST-segment elevation ACS.
CAPTIM [7]	840 ST-segment elevation ACS patients presenting within 6 hours of symptom onset (1,200 patients planned)	Patients were randomized to prehospital thrombolysis with alteplase (n = 419) vs primary PTCA (n = 421). Rescue PTCA was performed in 26% of alteplase group.	The average time from symptoms to alteplase was 130 minutes. In PCI group, the average time from symptoms to balloon inflation was 190 minutes. No difference was seen in the primary composite endpoint of 30-day mortality, reinfarction, or disabling stroke (8.2% with alteplase vs 6.2% with PCI, $P = 0.29$).	There is no difference in outcomes between prehospital thrombolysis and primary PCI. However, the study was underpowered and terminated prematurely due to lack of funding.

Trial	Patients	Treatment	Results	Conclusions
Stent-PAMI [8]	900 ST-segment elevation ACS patients undergoing emergency PTCA	Patients were randomized to PTCA (n = 448) vs PTCA with stenting (n = 452).	The PTCA/stent group had lower 6-month combined primary endpoint of death, reinfarction, disabling stroke, or TVR (12.6% vs 20.1%, $P<0.01$), due to a decrease in TVR. There was no difference in 6-month mortality.	PTCA/stent in ST-segment-elevation ACS results in less TVR than PTCA alone.
CADILLAC [9]	2,082 ST-segment elevation ACS patients	2×2 factorial design. Patients were randomized to: PTCA alone (n = 518), PTCA + abciximab (n = 528), stent alone (n = 512), or stent + abciximab (n = 524).	6-month composite rate of death, MI, disabling stroke, and TVR in PTCA, PTCA + abciximab, stent, and stent + abciximab groups was 20.0%, 16.5%, 11.5%, and 10.2%; ($P<0.001$), driven solely by difference in TVR.	In ST-segment elevation ACS, stents, as compared with PTCA, result in lower short-term and long-term TVR rates.
C-PORT [13]	451 ST-segment elevation ACS patients who were eligible for thrombolytics	The goal was to determine whether primary PCI is safe without surgical backup. Primary PCI programs were developed at 11 community hospitals lacking cardiac surgery. Treatment was either primary PCI (n = 225) or tPA (n = 226). In PCI group, 63% received stents and 76% received GPIIb/IIIa inhibitors.	The primary endpoint of 6-month composite of death, recurrent MI, and stroke was lower in the PCI group (12.4% vs 19.9%, $P = 0.03$), primarily due to lower reinfarction rate. Also, PCI group had decreased length of stay (4.5 vs 6.0 days, $P = 0.02$).	Primary PCI at facilities without cardiac surgery backup is safe and results in improved 6-month outcomes as compared with thrombolytics.

Table 3 continues on page 162

Trial	Patients	Treatment	Results	Conclusions
Air PAMI [20]	138 high-risk ST-segment elevation ACS patients	Patients were randomized to transfer for primary PCI (n = 71) vs on-site thrombolysis (n = 67).	The primary endpoint of 30-day death, nonfatal reinfarction, or disabling stroke occurred in 8.4% of PCI group compared with 13.6% of thrombolytic group (P = 0.33). However, the trial failed to recruit the necessary sample size.	In an underpowered trial, a nonsignificant trend towards improved outcomes was found with transfer for PCI vs on-site thrombolysis in ST-segment elevation ACS.
DANAMI-2 [21]	1,572 patients with ST-segment elevation ACS presenting within 12 hours	Patients (n = 1,129) presenting to referral hospitals were randomized to transfer for primary PCI or tPA and no transfer. Patients (n = 443) presenting to invasive centers were randomized to PCI or tPA. 96% of patients were transferred within 2 hours. The time from symptoms to balloon inflation was 224 minutes in transfer patients and 188 minutes for patients presenting to invasive center.	The primary endpoint of 30-day death, reinfarction, or disabling stroke was lower in PCI group (8.0% vs 13.7%, $P<0.001$) due to lower reinfarction rate. In patients presenting to referral hospitals, the primary endpoint occurred less frequently in subgroup of patients transferred for PCI (8.5% vs 14.2% in tPA patients, P = 0.002).	Primary PCI is superior to thrombolytics at invasive centers. For patients presenting to noninvasive centers, transfer for primary PCI is superior to on-site thrombolytics, provided transfer time is <2 hours.

Trial	Patients	Treatment	Results	Conclusions
PRAGUE [22]	300 ST-segment elevation ACS patients presenting within 6 hours of symptom onset to hospitals without catheterization laboratories	Patients were randomized to: IV SK (n = 99), transfer for primary PTCA with thrombolytics during transfer (n = 100), or transfer for primary PTCA (n = 101).	The combined endpoint of 30-day death, reinfarction, or stroke occurred in 23% of the SK group, 15% of the transfer group for PTCA with thrombolytics during transfer, and 8% of the transfer for PTCA-only group (P<0.02) due to less reinfarction in primary PTCA-only group.	Transfer for primary PTCA resulted in better 30-day outcomes due to lower reinfarction rates. Thrombolytics showed no benefit during transfer for primary PTCA.
PRAGUE-2 [23]	850 patients with ST-segment elevation presenting to hospitals without catheterization laboratories	Patients were randomized to on-site thrombolysis (n = 421) or transport for primary PCI (n = 429).	The primary endpoint of 30-day mortality was 6.8% with PCI compared with 10.0% with thrombolysis (P = 0.12). The secondary endpoint of combined 30-day death, reinfarction, or stroke occurred in 8.4% of patients after PCI compared with 15.2% after thrombolytics (P<0.003). Patients randomized within 3 hours of symptom onset had equivalent 30-day mortality (7.3% with PCI, 7.4% with thrombolysis), but patients randomized >3 hours after symptoms had lower mortality with PCI (6% vs 15%, P<0.02).	In ST-segment elevation ACS, transfer for primary PCI is superior to thrombolytics. The benefit was most pronounced in patients presenting >3 hours after symptom onset.

Table 3 continues on page 164

Trial	Patients	Treatment	Results	Conclusions
SHOCK [24,25]	302 patients with acute MI and cardiogenic shock	Patients were randomized to emergency revascularization (n = 152), PTCA (64%) or CABG (36%), or intensive medical therapy (n = 150). IABP was recommended in both groups and thrombolytics recommended in medical therapy group.	The primary endpoint of 30-day all-cause mortality was nonsignificantly lower in revascularization group (46.7% vs 56.0%, $P = 0.11$). However, 6-month (50.3% vs 63.1%, $P = 0.027$) and 1-year mortality (53.3% vs 66.4%, $P < 0.03$) were significantly lower in revascularization group.	For patients with MI and cardiogenic shock, early revascularization reduces long-term mortality. One caveat is that elderly patients (>74 years old) did not appear to benefit from revascularization.
RAPPORT [60]	483 patients with ST-segment elevation ACS referred for primary PTCA	Patients were randomized to abciximab bolus followed by 12-hour infusion (n = 241) vs placebo (n = 242). Intent was for all patients to undergo PTCA.	There was no difference in primary endpoint of composite of death, MI, or any repeat TVR at 6 months (28.1% placebo, 28.2% abciximab). However, rate of death, MI, or urgent TVR was lower at 30 days and 6 months with abciximab (11.6% vs 17.8% at 6 months, $P = 0.048$). Higher major bleeding with abciximab (16.6% vs 9.5%, $P = 0.02$).	In primary PTCA, abciximab decreases composite of 6-month death, MI, or urgent TVR, at the expense of increased bleeding.
STOPAMI [63]	140 patients with ST-segment elevation ACS	Patients were randomized to stent with abciximab (n = 71) vs alteplase (n = 69). The primary endpoint of myocardial salvage index was based on technetium-99m sestamibi SPECT.	The stent group had smaller infarcts (14% of LV vs 19%, $P = 0.02$) and a lower rate of composite of death, reinfarction, or stroke at 6 months (8.5% vs 23.2%, $P = 0.02$).	In ST-segment elevation ACS, stents plus abciximab resulted in smaller infarct size and improved 6-month outcomes.

Trial	Patients	Treatment	Results	Conclusions
STOPAMI-2 [64]	162 patients with ST-segment elevation ACS	Patients were randomized to stent with abciximab (n = 81) vs alteplase with abciximab (n = 81). Primary endpoint of myocardial salvage index based on technetium-99m sestamibi SPECT.	Stenting with abciximab resulted in the salvage of 13.6% of LV as compared with 8.0% with alteplase and abciximab (P = 0.007).	Stenting with abciximab results in more myocardial salvage in ST-segment elevation ACS than alteplase with abciximab.
ADMIRAL [65]	300 patients with ST-segment elevation ACS	Primary stenting was carried out in all patients. Patients were randomized to abciximab bolus followed by 12-hour infusion (n = 149) vs placebo (n = 151).	The abciximab group had lower 30-day (6.0% vs 14.6%, P = 0.01) and 6-month (7.4% vs 15.9%, P = 0.02) composite rates of death, MI, or urgent TVR. This was driven by differences in rates of TVR.	Stenting with abciximab is superior to stenting alone for ST-segment elevation ACS, primarily due to less urgent TVR.

Table 3. Pivotal clinical trials in interventional approaches to ST-segment elevation acute coronary syndromes (ACS). CABG: coronary artery bypass graft; GP: glycoprotein; IABP: intra-aortic balloon pump; IV: intravenous; LV: left ventricle; MI: myocardial infarction; PCI: percutaneous coronary intervention; PTCA: percutaneous transluminal coronary angioplasty; SK: streptokinase; SPECT: single-photon emission computed tomography; tPA: tissue plasminogen activator; TVR: target-vessel revascularization.

A theoretical complication of the use of stents in ST-segment elevation ACS is that stents, by virtue of their exposed metal surface, might serve as a thrombotic nidus. However, the Stent-PAMI [8] and CADILLAC [9] trials (see **Table 3**) provided evidence that ST-segment elevation ACS patients undergoing stent implantation fare better than patients undergoing PTCA alone, with a reduced need for repeat revascularization and no increase in thrombotic complications.

Facilitated PCI – a treatment of the future?

Despite advances in ACS therapy, the 30-day mortality rate for ST-segment elevation ACS remains ~7%. Facilitated PCI is one approach employed in attempts to improve outcomes. In this procedure, GPIIb/IIIa inhibitors and/or reduced-dose thrombolytics are given prior to primary PCI. Theoretically, earlier administration of such agents should lead to earlier thrombus resolution and improved coronary perfusion prior to PCI. However, a major disadvantage with facilitated PCI is increased bleeding.

Evidence suggesting that facilitated PCI may be efficacious primarily pertains to surrogate outcomes derived from subgroup analyses in nonrandomized comparisons. In the nonrandomized SPEED pilot trial, facilitated PCI resulted in an 86% rate of TIMI 3 flow at 90 minutes in the subgroup that underwent PCI after receiving reduced-dose reteplase and abciximab [10]. In addition, subgroup analysis of the TIMI 14 trial found that facilitated PCI resulted in a higher percentage of patients with resolution of ST-segment elevation [11]. The ongoing FINESSE trial, which is enrolling 3,000 patients with ST-segment elevation ACS, will randomize patients to abciximab and low-dose thrombolytics pre-PCI, abciximab pre-PCI, or abciximab during PCI [12]. The ADVANCE-MI trial is a similar trial of 6,000 patients testing facilitated PCI with eptifibatide. FINESSE and ADVANCE-MI will help to determine whether facilitated PCI confers additional benefits.

Primary PCI – operational issues

Traditionally, primary PCI for the treatment of ST-segment elevation ACS has been discouraged when cardiothoracic surgery (CTS) backup is not available. Yet the demonstrated efficacy of primary PCI, in conjunction with the fact that CTS is not available at all primary PCI facilities, makes it necessary to determine the safety and efficacy of primary PCI without surgical backup. Validation of such an approach would expand the number of ST-segment elevation ACS patients who could receive primary PCI. In the Atlantic C-PORT trial, primary PCI programs were implemented in 11 community hospitals without CTS backup [13]. In this setting, primary PCI still resulted in superior 6-month outcomes as compared with thrombolytics [13].

Another operational issue pertaining to primary PCI is the relationship between procedure volume and outcomes. Several studies have found that high-volume primary PTCA centers have lower in-hospital mortality than low-volume centers [14,15]. The largest study involves the National Registry of Myocardial Infarction, which included 257,602 patients receiving primary angioplasty for MI at 450 different hospitals [14]. In-hospital mortality was 28% lower at high-volume PTCA hospitals than at low-volume hospitals (relative risk 0.72, 95% confidence interval [CI] 0.60–0.87, $P<0.001$).

The notion of higher volumes translating into better outcomes also holds true at the physician level. In a study of 1,342 patients from the New York Coronary Angioplasty Reporting System Registry, a 57% decrease in in-hospital mortality was noted after primary PTCA for interventional cardiologists who performed a high volume of procedures, compared to those who performed a lower volume (95% CI 0.21–0.83) [16].

Less is known about the relationship between procedure volume and stent implantation. In elective procedures, improved outcomes with stents have been demonstrated at high-volume centers [17], and the volume–outcome relationship will likely persist with stenting in ACS. When possible, primary PCI should be performed by high-throughput cardiologists in high-volume hospitals.

Transfer for primary PCI

Although primary PCI is the preferred therapy for ST-segment elevation ACS, few hospitals have catheterization laboratories available around the clock. One key question is whether transfer of patients to another institution for primary PCI is superior to thrombolytics at the original institution. Door-to-balloon times above 2 hours have been associated with increased mortality [18]. Predictors of door-to-balloon time over 2 hours include hospital transfer, presentation in the evening or at night, and presentation to a low-volume facility [19].

The Air PAMI study was underpowered as a result of poor patient recruitment, but found that a strategy of transfer for primary PCI, when compared with on-site thrombolysis, resulted in a nonsignificant trend towards improved clinical outcomes in high-risk ST-segment elevation ACS patients [20]. The DANAMI-2 trial, which enrolled ST-segment elevation ACS patients presenting within 12 hours of symptom onset, demonstrated that transfer to another hospital for primary PCI within 3 hours resulted in better outcomes than thrombolytics at the original hospital [21].

Similarly, the PRAGUE trial found improved outcomes in ST-segment elevation ACS patients presenting within 6 hours who were transferred for primary PCI as compared with those who received thrombolytics at the original hospital [22]. This trial also considered the issue of prehospital thrombolytics with planned primary PCI and found no benefit with thrombolytics during transfer. PRAGUE-2 reinforced the superiority of transfer for primary PCI over on-site thrombolytics, demonstrating a reduction in the 30-day combined outcome of death, reinfarction, and stroke in the PCI group [23]. PRAGUE-2 found a mortality benefit of PCI in the subgroup of patients who were randomized at least 3 hours after symptom onset, whereas those randomized within 3 hours of symptom onset had equivalent mortality outcomes with either treatment. Overall, the evidence indicates that rapid transfer for primary PCI is preferred over thrombolytics at the presenting hospital.

Cardiogenic shock

Patients with MI who develop cardiogenic shock represent the most critically ill ACS patients. The SHOCK trial demonstrated that patients in cardiogenic shock benefit from revascularization as compared with thrombolytics, with significantly higher survival rates at 6 months and 1 year [24,25]. One caveat to these results is that, in patients over 75 years old, subgroup analysis revealed that the elderly did not fare as well with emergent revascularization as younger patients did [24,25].

Revascularization of infarct-related artery versus complete revascularization

If multivessel disease is found during ST-segment elevation ACS, the classic teaching has been that revascularization of only the infarct-related artery, rather than complete revascularization, should be performed at the time of emergent catheterization. PCI of non-infarct-related arteries has generally then been performed later as a staged procedure. The ACC/AHA guidelines state that "elective angioplasty of a non-infarct–related artery at the time of [acute] MI" is a class III recommendation (see **Table 2**) [3]. However, little clinical evidence exists to address this issue.

The most extensive analysis to date is an underpowered case-control study of 158 patients [26]. The study concluded that patients receiving complete revascularization during ST-segment elevation ACS fared worse than those receiving PCI of the infarct-related artery only. The complete revascularization patients had significantly higher stroke rates and showed a nonsignificant trend towards higher mortality at 30 days and 6 months.

Yet the theoretical advantages of complete revascularization include cost savings, patient convenience, and less residual ischemic burden. With advances in PCI (including GPIIb/IIIa inhibitors, clopidogrel, and stents) overall success rates have increased. As a result, cardiologists are more aggressive in performing complete revascularization for multivessel disease at the time of emergent catheterization for ST-segment elevation ACS. The correct approach remains a matter of debate and further study is needed.

Drug-eluting stents

A major advance in PCI has been the development of drug-eluting stents (DES). These decrease in-stent intimal hyperplasia and restenosis and lower the rate of major adverse cardiac events at 1 year after PCI [27–30]. However, given the higher cost of DES, interventional cardiologists often struggle with the issue of when to use DES rather than bare metal stents. Many cardiologists select DES for lesions at high risk of restenosis (such as small-caliber vessels, lesions in diabetics, and bifurcation lesions).

Few data exist on DES in ST-segment elevation ACS. Since the main advantage of DES is a decrease in neointimal proliferation, DES are unlikely to improve periprocedural outcomes in ST-segment elevation ACS, but might result in decreased restenosis rates. The RESEARCH registry appears to support the safety of DES in ST-segment elevation ACS when compared with historic controls [31]. However, concerns have recently emerged regarding the possibility of increased rates of thrombosis with DES, emphasizing the importance of appropriate antithrombotic therapy and operator technique.

Non-ST-segment elevation ACS

Non-ST-segment elevation ACS encompasses a broad spectrum of patients. Certain features define patients with ACS as being at higher risk, including new ST-segment depression and elevated troponin, B-natriuretic peptide, and C-reactive protein [32–35]. Minor elevations of creatine kinase isoenzyme MB (CK-MB) also confer an increased risk of 30-day and 6-month mortality [36].

Another means of risk stratification is the TIMI risk score [37]. Analysis of patients from the TACTICS-TIMI 18 trial revealed that patients with intermediate or high TIMI risk scores derived significant benefit from an early invasive strategy, whereas those with a low TIMI risk score did not [38]. Likewise, patients with either elevated troponins or ECG abnormalities derived substantial benefit from an invasive approach. Thus, risk stratification is imperative, especially in deciding which patients to refer for coronary angiography. **Table 4** provides a useful summary of the pivotal clinical trials of interventional approaches in non-ST-segment elevation ACS.

Invasive versus conservative strategy

Two fundamental questions in non–ST-segment elevation ACS are whether, and when, to pursue coronary angiography. Several randomized trials have compared invasive and conservative strategies. One of the earliest was TIMI 3B, which found that thrombolytics resulted in an increased incidence of MI [39] and that a small increase in 1-year revascularization was offset by a decrease in repeat hospitalization with an early invasive management strategy (coronary angiography at 18–48 hours, followed by revascularization as soon as possible if appropriate) [40]. The VANQWISH trial found that an early invasive strategy had a higher mortality rate than a conservative strategy [41].

Trial	Patients	Treatment	Results	Conclusions
TIMI IIIb [39,40]	1,473 patients with non-ST-segment elevation ACS	A 2×2 factorial design was used: tPA vs placebo and early invasive (angiography at 18–48 hours) vs conservative (angiography only for recurrent ischemia) strategies.	The tPA group had more MI (7.4% vs 4.9%, $P = 0.04$). There was no difference in 1-year composite of death or nonfatal MI for invasive vs conservative groups (10.8% vs 12.2%, $P = 0.42$). In the invasive group, the 1-year revascularization rate was higher (64% vs 58%, $P < 0.001$), but the repeat hospitalization rate was lower (26% vs 33%, $P < 0.001$).	This early trial demonstrated that there was no role for thrombolytics in non-ST-segment elevation ACS: either an early invasive or a conservative strategy was appropriate.
VANQWISH [41]	920 patients with non-ST-segment elevation ACS (all with CK-MB 1.5 times normal)	Patients were randomized to invasive (angiography at 3–7 days, n = 462) vs conservative strategy (stress test, with angiography if evidence for ischemia, n=458). There was low use of GPIIb/IIIa inhibitors and stents.	The invasive strategy had more in-hospital deaths (21 vs 6, $P = 0.007$) at 1 month (23 vs 9, $P = 0.021$) and at 1 year (58 vs 36, $P = 0.025$).	The authors concluded that the conservative strategy was superior. However, the invasive strategy had a higher rate of CABG, and the 30-day CABG mortality rate in the invasive group (11.6%) was quite high.

Trial	Patients	Treatment	Results	Conclusions
FRISC-II [42,43]	2,457 patients with non-ST-segment elevation ACS, initially treated with dalteparin	Patients were randomized to: dalteparin for 3 months + noninvasive, placebo for 3 months + noninvasive, dalteparin for 3 months + invasive, or placebo for 3 months + invasive. In the noninvasive strategy, angiography was performed for symptoms or ischemia on stress test.	Angiography was performed in 96% of the invasive and 10% of the noninvasive group within 7 days. The invasive group, regardless of dalteparin, had lower 6-month composite rate of death or MI (9.4% vs 12.1%, $P = 0.03$), driven by a significant decrease in MI (7.8 vs 10.1%, $P = 0.045$). At 1 year, the invasive group had lower mortality (2.2% vs 3.9%, $P = 0.016$) and less MI (8.6% vs 11.6 %, $P = 0.015$).	An early invasive strategy is preferred for non-ST-segment elevation ACS, as evident by a lower mortality rate at 1 year. Note that the median time to angiography of 4 days in the invasive group was longer than contemporary practice, raising the question of whether earlier angiography would be more beneficial.
RITA-3 [44]	1,810 patients with non-ST-segment elevation ACS receiving enoxaparin	Patients randomized to early invasive (n = 895) vs conservative (n = 915) groups. In the conservative group, angiography was performed for refractory angina or ischemia on stress test. The median time to angiography in the invasive group was 2 days.	The 4-month composite of death/MI/refractory angina rate was lower in the invasive group (9.6% vs 14.5%, $P = 0.001$), driven by a decrease in refractory angina. There was no significant difference in death or MI at 1 year.	Early invasive strategy for non-ST-segment elevation ACS results in improved 4-month clinical outcomes, manifested primarily by decreases in refractory angina.

Table 4 continues on page 174

Trial	Patients	Treatment	Results	Conclusions
TACTICS-TIMI 18 [45]	2,220 patients with non-ST-segment elevation ACS receiving tirofiban and UFH	Patients were randomized to early invasive (angiography at 4–48 hours) (n = 1,114) or conservative strategy (angiography only if abnormal stress test or objective evidence of recurrent ischemia (n = 1,106).	The primary endpoint of 6-month death, MI, or rehospitalization for ACS was lower with an early invasive strategy (15.9% vs 19.4%, $P = 0.025$). There was also significant decrease in death or MI at 6 months with the early invasive strategy (7.3% vs 9.5%, $P < 0.05$).	This trial again demonstrated superiority of an early invasive strategy for non-ST-segment elevation ACS, including benefit in the "harder" endpoints of death or MI at 6 months.
VINO [46]	131 patients with non-ST-segment elevation ACS	Patients were randomized to angiography on day 1 (n = 64) or early conservative approach (n = 67), with angiography only with recurrent ischemia or positive stress test. Mean time from randomization to angiography in invasive group was 6.2 hours.	The invasive group had lower 6-month mortality (3.1% vs 13.4%, $P < 0.03$) and 6-month recurrent MI (3.1% vs 14.9%, $P < 0.02$).	This small trial demonstrated the impressive benefit for very early angiography over conservative therapy. However, the lack of a traditional early angiography (1–3 days) group precludes any comparison between angiography on day 1 and angiography within 1–3 days.
ISAR-COOL [47]	410 patients with non-ST-segment elevation ACS (elevated troponin or ST-segment depression) on clopidogrel and GPIIb/IIIa inhibitors	Patients randomized to immediate invasive strategy (n = 203, median time to angiography 2.4 hours) vs delayed invasive strategy (n = 207, median time 86 hours).	Patients treated with the immediate invasive strategy had decreased 30-day composite endpoint of death or MI (5.9% vs 11.6%, $P = 0.04$).	This trial suggested benefit with an immediate invasive strategy.

Trial	Patients	Treatment	Results	Conclusions
TARGET [71]	4,809 patients undergoing elective or urgent PCI. Cardiogenic shock and ST-segment elevation ACS patients were excluded.	Patients randomized to tirofiban bolus and infusion for 18–24 hours vs abciximab bolus and infusion for 12 hours; GPIIb/IIIa inhibitor was given just prior to PCI; 95% were stented.	The primary endpoint of 30-day death, MI, or urgent TVR occurred in 7.6% of the tirofiban and in 6.0% of the abciximab group ($P = 0.038$). The abciximab group had a significant decrease in MI (5.4% vs 6.9%, $P = 0.04$).	Abciximab is preferred over tirofiban when a GPIIb/IIIa inhibitor is given at the time of PCI.

Table 4. Pivotal clinical trials in interventional approaches to non-ST-segment elevation acute coronary syndromes (ACS). All trials are randomized controlled trials unless otherwise specified. CABG: coronary artery bypass graft; CK: creatine kinase; GP: glycoprotein; IV: intravenous; MI: myocardial infarction; PCI: percutaneous coronary intervention; tPA: tissue plasminogen activator; TVR: target-vessel revascularization; UFH: unfractionated heparin.

However, in VANQWISH, the 30-day mortality rate for the subset of patients in the invasive group who underwent CABG was high (11.6% as compared with 3.4% in the subset of patients in the conservative group who underwent CABG), skewing the outcomes against the invasive group. Overall, initial trials favored conservative strategies for the treatment of non–ST-segment elevation ACS.

However, subsequent trials have demonstrated superiority with an invasive strategy. The FRISC-II trial randomized 2,457 patients to an early invasive strategy versus a conservative one and to 3 months of dalteparin versus placebo [42]. The goal of the invasive strategy was revascularization by 7 days. In FRISC-II, an early invasive strategy resulted in a significantly lower 6-month composite rate of death or MI. This was driven by a statistically significant decrease in 6-month MI as well as a significantly lower rate of death at 1 year [42,43]. The RITA-3 trial randomized 1,810 non–ST-segment elevation ACS patients on enoxaparin to either an early invasive strategy or a conservative strategy. The early invasive strategy resulted in less severe ischemia at 4 months, but similar rates of death and MI [44]. TACTICS-TIMI 18 provided conclusive evidence of a benefit of an early invasive strategy: angioplasty within 48 hours resulted in a significant decrease in the composite endpoint of death or MI at 6 months in ACS patients on tirofiban [45].

In non–ST-segment elevation ACS, early invasive strategies still result in a wait of 1–3 days before angiography. Two small randomized trials (VINO and ISAR-COOL) addressed whether even earlier angiography would improve outcomes. In the VINO trial, coronary angiography on day 1 resulted in significant decreases in 6-month mortality and MI (as compared with conservative therapy) [46]. However, the 6-month mortality rate of 13.4% in the conservative group is high compared with other trials. Also, since VINO compared conservative management with angiography on day 1, it is not clear whether very early angiography (ie, day 1) yields incremental benefits when compared with a more typical early invasive approach (ie, angiography within 2–3 days). The ISAR-COOL trial enrolled non–ST-segment elevation ACS patients with high-risk features (elevated troponin or ST-segment depression) and administered aspirin, heparin, clopidogrel, and tirofiban to all patients on study entry. Patients were then randomized to either an immediate invasive strategy (with a median time to angiography of 2.4 hours from presentation) or a delayed invasive strategy (with a median time to angiography of 86 hours). Immediate angiography resulted in a significantly lower composite rate of death or MI [47].

For non–ST-segment elevation ACS, an early invasive strategy is the preferred management. **Figure 2** combines the results from eight major trials comparing an invasive with a conservative strategy and illustrates the superiority of an invasive strategy. The ACC and AHA recently updated their practice guidelines for non–ST-segment elevation ACS (see **Table 2**) [48]. Class I indications for an early invasive strategy have been expanded to include elevated troponin, recurrent ischemia on maximum medical management, and new ST-segment depression. A fundamental question, which was raised by ISAR-COOL but requires further investigation, is whether immediate angiography provides added benefit over angiography within the first 24–72 hours of presentation. Finding a benefit from immediate angiography would fundamentally shift the current management paradigm for non–ST-segment elevation ACS.

Underutilization of coronary angiography

Despite evidence favoring an early invasive strategy in non–ST-segment elevation ACS, actual practice patterns lag behind. In the CRUSADE registry [48], which now consists of over 40,000 high-risk ACS patients presenting to more than 300 US hospitals, only two thirds of patients with positive cardiac enzymes or ST-segment depression have undergone cardiac catheterization prior to discharge, despite such criteria being class I indications for an early invasive strategy in the ACC/AHA ACS guidelines [49].

Underutilization of coronary angiography and PCI is not confined to the US. The GRACE registry consists of 11,543 patients from 14 countries (30% ST-segment elevation ACS, 25% non-ST-segment elevation ACS, 38% unstable angina) [50]. Only 40% of all patients received PCI during the initial hospitalization, reflecting a suboptimal rate of revascularization [51]. The ENACT registry, a multi-country European registry of ACS patients, found that most of the difference in revascularization rates was due to the availability of PCI at the presenting hospital and local practice patterns, rather than differences in patient characteristics [52]. Considerable opportunity exists for increasing revascularization rates in high-risk ACS patients.

Figure 2. Invasive versus conservative strategy outcomes in non-ST-segment elevation acute coronary syndromes (ACS). The risk ratio for death or myocardial infarction (MI) with an invasive versus a conservative strategy for non-ST-segment elevation ACS; an invasive strategy is superior. CI: confidence interval. (Reprinted with permission from *Lancet*, 2003;360:743–51).

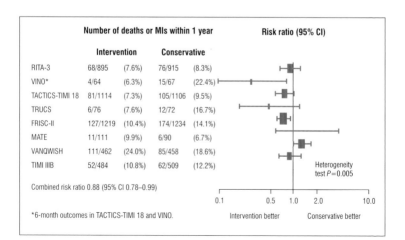

	Number of deaths or MIs within 1 year				Risk ratio (95% CI)
	Intervention		Conservative		
RITA-3	68/895	(7.6%)	76/915	(8.3%)	
VINO*	4/64	(6.3%)	15/67	(22.4%)	
TACTICS-TIMI 18	81/1114	(7.3%)	105/1106	(9.5%)	
TRUCS	6/76	(7.6%)	12/72	(16.7%)	
FRISC-II	127/1219	(10.4%)	174/1234	(14.1%)	
MATE	11/111	(9.9%)	6/90	(6.7%)	
VANQWISH	111/462	(24.0%)	85/458	(18.6%)	
TIMI IIIB	52/484	(10.8%)	62/509	(12.2%)	

Heterogeneity test $P = 0.005$

Combined risk ratio 0.88 (95% CI 0.78–0.99)

0.1   0.5   1.0   2.0   10.0

Intervention better   Conservative better

*6-month outcomes in TACTICS-TIMI 18 and VINO.

Adjunctive pharmacotherapy

Regimens of adjunctive pharmacotherapy in ACS differ depending on the presence or absence of ST-segment elevation. Other chapters of this handbook cover guidelines for pharmacotherapy for antiplatelets and GPIIb/IIIa inhibitors (see **Chapter 4**) and antithrombins (see **Chapter 6**), so in this section we highlight issues of adjunctive pharmacotherapy for ACS pertinent to PCI.

Clopidogrel

Clopidogrel is generally given in both ST-segment elevation and non–ST-segment elevation ACS once the decision has been made to proceed with PCI. ACC/AHA guidelines consider non–ST-segment elevation ACS to be a class I indication for the use of clopidogrel, regardless of whether an invasive or noninvasive strategy is planned [49]. The subset of ACS patients from the CURE trial [53] who underwent PCI was examined in PCI-CURE [54]. Compared with placebo, patients receiving clopidogrel had significantly decreased 30-day and long-term (mean 8 months) composite endpoints of death or MI. However, the patients received clopidogrel for a median of 10 days pre-PCI. Such an extended length of pretreatment is not practical if an early invasive strategy for non–ST-segment elevation ACS has been chosen.

The CREDO trial investigated whether shorter pretreatment periods of clopidogrel provide benefit [55]. Although performed in a largely elective PCI population, CREDO found that 300 mg of clopidogrel, given at least 6 hours prior to catheterization, resulted in a significant decrease in the 28-day composite of death, MI, or urgent target-vessel revascularization (TVR). In ACS, treatment with clopidogrel prior to PCI and continued for at least 3 months improves outcomes [54,56,57].

Whether to give clopidogrel prior to catheterization or to wait until after angiography is a contentious decision. The benefit of clopidogrel pretreatment must be balanced against the possibility of a delay in CABG should surgery be required. In CURE, CABG patients who received clopidogrel within 4 days of surgery had a higher rate of bleeding [53]. Similarly, Hongo and colleagues studied 224 consecutive patients undergoing CABG, and found that patients receiving clopidogrel within the past 7 days had a significantly higher rate of blood transfusions and reoperation for bleeding [58]. In our center, we generally withhold clopidogrel until the coronary anatomy has been defined, to ensure that CABG will not be delayed. However, in centers where early CABG is not a realistic possibility, clopidogrel pretreatment should be uniformly employed.

Glycoprotein IIb/IIIa inhibitors

In ST-segment elevation ACS, GPIIb/IIIa inhibitors are routinely started in the catheterization lab and continued for 12–18 hours after primary PCI. A distinction should be made between *periprocedural* use of GPIIb/IIIa inhibitors and their use in *facilitated* PCI, in which GPIIb/IIIa inhibitors and/or reduced-dose thrombolytics are given *prior* to primary PCI. GPIIb/IIIa inhibitors given *during* PCI for ST-segment elevation ACS do provide clinical benefit, primarily by decreasing urgent revascularization [59].

In the CADILLAC trial, abciximab added to stenting decreased 6-month revascularization rates [9]. In the RAPPORT trial, abciximab given in conjunction with primary PTCA resulted in a significant decrease in urgent TVR at 30 days [60]. In the ISAR-2 trial, ST-segment elevation ACS patients undergoing coronary stenting were randomized to either abciximab with reduced-dose heparin or heparin alone. The abciximab group had a significantly decreased rate of major adverse cardiac events at 30 days [61].

Abciximab with low-dose heparin in primary PCI for ST-segment elevation ACS also results in improved left ventricular function [62].

Finally, in the STOPAMI trial, abciximab with stenting, as compared with thrombolytics, resulted in more myocardial salvage in ST-segment elevation ACS [63]. STOPAMI-2 extended this concept one step further and found that primary PCI with abciximab, as compared with thrombolytics with abciximab, resulted in greater myocardial salvage [64]. Thus, a substantial benefit of GPIIb/IIIa inhibitors exists in primary PCI.

A logical extension would be to see whether abciximab prior to PCI for ST-segment elevation ACS would further improve outcomes. The ADMIRAL trial demonstrated that, when compared with stenting alone, administering abciximab prior to angiography in acute MI resulted in a lower rate of the composite endpoint, at 30 days and 6-months, of death, MI, or urgent TVR. This was primarily driven by less TVR [65]. While the ADMIRAL results suggest that earlier administration of GPIIb/IIIa inhibitors is efficacious, the control group in that study was stenting alone, and not abciximab *during* stenting. Thus, from ADMIRAL, one cannot conclude with absolute certainty that abciximab prior to PCI in ST-segment elevation ACS is better than abciximab during PCI, although preprocedural abciximab certainly improved preprocedural TIMI-3 flow rates.

In non-ST-segment ACS patients on aspirin and heparin, the ACC/AHA guidelines consider planned coronary angiography and PCI to be a class I indication for the use of GPIIb/IIIa inhibitors, administered either on admission or just prior to PCI [49]. Pooled data comprising 13,166 patients from 10 clinical trials involving GPIIb/IIIa inhibitors for PCI demonstrated significant decreases in short-term (48–96 hours), 30-day, and 6-month composite death and MI rates [66]. By combining data from three randomized, controlled trials (EPIC [67], EPILOG [68], and EPISTENT [69]), Topol and colleagues showed that the benefit of GPIIb/IIIa inhibitors persists long-term: they demonstrated a 20% mortality reduction at 3 years with abciximab given at the time of PCI as compared with placebo [70].

Only one trial has directly compared two GPIIb/IIIa inhibitors. The TARGET trial [71] compared tirofiban and abciximab in patients undergoing PCI, either electively or for non–ST-segment elevation ACS. Subgroup analysis of these patients based on clinical acuity (ACS versus non-ACS [stable angina or asymptomatic ischemia]) revealed that abciximab resulted in significant decreases in 30-day (5.8% versus 8.5%, $P = 0.004$) and 6-month MI rates (7.2% versus 9.8%, $P = 0.013$) in patients with ACS [72]. Thus, abciximab may be the preferred agent when a GPIIb/IIIa inhibitor is started at the time of PCI. How this compares with a strategy of "upstream" therapy with eptifibatide or tirofiban is unknown and requires further study.

Heparins and bivalirudin

Controversy exists concerning the choice of unfractionated heparin (UFH) or low molecular weight heparin (LMWH) in ACS patients in whom coronary angiography is planned. For ACS in general, enoxaparin is gaining favor, demonstrating superiority to UFH in both ST-segment ACS (ASSENT-3 [73]) and non–ST-segment ACS (ESSENCE [74,75]). ASSENT-3 compared full-dose tenecteplase with UFH, full-dose tenecteplase with LMWH, and half-dose tenecteplase with abciximab, and found that both the LMWH and the abciximab regimens were superior to the UFH regimen. The ESSENCE study compared subcutaneous enoxaparin with intravenous UFH. It found that enoxaparin resulted in a decreased need for revascularization at 30 days, with persistence of this trend at 1 year.

However, in ASSENT-3 and ESSENCE, an invasive strategy, which is now preferred, was not routinely performed. Despite evidence indicating enoxaparin's benefit over UFH in ACS, enoxaparin has yet to supplant UFH as the mainstay of treatment for the invasive management of ACS. Major issues limiting enoxaparin's acceptance include the uncertainty of transferring the use of enoxaparin to the catheterization laboratory, and the fact that there are fewer data concerning the combination of enoxaparin with other ACS therapies, such as GPIIb/IIIa inhibitors and clopidogrel. Most trials establishing the safety and efficacy of GPIIb/IIIa inhibitors and clopidogrel used UFH. Also, many interventional cardiologists are more comfortable with UFH than LMWH. This is a result of both their greater experience with following activated clotting times with heparin and the fact that UFH can be turned off and quickly reversed. Collet and colleagues reported a case series of 132 patients with non–ST-segment elevation ACS undergoing PCI after at least 48 hours on subcutaneous enoxaparin. They concluded that enoxaparin was safe and effective [76]. However, only a minority of patients in this series concurrently received GPIIb/IIIa inhibitors.

Early data concerning the combination of enoxaparin and GPIIb/IIIa inhibition appear favorable. The NICE-4 observational study concluded that intravenous enoxaparin with intravenous GPIIb/IIIa inhibitors had low rates of bleeding and reasonable efficacy at 30 days [77]. Caveats to this conclusion include the lack of a placebo arm and the administration route of enoxaparin, which was intravenous in NICE-4, unlike the standard subcutaneous dosing. The CRUISE study, a trial of 261 patients undergoing elective or urgent PCI with eptifibatide who were randomized to enoxaparin or UFH, reassuringly found no increase in bleeding complications with enoxaparin [78]. The ongoing SYNERGY trial is randomizing 10,000 high-risk ACS patients treated with an early invasive strategy to UFH versus enoxaparin. This trial should provide more definitive answers [79].

One alternative to heparin that is gaining popularity in PCI is the direct thrombin inhibitor bivalirudin. Recent data on bivalirudin from the REPLACE-2 trial suggest that, during PCI, bivalirudin with provisional GPIIb/IIIa inhibition is not inferior to UFH with planned GPIIb/IIIa inhibition [80]. Furthermore, bivalirudin was associated with significantly less in-hospital major bleeding. Some interventional cardiologists now use bivalirudin as an alternative to heparin for either low-risk ACS patients or for patients at high risk of bleeding. The ACUITY trial is randomizing ACS patients to bivalirudin or enoxaparin prior to PCI. This will help to determine the optimal antithrombotic regimen in non-ST-segment elevation ACS.

Role of CABG in ACS

ST-segment elevation ACS

CABG is generally deferred in ST-segment elevation ACS since the priority is to quickly re-establish flow in the occluded artery, preferably by PCI to perfuse jeopardized myocardium. An acute mechanical complication of MI, such as ventricular septal defect or papillary muscle rupture, would warrant emergency open-heart surgery. Emergent CABG is only contemplated if maximum nonsurgical management, including PCI and intra-aortic balloon pump, fails to stabilize the patient. **Table 2** outlines the ACC/AHA recommendations for emergent CABG in ST-segment elevation ACS.

Discovering surgical coronary artery disease such as left main or triple-vessel disease at the time of diagnostic catheterization for ST-segment elevation ACS poses a difficult dilemma. Cardiothoracic surgeons are appropriately reluctant to perform emergency CABG during acute MI. In patients with ST-segment elevation ACS with surgical disease, we generally perform PCI on the infarct-related artery to salvage jeopardized myocardium until CABG is performed. The timing of CABG depends on patient stability. It varies from emergent CABG in the next 1–2 days, while the patient is still in the intensive care unit, to CABG several days later, after the patient has been transferred to the cardiac ward. DES may further shift the approach to staged multivessel PCI in the future.

A further dilemma is whether to stent or perform PTCA only on the infarct-related artery. If stenting is performed, then clopidogrel is strongly recommended for at least 1 month. Clopidogrel administration delays

CABG due to increased bleeding risk. Thus, in patients with ST-segment elevation ACS who require surgical revascularization, we sometimes perform balloon angioplasty alone in the infarct-related artery, accepting a higher rate of restenosis in the native vessel in exchange for an earlier CABG date. Again, with the advent of DES, multivessel, complex, staged PCI may further decrease the need for CABG.

Non-ST-segment elevation ACS

In contrast to patients with ST-segment elevation ACS, those with non-ST-segment elevation ACS found to have surgical disease during angiography are more likely to undergo CABG without bridging PCI. The ACC/AHA guidelines regarding the use of CABG or PCI in non-ST-segment elevation ACS are summarized in **Table 2**. When coronary angiography is performed in non-ST-segment elevation ACS, the patient is usually not actively infarcting and there is not as pressing a need to revascularize the myocardium emergently. In our center, provided these patients are hemodynamically stable and not actively infarcting, we tend not to perform culprit vessel PCI. Instead we refer the patient for urgent CABG, to be performed in the next few days. However, future data supporting any time-dependent benefit of very early revascularization (as well as expanded indications for DES) may further diminish the need for CABG.

Conclusions

In ST-segment elevation ACS, primary PCI is preferred over thrombolytics. In non-ST-segment elevation ACS, risk stratification is imperative. For intermediate and high-risk non-ST-segment elevation ACS patients (manifested as elevated cardiac markers or ST-segment-segment depression) an early invasive strategy is superior to conservative management. Low-risk non-ST-segment elevation ACS patients may be suitable for an initial noninvasive approach, though an invasive approach appears to be cost-effective across all risk strata [81].

In all ACS patients, minimizing the time to PCI is paramount. Shorter door-to-balloon times are associated with improved outcomes in ST-segment elevation ACS. Recent evidence suggests that very early revascularization in non-ST-segment elevation ACS may provide added benefit. If the benefits of very early revascularization in non-ST-segment elevation ACS patients are validated by larger clinical trials, their management may change dramatically and propel the development of acute chest pain centers, analogous to trauma centers [82,83].

Finally, despite the demonstrated benefit of PCI in ACS, revascularization rates are lower than desired [48]. To expand access to PCI in ACS and decrease the time to coronary angiography, protocols for routing or rapid transfer of patients to high-volume invasive heart centers that provide around-the-clock PCI need to be established. Such efforts are requisite to improving outcomes in ACS.

References

1. Chen MS, Bhatt DL. Highlights of the 2002 Update to the 2000 American College of Cardiology/American Heart Association Acute Coronary Syndrome Guidelines. *Cardiol Rev* 2003;11:113–21.
2. Smith SC Jr, Dove JT, Jacobs AK, et al. ACC/AHA guidelines for percutaneous coronary intervention (revision of the 1993 PTCA guidelines)-executive summary: a report of the American College of Cardiology/American Heart Association task force on practice guidelines (Committee to revise the 1993 guidelines for percutaneous transluminal coronary angioplasty) endorsed by the Society for Cardiac Angiography and Interventions. *Circulation* 2001;103:3019–41.
3. Ryan TJ, Antman EM, Brooks NH, et al. 1999 update: ACC/AHA guidelines for the management of patients with acute myocardial infarction. A report of the American College of Cardiology/American Heart Association Task Force on Practice Guidelines (Committee on Management of Acute Myocardial Infarction). Available at http://www.acc.org/clinical/guidelines/miguide.pdf and http://www.americanheart.org. Accessed on October 2, 2003.
4. Weaver WD, Simes RJ, Betriu A, et al. Comparison of primary coronary angioplasty and intravenous thrombolytic therapy for acute myocardial infarction: a quantitative review. *JAMA* 1997;278:2093–8.
5. Keeley EC, Boura JA, Grines CL. Primary angioplasty versus intravenous thrombolytic therapy for acute myocardial infarction: a quantitative review of 23 randomised trials. *Lancet* 2003;361:13–20.
6. Berger AK, Schulman KA, Gersh BJ, et al. Primary coronary angioplasty vs thrombolysis for the management of acute myocardial infarction in elderly patients. *JAMA* 1999;282:341–8.

7. Bonnefoy E, Lapostolle F, Leizorovicz A, et al. Primary angioplasty versus prehospital fibrinolysis in acute myocardial infarction: a randomised study. *Lancet* 2002;360:825–9.

8. Grines CL, Cox DA, Stone GW, et al. Coronary angioplasty with or without stent implantation for acute myocardial infarction. Stent Primary Angioplasty in Myocardial Infarction Study Group. *N Engl J Med* 1999;341:1949–56.

9. Stone GW, Grines CL, Cox DA, et al. Comparison of angioplasty with stenting, with or without abciximab, in acute myocardial infarction. *N Engl J Med* 2002;346:957–66.

10. Herrmann HC, Moliterno DJ, Ohman EM, et al. Facilitation of early percutaneous coronary intervention after reteplase with or without abciximab in acute myocardial infarction: results from the SPEED (GUSTO-4 Pilot) Trial. *J Am Coll Cardiol* 2000;36:1489–96.

11. de Lemos JA, Gibson CM, Antman EM, et al. Abciximab and early adjunctive percutaneous coronary intervention are associated with improved ST-segment resolution after thrombolysis: Observations from the TIMI 14 Trial. *Am Heart J* 2001;141:592–8.

12. Herrmann HC, Kelley MP, Ellis SG. Facilitated PCI: rationale and design of the FINESSE trial. *J Invasive Cardiol* 2001;13 (Suppl A):10A–15A.

13. Aversano T, Aversano LT, Passamani E, et al. Thrombolytic therapy vs primary percutaneous coronary intervention for myocardial infarction in patients presenting to hospitals without on-site cardiac surgery: a randomized controlled trial. *JAMA* 2002;287:1943–51.

14. Canto JG, Every NR, Magid DJ, et al. The volume of primary angioplasty procedures and survival after acute myocardial infarction. National Registry of Myocardial Infarction 2 Investigators. *N Engl J Med* 2000;342:1573–80.

15. Magid DJ, Calonge BN, Rumsfeld JS, et al. Relation between hospital primary angioplasty volume and mortality for patients with acute MI treated with primary angioplasty vs thrombolytic therapy. *JAMA* 2000;284:3131–8.

16. Vakili BA, Kaplan R, Brown DL. Volume-outcome relation for physicians and hospitals performing angioplasty for acute myocardial infarction in New York state. *Circulation* 2001;104:2171–6.

17. McGrath PD, Wennberg DE, Dickens JD Jr, et al. Relation between operator and hospital volume and outcomes following percutaneous coronary interventions in the era of the coronary stent. *JAMA* 2000;284:3139–44.

18. Cannon CP, Gibson CM, Lambrew CT, et al. Relationship of symptom-onset-to-balloon time and door-to-balloon time with mortality in patients undergoing angioplasty for acute myocardial infarction. *JAMA* 2000;283:2941–7.

19. Angeja BG, Gibson CM, Chin R, et al. Predictors of door-to-balloon delay in primary angioplasty. *Am J Cardiol* 2002;89:1156–61.

20. Grines CL, Westerhausen DR Jr, Grines LL, et al. A randomized trial of transfer for primary angioplasty versus on-site thrombolysis in patients with high-risk myocardial infarction: the Air Primary Angioplasty in Myocardial Infarction study. *J Am Coll Cardiol* 2002;39:1713–9.

21. Andersen HR, Nielsen TT, Rasmussen K, et al. A comparison of coronary angioplasty with fibrinolytic therapy in acute myocardial infarction. *N Engl J Med* 2003;349:733–42.

22. Widimsky P, Groch L, Zelizko M, et al. Multicentre randomized trial comparing transport to primary angioplasty vs immediate thrombolysis vs combined strategy for patients with acute myocardial infarction presenting to a community hospital without a catheterization laboratory. The PRAGUE study. *Eur Heart J* 2000;21:823–31.

23. Widimsky P, Budesinsky T, Vorac D, et al. Long distance transport for primary angioplasty vs immediate thrombolysis in acute myocardial infarction. Final results of the randomized national multicentre trial–PRAGUE-2. *Eur Heart Jl* 2003;24:94–104.

24. Hochman JS, Sleeper LA, Webb JG, et al. Early revascularization in acute myocardial infarction complicated by cardiogenic shock. SHOCK Investigators. Should We Emergently Revascularize Occluded Coronaries for Cardiogenic Shock. *N Engl J Med* 1999;341:625–34.

25. Hochman JS, Sleeper LA, White HD, et al. One-year survival following early revascularization for cardiogenic shock. *JAMA* 2001;285:190–2.

26. Roe MT, Cura FA, Joski PS, et al. Initial experience with multivessel percutaneous coronary intervention during mechanical reperfusion for acute myocardial infarction. *Am J Cardiol* 2001;88:170–3, A6.

27. Hong MK, Mintz GS, Lee CW, et al. Paclitaxel coating reduces in-stent intimal hyperplasia in human coronary arteries: a serial volumetric intravascular ultrasound analysis from the ASian Paclitaxel-Eluting Stent Clinical Trial (ASPECT). *Circulation* 2003;107:517–20.

28. Sousa JE, Costa MA, Sousa AG, et al. Two-year angiographic and intravascular ultrasound follow-up after implantation of sirolimus-eluting stents in human coronary arteries. *Circulation* 2003;107:381–3.

29. Grube E, Silber S, Hauptmann KE, et al. TAXUS I: six- and twelve-month results from a randomized, double-blind trial on a slow-release paclitaxel-eluting stent for de novo coronary lesions. *Circulation* 2003;107:38–42.

30. Morice MC, Serruys PW, Sousa JE, et al. A randomized comparison of a sirolimus-eluting stent with a standard stent for coronary revascularization. *N Engl J Med* 2002;346:1773–80.

31. Lee CH, Lemos PA, van Domburg RT, et al. Safety and Efficacy of Sirolimus-Eluting Stent (cypher) in Acute Myocardial Infarction: A substudy of the Rapamycin-Eluting Stent Evaluation at Rotterdam Cardiology Hospital (RESEARCH) Study. *J Am Coll Cardiol* 2003;41:21A (Abstract).

32. Antman EM, Tanasijevic MJ, Thompson B, et al. Cardiac-specific troponin I levels to predict the risk of mortality in patients with acute coronary syndromes. *N Engl J Med* 1996;335:1342–9.

33. Sabatine MS, Morrow DA, de Lemos JA, et al. Multimarker approach to risk stratification in non-ST elevation acute coronary syndromes: simultaneous assessment of troponin I, C-reactive protein, and B-type natriuretic peptide. *Circulation* 2002;105:1760–3.

34. Haverkate F, Thompson SG, Pyke SD, et al. Production of C-reactive protein and risk of coronary events in stable and unstable angina. European Concerted Action on Thrombosis and Disabilities Angina Pectoris Study Group. *Lancet* 1997;349:462–6.

35. Morrow DA, Rifai N, Antman EM, et al. C-reactive protein is a potent predictor of mortality independently of and in combination with troponin T in acute coronary syndromes: a TIMI 11A substudy. Thrombolysis in Myocardial Infarction. *J Am Coll Cardiol* 1998;31:1460–5.

36. Alexander JH, Sparapani RA, Mahaffey KW, et al. Association between minor elevations of creatine kinase-MB level and mortality in patients with acute coronary syndromes without ST-segment elevation. PURSUIT Steering Committee. Platelet Glycoprotein IIb/IIIa in Unstable Angina: Receptor Suppression Using Integrilin Therapy. *JAMA* 2000;283:347–53.

37. Antman EM, Cohen M, Bernink PJ, et al. The TIMI risk score for unstable angina/non-ST elevation MI: A method for prognostication and therapeutic decision making. *JAMA* 2000;284:835–42.

38. Cannon CP, Weintraub WS, Demopoulos LA, et al. Comparison of early invasive and conservative strategies in patients with unstable coronary syndromes treated with the glycoprotein IIb/IIIa inhibitor tirofiban. *N Engl J Med* 2001;344:1879–87.

39. Effects of tissue plasminogen activator and a comparison of early invasive and conservative strategies in unstable angina and non-Q-wave myocardial infarction. Results of the TIMI IIIB Trial. Thrombolysis in Myocardial Ischemia. *Circulation* 1994;89:1545–56.

40. Anderson HV, Cannon CP, Stone PH, et al. One-year results of the Thrombolysis in Myocardial Infarction (TIMI) IIIB clinical trial. A randomized comparison of tissue-type plasminogen activator versus placebo and early invasive versus early conservative strategies in unstable angina and non-Q wave myocardial infarction. *J Am Coll Cardiol* 1995;26:1643–50.

41. Boden WE, O'Rourke RA, Crawford MH, et al. Outcomes in patients with acute non-Q-wave myocardial infarction randomly assigned to an invasive as compared with a conservative management strategy. Veterans Affairs Non-Q-Wave Infarction Strategies in Hospital (VANQWISH) Trial Investigators. *N Engl J Med* 1998;338:1785–92.

42. Invasive compared with non-invasive treatment in unstable coronary-artery disease: FRISC II prospective randomised multicentre study. FRagmin and Fast Revascularisation during InStability in Coronary artery disease Investigators. *Lancet* 1999;354:708–15.

43. Wallentin L, Lagerqvist B, Husted S, et al. Outcome at 1 year after an invasive compared with a non-invasive strategy in unstable coronary-artery disease: the FRISC II invasive randomised trial. FRISC II Investigators. Fast Revascularisation during Instability in Coronary artery disease. *Lancet* 2000;356:9–16.

44. Fox KA, Poole-Wilson PA, Henderson RA, et al. Interventional versus conservative treatment for patients with unstable angina or non-ST-elevation myocardial infarction: the British Heart Foundation RITA 3 randomised trial. Randomized Intervention Trial of unstable Angina. *Lancet* 2002;360:743–51.

45. Cannon CP, Weintraub WS, Demopoulos LA, et al. Comparison of early invasive and conservative strategies in patients with unstable coronary syndromes treated with the glycoprotein IIb/IIIa inhibitor tirofiban. *N Engl J Med* 2001;344:1879–87.

46. Spacek R, Widimsky P, Straka Z, et al. Value of first day angiography/angioplasty in evolving non-ST segment elevation myocardial infarction: an open multicenter randomized trial. The VINO Study. *Eur Heart J.* 2002;23:230–8.

47. Neumann FJ, Kasrati A, Pogatsa-Murray G, et al. Evaluation of prolonged antithrombotic pretreatment (Cooling-Off Strategy) before intervention in patients with unstable coronary syndromes. *JAMA* 2003;290:1593–9.

48. Bhatt DL, Greenbaum A, Roe MT, et al. An early invasive approach to acute coronary syndromes in CRUSADE: A dissociation between clinical guidelines and current practice. *Circulation* 2002:II-494.

49. Braunwald E, Antman EM, Beasley JW, et al. ACC/AHA 2002 guideline update for the management of patients with unstable angina and non-ST-segment elevation myocardial infarction: a report of the American College of Cardiology/American Heart Association Task Force on Practice Guidelines (Committee on the Management of Patients With Unstable Angina). Available at http://www.acc.org/clinical/guidelines/unstable/unstable.pdf. Accessed on October 2, 2003.

50. Steg PG, Goldberg RJ, Gore JM, et al. Baseline characteristics, management practices, and in-hospital outcomes of patients hospitalized with acute coronary syndromes in the Global Registry of Acute Coronary Events (GRACE). *Am J Cardiol* 2002;90:358–63.

51. Eagle KA, Goodman SG, Avezum A, et al. Practice variation and missed opportunities for reperfusion in ST-segment-elevation myocardial infarction: findings from the Global Registry of Acute Coronary Events (GRACE). *Lancet* 2002;359:373–7.

52. Gabriel Steg P, Iung B, Feldman LJ, et al. Determinants of use and outcomes of invasive coronary procedures in acute coronary syndromes: results from ENACT. *Eur Heart J* 2003;24:613–22.

53. Yusuf S, Zhao F, Mehta SR, et al. Effects of clopidogrel in addition to aspirin in patients with acute coronary syndromes without ST-segment elevation. *N Engl J Med* 2001;345:494–502.

54. Mehta SR, Yusuf S, Peters RJ, et al. Effects of pretreatment with clopidogrel and aspirin followed by long-term therapy in patients undergoing percutaneous coronary intervention: the PCI-CURE study. *Lancet* 2001;358:527–33.

55. Steinhubl SR, Berger PB, Mann JT 3rd, et al. Early and sustained dual oral antiplatelet therapy following percutaneous coronary intervention: a randomized controlled trial. *JAMA* 2002;288:2411–20.

56. Chew DP, Bhatt DL, Robbins MA, et al. Effect of clopidogrel added to aspirin before percutaneous coronary intervention on the risk associated with C-reactive protein. *Am J Cardiol* 2001;88:672–4.

57. Assali AR, Salloum J, Sdringola S, et al. Effects of clopidogrel pretreatment before percutaneous coronary intervention in patients treated with glycoprotein IIb/IIIa inhibitors (abciximab or tirofiban). *Am J Cardiol* 2001;88:884–6.

58. Hongo RH, Ley J, Dick SE, et al. The effect of clopidogrel in combination with aspirin when given before coronary artery bypass grafting. *J Am Coll Cardiol* 2002;40:231–7.

59. Eisenberg M, Jamal S. Glycoprotein IIb/IIIa inhibition in the setting of acute ST-segment elevation myocardial infarction. *J Am Coll Cardiol* 2003;42:1–6.

60. Brener SJ, Barr LA, Burchenal JE, et al. Randomized, placebo-controlled trial of platelet glycoprotein IIb/IIIa blockade with primary angioplasty for acute myocardial infarction. ReoPro and Primary PTCA Organization and Randomized Trial (RAPPORT) Investigators. *Circulation* 1998;98:734–41.

61. Neumann FJ, Kastrati A, Schmitt C, et al. Effect of glycoprotein IIb/IIIa receptor blockade with abciximab on clinical and angiographic restenosis rate after the placement of coronary stents following acute myocardial infarction. *J Am Coll Cardiol* 2000;35:915–21.

62. Neumann FJ, Blasini R, Schmitt C, et al. Effect of glycoprotein IIb/IIIa receptor blockade on recovery of coronary flow and left ventricular function after the placement of coronary-artery stents in acute myocardial infarction. *Circulation* 1998;98:2695–701.

63. Schomig A, Kastrati A, Dirschinger J, et al. Coronary stenting plus platelet glycoprotein IIb/IIIa blockade compared with tissue plasminogen activator in acute myocardial infarction. Stent versus Thrombolysis for Occluded Coronary Arteries in Patients with Acute Myocardial Infarction Study Investigators. *N Engl J Med* 2000;343:385–91.

64. Kastrati A, Mehilli J, Dirschinger J, et al. Myocardial salvage after coronary stenting plus abciximab versus fibrinolysis plus abciximab in patients with acute myocardial infarction: a randomised trial. *Lancet* 2002;359:920–5.

65. Montalescot G, Barragan P, Wittenberg O, et al. Platelet glycoprotein IIb/IIIa inhibition with coronary stenting for acute myocardial infarction. *N Engl J Med* 2001;344:1895–903.

66. Kong DF, Califf RM, Miller DP, et al. Clinical outcomes of therapeutic agents that block the platelet glycoprotein IIb/IIIa integrin in ischemic heart disease. *Circulation* 1998;98:2829–35.

67. Topol EJ, Califf RM, Weisman HF, et al. Randomised trial of coronary intervention with antibody against platelet IIb/IIIa integrin for reduction of clinical restenosis: results at six months. The EPIC Investigators. *Lancet* 1994;343:881–6.

68. Platelet glycoprotein IIb/IIIa receptor blockade and low-dose heparin during percutaneous coronary revascularization. The EPILOG Investigators. *N Engl J Med* 1997;336:1689–96.

69. Randomised placebo-controlled and balloon-angioplasty-controlled trial to assess safety of coronary stenting with use of platelet glycoprotein-IIb/IIIa blockade. The EPISTENT Investigators. Evaluation of Platelet IIb/IIIa Inhibitor for Stenting. *Lancet* 1998;352:87–92.

70. Topol EJ, Lincoff AM, Kereiakes DJ, et al. Multi-year follow-up of abciximab therapy in three randomized, placebo-controlled trials of percutaneous coronary revascularization. *Am J of Med* 2002;113:1–6.

71. Topol EJ, Moliterno DJ, Herrmann HC, et al. Comparison of two platelet glycoprotein IIb/IIIa inhibitors, tirofiban and abciximab, for the prevention of ischemic events with percutaneous coronary revascularization. *N Engl J Med* 2001;344:1888–94.

72. Stone GW, Moliterno DJ, Bertrand M, et al. Impact of clinical syndrome acuity on the differential response to 2 glycoprotein IIb/IIIa inhibitors in patients undergoing coronary stenting: the TARGET Trial. *Circulation* 2002;105:2347–54.

73. Efficacy and safety of tenecteplase in combination with enoxaparin, abciximab, or unfractionated heparin: the ASSENT-3 randomised trial in acute myocardial infarction. *Lancet* 2001;358:605–13.

74. Cohen M, Demers C, Gurfinkel EP, et al. A comparison of low-molecular-weight heparin with unfractionated heparin for unstable coronary artery disease. Efficacy and Safety of Subcutaneous Enoxaparin in Non-Q-Wave Coronary Events Study Group. *N Engl J Med* 1997;337:447–52.

75. Goodman SG, Cohen M, Bigonzi F, et al. Randomized trial of low molecular weight heparin (enoxaparin) versus unfractionated heparin for unstable coronary artery disease: one-year results of the ESSENCE Study. Efficacy and Safety of Subcutaneous Enoxaparin in Non-Q Wave Coronary Events. *J Am Coll Cardiol* 2000;36:693–8.

76. Collet JP, Montalescot G, Lison L, et al. Percutaneous coronary intervention after subcutaneous enoxaparin pretreatment in patients with unstable angina pectoris. *Circulation* 2001;103:658–63.

77. Young JJ, Kereiakes DJ, Grines CL. Low-molecular-weight heparin therapy in percutaneous coronary intervention: the NICE 1 and NICE 4 trials. National Investigators Collaborating on Enoxaparin Investigators. *J Invasive Cardiol* 2000;12(Suppl E):E14–8;discussion E25–8.

78. Bhatt DL, Lee BI, Casterella PJ, et al. Safety of concomitant therapy with eptifibatide and enoxaparin in patients undergoing percutaneous coronary intervention: Results of the coronary revascularization using integrilin and single bolus enoxaparin study. *J Am Coll Cardiol* 2003;41:20–5.

79. The Synergy Executive Committee. Superior Yield of the New strategy of Enoxaparin, Revascularization, and GlYcoprotein IIb IIIa inhibitors. The SYNERGY trial: study design and rationale. *Am Heart J* 2002;143:952–60.

80. Lincoff AM, Bittl JA, Harrington RA, et al. Bivalirudin and provisional glycoprotein IIb/IIIa blockade compared with heparin and planned glycoprotein IIb/IIIa blockade during percutaneous coronary intervention: REPLACE-2 randomized trial. *JAMA* 2003;289:853–63.

81. Mahoney EM, Jurkovitz CT, Chu H, et al. Cost and cost-effectiveness of an early invasive vs conservative strategy for the treatment of unstable angina and non-ST-segment elevation myocardial infarction. *JAMA* 2002;288:1851–8.

82. Topol EJ, Kereiakes DJ. Regionalization of care for acute ischemic heart disease: a call for specialized centers. *Circulation* 2003;107:1463–6.

83. Califf RM, Faxon DP. Need for centers to care for patients with acute coronary syndromes. *Circulation* 2003;107:1467–70.

9

Mechanical and electrical complications

Mauricio G Cohen & E Magnus Ohman

Introduction: identifying high-risk patients

The definition of high-risk acute coronary syndromes (ACS) patients encompasses a wide spectrum of clinical syndromes, from unstable angina at higher risk of developing potentially fatal complications to cardiogenic shock or life-threatening ventricular arrhythmias. In general, major complications of ACS develop several hours after hospital admission. Therefore, defining an individual patient's risk during the early hours after hospital presentation is crucial both to determining how intensive their care should be and to preventing downstream complications.

Risk stratification can be achieved using simple clinical data, a 12-lead electrocardiogram (ECG), and biochemical markers of myocardial injury. The use of multivariable modeling techniques in large trial databases can combine these simple clinical variables, providing >80% of the prognostic information. These models have been developed for two distinct ACS populations based on the presence or absence of ST-segment elevation on the admission ECG. In fact, the presence of ST-segment elevation mandates immediate coronary reperfusion, whereas its absence allows for initial medical stabilization and a longer time frame for interventional catheterization procedures.

ST-segment elevation MI		
Clinical trial	GUSTO-I	TIMI risk score (In-Time II)
Number of patients	41,021	13,253
Predicted outcome	30-day death	30-day death
C-index	0.836	0.78
Clinical history	Age; prior MI	Age; diabetes; hypertension; recent angina; time to treatment
Hospital presentation	Systolic BP Heart rate Killip class	Systolic BP Heart rate Killip class Low body weight
ECG	Infarct location	Infarct location LBBB
Biochemical markers	–	–
Non-ST-segment elevation ACS		
Clinical trial	PURSUIT	PURSUIT	TIMI risk score (TIMI 11B)
Number of patients	9,461		1,957
Predicted outcome	30-day death	30-day death/MI	14-day death/MI/ revascularization
C-index	0.814	0.669	0.65
Clinical history	Age; recent angina; gender (male); heart failure	Age; recent angina; gender (male); heart failure	Age; recent angina; family history of CAD; diabetes; current smoking; hypertension; previous aspirin; CAD >50%
Hospital presentation	Systolic BP Heart rate Rales	Rales	–
ECG	ST-segment depression	ST-segment depression	ST-segment elevation or depression
Biochemical markers	↑ CK-MB	↑ CK-MB	↑ CK-MB or troponin

Table 1. Variables included in risk scores for the prediction of unfavorable outcomes in acute coronary syndromes (ACS). BP: blood pressure; CAD: coronary artery disease; CK-MB: creatine kinase isoenzyme MB; ECG: electrocardiogram; LBBB: left bundle branch block; MI: myocardial infarction. The c-index measures the ability of the model to predict actual outcomes. A c-index of 0.6–0.7 has limited value, 0.7–0.8 has modest value, and >0.8 allows sufficient discrimination to be utilized in clinical scenarios.

Table 1 compares multivariable models developed from large clinical trials enrolling patients with ST-segment elevation myocardial infarction (MI) and non-ST-segment elevation ACS [1–4].

Table 2 summarizes the risk stratification proposed by the American College of Cardiology (ACC)/

Table 2. Short-term risk of death or nonfatal myocardial infarction in patients with unstable angina (adapted from *J Am Coll Cardiol* 2002; 40:1366–74, with permission).

	High risk	Intermediate risk	Low risk
	At least one of the following features must be present:	No high-risk feature but must have one of the following:	No high- or intermediate-risk feature but may have any of the following:
History	Accelerating tempo of ischemic symptoms in preceding 48 hours	Prior myocardial infarction, peripheral or cerebrovascular disease, or coronary artery bypass graft, prior aspirin use	Increased angina frequency, severity, or duration Angina provoked at a lower threshold
Character of pain	Prolonged ongoing (>20 mins) rest pain	Prolonged (>20 mins) rest angina, now resolved, with moderate or high likelihood of CAD Rest angina (<20 mins) or angina relieved with rest or nitroglycerin	New-onset angina within 2 weeks to 2 months
Clinical findings	Pulmonary edema, most likely due to ischemia New or worsening mitral regurgitation murmur S2 or new/worsening rales Hypotension, bradycardia, tachycardia Age >75 years	Age >70 years	–
Electrocardiogram	Angina at rest with transient ST-segment changes >0.05 mV Bundle branch block, new or presumed new Sustained ventricular tachycardia	T-wave inversion >0.2 mV Pathological Q waves	Normal or unchanged ECG during an episode of chest discomfort
Cardiac markers	Elevated (troponin T or troponin I)	Slightly elevated (troponin T >0.01 but <0.1 ng/mL)	Normal

American Heart Association (AHA) guidelines for patients with unstable angina [5].

Cardiogenic shock

Cardiogenic shock is the most common cause of death in patients hospitalized for ACS (with or without ST-segment elevation). It is characterized by inadequate tissue perfusion due to reduced cardiac output in the absence of hypovolemia [6]. In ~80% of the cases, it is the result of severe left ventricular (LV) failure associated with MI; see **Figure 1** for other causes of cardiogenic shock and **Figure 2** for their respective mortality rates [7]. The incidence of cardiogenic shock has remained stable at ~7% over

Figure 1. Etiologies of cardiogenic shock. (adapted from *QJM* 2001;94:57–67). LV: left ventricular; MR: mitral regurgitation; RV: right ventricular; VSR: ventricular septal rupture.

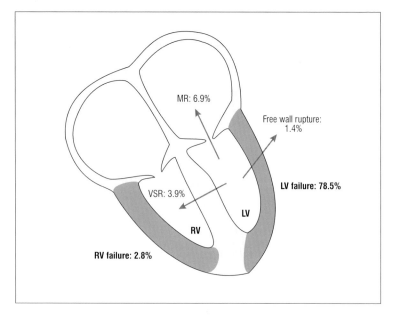

MR: 6.9%

Free wall rupture: 1.4%

LV failure: 78.5%

VSR: 3.9%

LV

RV

RV failure: 2.8%

the last 25 years, despite major advances in MI management [8].

The time course of cardiogenic shock is variable, depending on whether the initial presentation is with or without ST-segment elevation. The median time from MI to shock in ST-segment elevation patients is 5–8 hours, whereas in non-ST-segment elevation patients this period is substantially longer (76–94 hours). Of note, only 11% of ACS patients enrolled in clinical trials presented with shock at hospital admission [9–12].

The serious consequences of cardiogenic shock mean that identifying patients at risk of developing this complication is necessary for early detection and aggressive management. In a multivariable model of cardiogenic shock in ST-segment elevation ACS, simple clinical variables such as advanced age,

Figure 2. Mortality according to major categories in the SHOCK trial and registry combined. LV: left ventricular; MR: mitral regurgitation; RV: right ventricular; VSR: ventricular septal rupture.

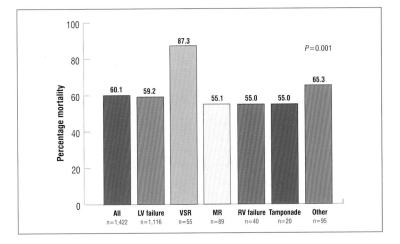

Figure 3. Pathophysiology of cardiogenic shock (adapted from *Circulation* 2003;107:2998–3002, with permission). iNOS: inducible macrophage-type nitric oxide synthase; LVEDP: left ventricular end diastolic pressure; NO: nitric oxide.

hypotension, tachycardia, and Killip class provided >85% of the predictive information [13]. Non-ST-segment elevation ACS patients who develop shock are more likely to be older and have had MI, coronary artery bypass graft (CABG), or congestive heart failure, compared with ST-segment elevation patients. In addition to the predictors indicated for ST-segment elevation ACS, elevated cardiac enzymes and the presence of ST-segment depression on the admission ECG are major risk factors for shock in non-ST-segment elevation ACS [12].

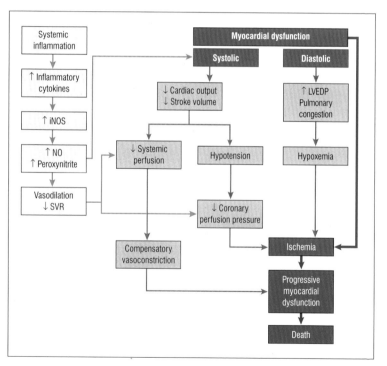

Pathophysiology

On the basis of autopsy studies, it is classically accepted that the development of cardiogenic shock is directly related to the extent of myocardial necrosis. Thus, an infarct involving more than half of the LV myocardium would result in a vicious spiral consisting of a low cardiac output state, hypotension, pulmonary congestion, further myocardial ischemia, and further reduction in contractility and cardiac output, triggering compensatory mechanisms aimed at augmenting the systemic vascular resistance (SVR) with vasoconstriction [14,15].

However, recent observations from the SHOCK trial and registry have challenged this notion, indicating that patients in cardiogenic shock have moderate LV dysfunction with ejection fractions (EFs) of ~30% and SVR in the normal range [16,17]. A plausible explanation for these findings is the development of a systemic inflammatory response syndrome secondary to cardiogenic shock with fever and elevated white blood count, complement, interleukins, and C-reactive protein, with an inadequately low SVR despite vasopressors. It seems that the release of cytokines may trigger an excessive synthesis of nitric oxide, reaching toxic levels. It has been proposed that this is a major cause of refractory myocardial depression (see **Figure 3**) [18].

Clinical findings and diagnosis

Cardiogenic shock is a medical emergency; therefore, the initial clinical assessment should be accompanied by supportive measures to avoid irreversible end-organ damage. Major clinical manifestations of shock resulting from elevated LV filling pressures include dyspnea, pulmonary edema, and hypoxemia, and from decreased cardiac output include systemic hypotension, oliguria, altered mental status, lactic acidosis, cold clammy skin, and mottled extremities (see **Figure 4**). Nevertheless, these features may not always be present in patients with cardiogenic shock. Pulmonary congestion may be absent in a third of cases, and in a lower proportion of cases peripheral hypoperfusion may not be accompanied by hypotension (and *vice versa*) [19].

Timing of shock development has important clinical implications, as late shock (>36 hours) should raise suspicion of mechanical complications. Therefore, prompt echocardiographic examination is warranted for establishing the cause of shock and assessing the LV and right ventricular (RV) function.

Transesophageal echocardiography is particularly useful for the diagnosis of mechanical complications or aortic dissection. Independent echocardiographic predictors of death in the SHOCK trial were left ventricular ejection fraction (LVEF) and severity of mitral regurgitation (MR) [17]. Pulmonary artery catheterization should be performed by experienced physicians following specific guidelines established by the ACC. Major indications include differentiation between cardiogenic and other causes of shock after failure of initial therapy with vasopressors and fluids, guidance of pharmacologic therapy in

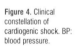

Figure 4. Clinical constellation of cardiogenic shock. BP: blood pressure.

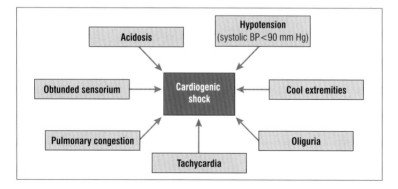

cardiogenic shock, and diagnosis and short-term monitoring of medical management of mechanical complications before corrective surgery [20].

Management
Initial medical stabilization
Initial medical stabilization should include proper oxygenation, with mechanical ventilation if necessary, correction of acidosis, treatment of arrhythmias, and maintenance of adequate mean arterial pressure using dopamine or epinephrine depending on the degree of hemodynamic compromise. Dobutamine can be used in association with other agents when hypotension is not severe. In addition, all patients should receive aspirin and intravenous heparin. The use of intravenous platelet glycoprotein (GP)IIb/IIIa inhibitors has been associated with a significant mortality reduction in patients presenting without ST-segment elevation [12]. Further understanding of the role of nitric oxide in the pathogenesis of shock has led to investigations testing the use of L-NAME (a nitric oxide synthase inhibitor) in a small group of cardiogenic shock patients, with promising results [21].

Intra-aortic balloon counterpulsation
The use of an intra-aortic balloon pump (IABP) is associated with improved cardiac function and diastolic blood pressure, a reduction in systemic acidosis, enhanced coronary perfusion, and less infarct-related artery reocclusion. In fact, registry data indicate improved survival with early IABP insertion in patients with cardiogenic shock [22,23]. The current ACC/AHA guidelines recommend early IABP insertion as a class I indication for patients with cardiogenic shock [24].

Revascularization
The temporal trends for cardiogenic shock outcomes in a population-based study have shown a significant survival improvement after 1990, when percutaneous revascularization for MI started to

gain acceptance (see **Figure 5**). More recently, the SHOCK trial has confirmed the superiority of emergency revascularization (within 18 hours) by either percutaneous coronary intervention (PCI) or CABG (as compared with aggressive medical stabilization). Even though the primary endpoint (overall survival at 30 days) did not reach statistical significance (53% vs 44%, $P = 0.109$), at 12-month follow-up there was a significant survival benefit with early revascularization (47% vs 34%, $P = 0.025$) with 132 lives saved per 1,000 patients [16,25]. Therefore, all initial management efforts, including IABP counterpulsation, should be aimed at patient stratification through coronary angiography followed by a preferred revascularization method according to coronary anatomy as depicted in **Figure 6**. The benefit appears to be greatest for patients <75 years of age.

Figure 5. Adjusted temporal trends of in-hospital mortality for cardiogenic shock (adjusted to age, gender, medical history, previous myocardial infarction, and type and location of acute myocardial infarction) [8]. CI: confidence interval.

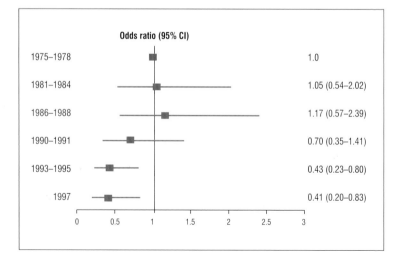

Based on the results of the SHOCK trial, the ACC/AHA guidelines for MI now recommend emergency revascularization for patients <75 years with cardiogenic shock [24]. However, early revascularization should not be systematically denied to the elderly, as observational studies have shown that these patients derive substantial benefit from the more aggressive approach [26,27]. Therefore, the decision of whether to treat elderly patients should be made on an individual basis from an assessment of their comorbidities and functional status. The use of

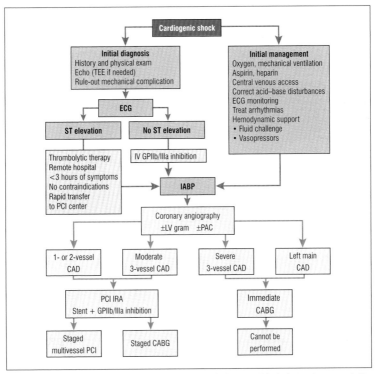

Figure 6. Algorithm for the management of cardiogenic shock. Early mechanical revascularization is strongly recommended for all suitable candidates <75 years of age; however, selected patients ≥75 years of age with preserved functional status should also be offered this strategy. CABG: coronary artery bypass grafting; CAD: coronary artery disease; ECG: electrocardiogram; GP: glycoprotein; IABP: intra-aortic balloon pump; IRA: infarct-related artery; IV: intravenous; LV: left ventricular; PAC: pulmonary artery catheterization; PCI: percutaneous coronary intervention; TEE: transesophageal echocardiography.

GPIIb/IIIa inhibitors and stents during PCI appears to be associated with improved outcomes in cardiogenic shock [28].

Patients presenting to sites without interventional facilities should be referred to a tertiary care center with IABP placement before transport. If the anticipated time to revascularization is >2 hours, thrombolytic therapy should be considered as a valid alternative. A substudy from the SHOCK registry suggested a synergistic effect of IABP counterpulsation and thrombolytic therapy. Patients treated with thrombolytic therapy and IABP had 47% in-hospital mortality (versus 52% with IABP alone, 63% with thrombolytic therapy alone, and 77% with neither [$P<0.0001$]) [22].

Right ventricular infarction

RV infarction is almost exclusively a complication of inferior MI, resulting from a proximal occlusion of the right coronary artery before the origin of the acute marginal branches (see **Table 3**) [29–32]. In general, RV involvement occurs in one third of inferior infarcts [31]. Possible explanations for the RV resistance to ischemia include:

- lower oxygen demand due to smaller muscle mass and workload
- coronary perfusion occurring in systole and diastole
- direct oxygen diffusion from intracavitary blood
- more extensive collateral flow from the left coronary system [33]

The development of RV ischemia causes dilatation and decreased compliance of the RV, which in turn leads to elevated right-sided pressures with reduced LV filling. This results in important hemodynamic changes, including decreased cardiac output and hypotension [29,30,34,35].

Clinically important hemodynamic abnormalities occur in only 10% of RV infarcts with the classic triad of hypotension, clear lung fields, and distended neck veins [36,37]. Because of important management and prognostic implications, all patients with inferior MI should be screened for RV ischemia with right precordial leads. The presence of doming ST-segment elevation ≥1 mm in lead V_{4R} is considered a reliable marker of RV infarction with a sensitivity and specificity of 80%–90% [38–40].

Major hemodynamic findings in RV infarction include a disproportionately elevated right atrial pressure (≥10 mm Hg), with a ratio of right atrial to pulmonary capillary pressure ≥0.8, and a characteristic right atrial waveform with a brisk systolic X and a blunted Y descent. Differential diagnoses include cardiac tamponade and constrictive pericarditis [36,41,42]. Two-dimensional echocardiography is useful to define the severity of RV

Table 3. Right ventricular infarction. ECG: electrocardiogram; PCWP: pulmonary capillary wedge pressure.

Incidence	One third of inferior myocardial infarctions, associated with proximal right coronary artery occlusion
Symptoms and signs	Hypotension, clear lungs, distended neck veins, and Kussmaul's sign
ECG	ST-segment elevation ≥1 mm in V4R
Hemodynamics	Increased right atrial pressure Right atrial/PCWP ≥0.8 Prominent X descent, blunted Y descent
Echocardiography	Right ventricular dilatation Leftward displacement of the interventricular septum during diastole
Management	Maintenance of ventricular preload Inotropic support Preservation of atrioventricular synchrony and sinus rhythm Reduction of left ventricular afterload Reperfusion therapy

infarction, with demonstration of RV dilatation and reversed interventricular septal curvature indicative of increased RV end-diastolic pressure [32,35].

Even though RV involvement in patients with inferior MI is not associated with larger LV infarct size, it is independently associated with a three-fold increase in mortality and other in-hospital complications such as shock, advanced atrioventricular (AV) block, and ventricular arrhythmias (see **Figure 7**) [40,43–45].

Figure 7. Pooled analysis of the incidence of complications in patients with inferior myocardial infarction with and without right ventricular (RV) involvement [44].
AV: atrioventricular;
VF: ventricular fibrillation;
VT: ventricular tachycardia.

Management

The management of RV infarction includes volume loading to maintain an adequate RV preload. Drugs commonly used in LV infarcts to reduce preload, such

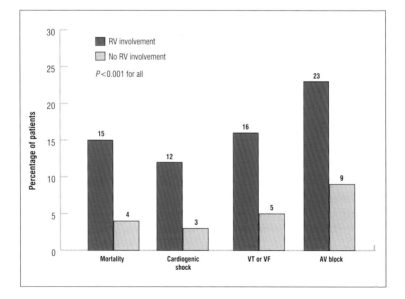

as diuretics and nitrates, are contraindicated in RV infarction. Inotropic support is warranted if hypotension and low output state do not resolve after 0.5–1.0 L of normal saline have been given. AV synchrony is also important for sustaining adequate RV preload and cardiac output. Sequential AV pacing and maintenance of sinus rhythm with cardioversion should be considered in patients with advanced AV block or atrial fibrillation, respectively.

Associated LV dysfunction should be managed by afterload reduction with IABP insertion or arterial vasodilators such as sodium nitroprusside [25,34,35]. Primary percutaneous intervention is the preferred reperfusion strategy, with prompt RV function recovery and excellent clinical outcome [46]. Thrombolytic therapy is associated with a high failure rate because of extensive clot burden in the proximal right coronary artery occlusion and impaired delivery of the thrombolytic agent attributable to hypotension [35].

Mitral incompetence

Acute and severe MR usually occur in association with relatively small inferior infarcts due to necrosis of a papillary muscle [47]. The posteromedial papillary muscle is particularly vulnerable to ischemia due to its single blood supply derived from the dominant coronary artery (right coronary artery or circumflex) [48–52]. Ischemia of the papillary muscle with severe dysfunction causes misalignment of the mitral valve apparatus, resulting in MR. Other mechanisms responsible for the occurrence of MR in the setting of MI include LV expansion with dilatation of the mitral annulus and, less frequently, rupture of the papillary muscle or chordae tendineae (see **Table 4**).

MR complicating acute MI has been reported in 14%–55% of cases and is associated with less favorable outcomes, whereas papillary muscle rupture (either of the entire trunk or a head) has been reported in ~1%

	Free wall rupture	Ventricular septal rupture	Papillary muscle rupture
Incidence	<1%	Without thrombolysis: 1%–3% With thrombolysis: <1%	1%
Time course	3–7 days	Without thrombolysis: 3–5 days With thrombolysis: <24 hours	2–7 days
Infarct location	Anterior or inferior	Anterior (65%) or inferior (35%)	Inferior–posterior
Clinical presentation	Pericardial chest pain, nausea, vomiting, restlessness	Chest pain, severe hypotension	Rapid-onset heart failure with pulmonary edema and hypotension
Physical exam	Sudden hypotension and shock, followed by pulseless electrical activity and death Jugular vein distension, pulsus paradoxus	Harsh holosystolic murmur at the left sternal border, usually accompanied by a thrill	Crescendo–decrescendo, soft, systolic murmur located in the apex
ECG	Persistent ST-segment elevation Low QRS voltage Pulseless electrical activity	Nonspecific	Inferior and/or posterior MI
Echocardiography	Pericardial effusion with high acoustic echoes consistent with clotted blood RA and RV collapse A pericardial effusion >5 mm is 100% sensitive	Color Doppler shows an area of turbulent transeptal flow with left-to-right shunt	TEE most useful. Flail mitral valve leaflet with systolic prolapse into the LA Mobile mass in the LA or LV Preserved LV volume and function
Catheterization	Equalization of diastolic pressures	Oxygen step-up from RA to RV or PA Large "v" waves Passage of contrast to the RV	Pulmonary capillary wedge pressure tracing with large "v" waves. High pulmonary pressures. Mitral regurgitation. Oxygen step up in the RA possible due to right-to-left shunting through a patent foramen ovale
Mortality	>90%	95% without surgery 30% (simple VSR) to 70% (complex VSR) with surgery	90% without surgery 40% with surgery

Table 4. Differential diagnosis of mechanical complications of acute myocardial infarction (MI). ECG: electrocardiogram; LA: left atrium; LV: left ventricle; PA: pulmonary artery; RA: right atrium; RV: right ventricle; TEE: transesophageal echocardiography; VSR: ventricular septal rupture.

of cases [49,53–57]. In general, acute MR occurs between day 2 and day 7 post-MI and is poorly tolerated [58].

The abrupt increase in left atrial volume in a nondilated, noncompliant chamber results in a marked elevation in pressure, leading to rapid development of refractory pulmonary edema and hemodynamic deterioration.

The heart sounds are usually soft and muffled or masked by pulmonary edema [59]. The mitral murmur associated with papillary muscle dysfunction is usually located in the apex and has the qualities of a soft ejection murmur with delayed onset and midsystolic accentuation as the papillary muscle fails to contract during systole. The murmur associated with a ruptured papillary muscle is louder and "diamond-shaped", but in up to 50% of cases it may not be clinically detected because of rapid equilibration of systolic LV and left atrial pressures [48,60].

Diagnosis

Prompt transesophageal echocardiographic examination with color Doppler is key to the diagnosis of acute MR. Major signs include the presence of a flail mitral valve leaflet with systolic prolapse into the left atrium and a mobile mass in the left atrium or the LV. A normal-sized LV with preserved or hyperdynamic function are useful indirect signs of papillary muscle rupture in a patient with cardiogenic shock and/or pulmonary edema [61]. Pulmonary artery catheterization with demonstration of abnormally tall "V" waves in the pulmonary muscle wedge pressure waveform can be utilized to monitor the effect of pharmacologic therapies.

Management

The initial management of acute MR is based on afterload reduction to decrease the regurgitant fraction, with sodium nitroprusside and IABP counterpulsation. Aggressive initial stabilization should be followed by immediate mitral valve replacement. In the SHOCK trial registry, surgery was associated with lower unadjusted mortality compared with conservative management (40% vs 71%, $P = 0.003$) [47]. Other series have reported a surgical mortality of 27%–55% with mitral valve replacement [24]. Mitral valve repair with reimplantation of the ruptured papillary muscle has also been attempted with good results [62].

Ventricular septal rupture

In the prethrombolytic era, the reported incidence of ventricular septal rupture (VSR) complicating acute MI was 1%–3% with a time course of 3–5 days [63–65]. More contemporary data demonstrate that thrombolytic-treated patients have a lower incidence of VSR (<1%), but a shorter time course (24 hours). Major clinical predictors for VSR include advanced age, female gender, anterior infarct location, hypertension, and absence of previous angina or MI [66,67]. In general, infarcts complicated by VSR are larger and more likely to have an occluded artery (TIMI 0–1 grade flow) with poor collateral blood flow. VSR occurs more frequently with anterior than inferior MI. However, VSR complicating inferior MI is morphologically more complex, compromising the basal inferoposterior septum and the right ventricle. In fact, RV involvement in the setting of VSR carries a greater risk of cardiogenic shock and death. VSR occurring with anterior MI is apical and simple [64–66,68–71].

Diagnosis

Color Doppler echocardiography is diagnostic, with visualization of a septal rupture with turbulent transseptal flow allowing the quantification of left-to-right shunt [72]. Right heart catheterization (with demonstration of an oxygen "step-up" from the right ventricle into the right atrium and large "V" waves) can be best used for pharmacologic therapy monitoring [71]. The indication of coronary angiography with left ventriculography should be carefully assessed in patients with hemodynamic instability, as it may correlate with further clinical deterioration [73].

Management

Patients with VSR should be aggressively stabilized with afterload reduction (vasodilators, diuretics) and IABP insertion to decrease the left-to-right shunt. Because of the unpredictable course of these patients, surgical closure of the defect with or without CABG should be performed immediately after the diagnosis [25,59]. Catheter-based techniques for septal occlusion are currently being assessed in selected cases [74,75].

Life-threatening ventricular arrhythmias associated with acute coronary syndromes

Ventricular fibrillation

Primary ventricular fibrillation (VF) is the most frequent cause of out-of-hospital death in the setting of acute MI. Pathophysiologic mechanisms include increased adrenergic tone and rapid ion fluxes with subsequent electrical instability in the ischemic myocardium. VF complicates MI in ~3%–5% of cases, usually during the first 4 hours after the onset of symptoms, and declines thereafter [76–80].

A meta-analysis has suggested that the incidence of VF during the first hospital day is the same in patients treated with or without thrombolytic therapy [80]. Patients with VF are at increased risk of death during hospitalization, especially if associated with low EF and heart failure. However, the long-term prognosis of hospital survivors does not appear to be affected [77–79].

Management

The management of VF includes immediate electric defibrillation with 200 J. Resistant VF can be managed with subsequent defibrillations at increasing levels of energy and additional adjunctive measures such as IV epinephrine (1 mg), and a bolus of lidocaine (1.5 mg/kg) or amiodarone (150 mg), followed by resuscitation according to the advanced cardiac life support (ACLS) guidelines [24]. The use of amiodarone in this setting is supported by data from randomized trials showing that its use in out-of-hospital VF arrest is associated with a significantly higher rate of survival to hospital admission compared with lidocaine (22.6% vs 12%, $P = 0.009$) [82]. Similar findings were observed in another randomized trial comparing amiodarone with placebo in the same patient population [83].

Ventricular tachycardia

Ventricular tachycardia (VT) complicates MI in up to 20% of cases [78–80,84–86]. VT is classically defined according to the timing of occurrence before or after the first 48 hours following MI (as "early" or "late") and according to its morphology (as "polymorphic" or "monomorphic") [87]. This classification also has clinical and prognostic implications.

Polymorphic VT is usually nonsustained and secondary to reversible causes such as active ischemia, reperfusion, or electrolyte imbalance. The increased adrenergic tone generated by the activation of myocardial receptors by ischemic or necrotic tissue, enhanced sympathetic activity, and the increased susceptibility of the ischemic myocardium to catecholamines have been proposed as major pathophysiologic mechanisms. In contrast, monomorphic VT typically has a fixed substrate as a result of a re-entry mechanism through patchy scar tissue at the edge of the infarcted area [88].

Patients who develop VT have a more complicated hospital course and increased short- and long-term mortality [79,80]. In addition, a longer time from presentation to the occurrence of the first arrhythmic event is associated with increased risk for adverse outcomes [87]. In fact, 1-year mortality of 30-day survivors is significantly greater in patients with late VT (>48 hours) than in those with early VT [79]. **Table 5** summarizes the current ACC/AHA recommendations for the management of ventricular arrhythmias complicating acute MI.

Patients with non-ST-elevation ACS are also at risk of developing life-threatening ventricular arrhythmias during hospitalization (with an incidence of 2% according to a pooled analysis of four clinical trials including 26,436 patients). Patients with VT/VF during hospitalization had a 5- to 15-fold higher mortality at 6 months, with most deaths occurring during the first month [90].

Table 5. Management of ventricular arrhythmias in acute coronary syndromes.

Arrhythmia	Management
Premature ventricular beats	Correction of possible causes, hypokalemia, hypomagnesemia, increased sympathetic tone (beta-blockers) No pharmacologic treatment indicated If symptomatic, amiodarone or lidocaine
Accelerated idioventricular rhythm	No treatment indicated If symptomatic, atropine to increase sinus node rate
Nonsustained ventricular tachycardia	Beta-blockers. No specific treatment indicated. If symptomatic, consider amiodarone or lidocaine
Sustained monomorphic ventricular tachycardia	If associated with angina, pulmonary edema, or hypotension: immediate direct-current cardioversion, starting at 100 J, followed by lidocaine (bolus and injection) or amiodarone Restoration of hemodynamic stability; if recurrent, amiodarone If the patient is stable: lidocaine or amiodarone
Polymorphic ventricular tachycardia	If related to recurrent ischemia, consider revascularization If related to QT prolongation, consider rapid override pacing and magnesium. Rule out drug toxicity.
Ventricular fibrillation	Immediate defibrillation. Restoration of hemodynamic stability. Follow advanced cardiac life support (ACLS) guidelines.

The presence of a depressed residual LV function is a strong predictor for sudden cardiac death post-MI and deserves special consideration. Randomized data indicate that patients with EFs of 31%–40% and inducible VT derive a survival benefit with implantable cardioverter defibrillators (ICD) [91,92], whereas patients with an EF of ≤ 30% benefit from prophylactic ICD insertion regardless of the presence of inducible arrhythmias [93]. **Figure 8** is a proposed management algorithm for patients with ventricular arrhythmias post-MI.

Figure 8. Algorithm for the management of ventricular arrhythmias in acute coronary syndromes.
EF: ejection fraction;
EP: electrophysiology;
ICD: implantable cardioverter defibrillator.

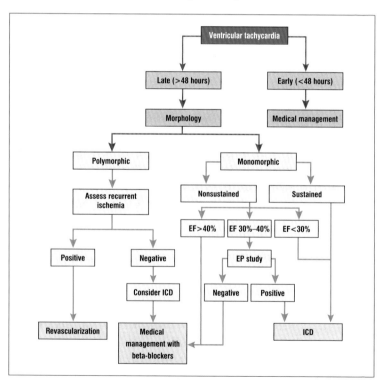

Prevention of ventricular tachyarrhythmias

It is well accepted that prophylactic administration of lidocaine reduces the incidence of in-hospital primary VF by ~30%, at the expense of increased mortality due to increased rates of bradyarrhythmias and asystole [94,95]. Amiodarone has also been tested in the acute and chronic phases of MI. A pooled analysis of these studies showed a trend towards increased survival among amiodarone-treated patients (odds ratio 0.87; 95% confidence interval 0.78–0.99) [96]. However, the only study performed in the early phase of acute MI showed a 19% nonsignificant increase in mortality [97]. Therefore, it appears that there is no role for antiarrhythmic therapy in the prevention of ventricular arrhythmias in the acute period post-MI. Currently, the only accepted prophylactic strategies include the early administration of beta-blockers and the correction of electrolyte imbalances [98,99].

Conclusions

Even though reperfusion therapy has significantly reduced the incidence and the time course of life-threatening mechanical and electrical complications in ACS patients, the risk is still significant. The clinician should rapidly assess an unstable ACS patient's risk and define the need for aggressive therapies based on simple clinical variables, an ECG, and cardiac marker data. Cardiogenic shock should be aggressively managed with IABP counterpulsation and primary PCI. Early diagnosis of mechanical complications is critical to preventing catastrophic outcomes. A high suspicion index is warranted for diagnosis and rapid institution of corrective therapies.

The timing and morphology of electrical instability complicating ACS are major determinants of outcomes. Beta-blockers play a central role in the management of ventricular arrhythmias. Patients with a low EF are at increased risk of sudden cardiac death and should be carefully evaluated in order to provide appropriate pharmacologic therapies or insert an ICD.

References

1. Lee KL, Woodlief LH, Topol EJ, et al. Predictors of 30-day mortality in the era of reperfusion for acute myocardial infarction. Results from an international trial of 41,021 patients. GUSTO-I Investigators. *Circulation* 1995;91:1659–68.

2. Boersma E, Pieper KS, Steyerberg EW, et al. Predictors of outcome in patients with acute coronary syndromes without persistent ST-segment elevation. Results from an international trial of 9461 patients. The PURSUIT Investigators. *Circulation* 2000;101:2557–67.

3. Antman EM, Cohen M, Bernink PJ, et al. The TIMI risk score for unstable angina/non-ST elevation MI: A method for prognostication and therapeutic decision making. *JAMA* 2000;284:835–42.

4. Morrow DA, Antman EM, Giugliano RP, et al. A simple risk index for rapid initial triage of patients with ST-elevation myocardial infarction: an InTIME II substudy. *Lancet* 2001;358:1571–5.

5. Braunwald E, Antman EM, Beasley JW, et al. ACC/AHA 2002 guideline update for the management of patients with unstable angina and non-ST-segment elevation myocardial infarction–summary article: a report of the American College of Cardiology/American Heart Association task force on practice guidelines (Committee on the Management of Patients With Unstable Angina). *J Am Coll Cardiol* 2002;40:1366–74.

6. Hasdai D, Topol EJ, Califf RM, et al. Cardiogenic shock complicating acute coronary syndromes. *Lancet* 2000;356:749–56.

7. Hochman JS, Buller CE, Sleeper LA, et al. Cardiogenic shock complicating acute myocardial infarction–etiologies, management and outcome: a report from the SHOCK Trial Registry. SHould we emergently revascularize Occluded Coronaries for cardiogenic shocK? *J Am Coll Cardiol* 2000;36(3 Suppl A):1063–70.

8. Goldberg RJ, Samad NA, Yarzebski J, et al. Temporal trends in cardiogenic shock complicating acute myocardial infarction. *N Engl J Med* 1999;340:1162–8.

9. Holmes DR Jr, Bates ER, Kleiman NS, et al. Contemporary reperfusion therapy for cardiogenic shock: the GUSTO-I trial experience. The GUSTO-I Investigators. Global Utilization of Streptokinase and Tissue Plasminogen Activator for Occluded Coronary Arteries. *J Am Coll Cardiol* 1995;26:668–74.

10. Holmes DR Jr, Berger PB, Hochman JS, et al. Cardiogenic shock in patients with acute ischemic syndromes with and without ST-segment elevation. *Circulation* 1999;100:2067–73.

11. Menon V, Hochman JS, Stebbins A, et al. Lack of progress in cardiogenic shock: lessons from the GUSTO trials. *Eur Heart J* 2000;21:1928–36.

12. Hasdai D, Harrington RA, Hochman JS, et al. Platelet glycoprotein IIb/IIIa blockade and outcome of cardiogenic shock complicating acute coronary syndromes without persistent ST-segment elevation. *J Am Coll Cardiol* 2000;36:685–92.

13. Hasdai D, Califf RM, Thompson TD, et al. Predictors of cardiogenic shock after thrombolytic therapy for acute myocardial infarction. *J Am Coll Cardiol* 2000;35:136–43.

14. Alonso DR, Scheidt S, Post M, et al. Pathophysiology of cardiogenic shock. Quantification of myocardial necrosis, clinical, pathologic and electrocardiographic correlations. *Circulation* 1973;48:588–96.

15. Hollenberg SM, Kavinsky CJ, Parrillo JE. Cardiogenic shock. *Ann Intern Med* 1999;131:47–59.

16. Hochman JS, Sleeper LA, Webb JG, et al. Early revascularization in acute myocardial infarction complicated by cardiogenic shock. SHOCK Investigators. Should We Emergently Revascularize Occluded Coronaries for Cardiogenic Shock. *N Engl J Med* 1999;341:625–34.

17. Picard MH, Davidoff R, Sleeper LA, et al. Echocardiographic predictors of survival and response to early revascularization in cardiogenic shock. *Circulation* 2003;107:279–84.

18. Hochman JS. Cardiogenic shock complicating acute myocardial infarction: expanding the paradigm. *Circulation* 2003;107:2998–3002.

19. Menon V, Slater JN, White HD, et al. Acute myocardial infarction complicated by systemic hypoperfusion without hypotension: report of the SHOCK trial registry. *Am J Med* 2000;108:374–80.

20. Mueller HS, Chatterjee K, Davis KB, et al. ACC expert consensus document. Present use of bedside right heart catheterization in patients with cardiac disease. American College of Cardiology. *J Am Coll Cardiol* 1998;32:840–64.

21. Cotter G, Kaluski E, Milo O, et al. LINCS: L–NAME (a NO synthase inhibitor) in the treatment of refractory cardiogenic shock: a prospective randomized study. *Eur Heart J* 2003;24:1287–95.

22. Sanborn TA, Sleeper LA, Bates ER, et al. Impact of thrombolysis, intra-aortic balloon pump counterpulsation, and their combination in cardiogenic shock complicating acute myocardial infarction: a report from the SHOCK Trial Registry. SHould we emergently revascularize Occluded Coronaries for cardiogenic shocK? *J Am Coll Cardiol* 2000;36(3 Suppl A):1123–9.

23. Chen EW, Canto JG, Parsons LS, et al. Relation between hospital intra-aortic balloon counterpulsation volume and mortality in acute myocardial infarction complicated by cardiogenic shock. *Circulation* 2003;108:951–7.

24. Ryan TJ, Antman EM, Brooks NH, et al. 1999 update: ACC/AHA guidelines for the management of patients with acute myocardial infarction. A report of the American College of Cardiology/American Heart Association Task Force on Practice Guidelines (Committee on Management of Acute Myocardial Infarction). *J Am Coll Cardiol* 1999;34:890–911.

25. Hochman JS, Sleeper LA, White HD, et al. One-year survival following early revascularization for cardiogenic shock. *JAMA* 2001;285:190–2.

26. Dzavik V, Sleeper LA, Cocke TP, et al. Early revascularization is associated with improved survival in elderly patients with acute myocardial infarction complicated by cardiogenic shock: a report from the SHOCK Trial Registry. *Eur Heart J* 2003;24:828–37.

27. Dauerman HL, Goldberg RJ, Malinski M, et al. Outcomes and early revascularization for patients > or = 65 years of age with cardiogenic shock. *Am J Cardiol* 2001;87:844–8.

28. Chan AW, Chew DP, Bhatt DL, et al. Long-term mortality benefit with the combination of stents and abciximab for cardiogenic shock complicating acute myocardial infarction: a 7-year prospective analysis. *Am J Cardiol* 2002;89:132–6.

29. Isner JM, Roberts WC. Right ventricular infarction complicating left ventricular infarction secondary to coronary heart disease. Frequency, location, associated findings and significance from analysis of 236 necropsy patients with acute or healed myocardial infarction. *Am J Cardiol* 1978;42:885–94.

30. Andersen HR, Falk E, Nielsen D. Right ventricular infarction: frequency, size and topography in coronary heart disease: a prospective study comprising 107 consecutive autopsies from a coronary care unit. *J Am Coll Cardiol* 1987;10:1223–32.

31. Zeymer U, Neuhaus KL, Wegscheider K, et al. Effects of thrombolytic therapy in acute inferior myocardial infarction with or without right ventricular involvement. HIT-4 Trial Group. Hirudin for Improvement of Thrombolysis. *J Am Coll Cardiol* 1998;32:876–81.

32. Bowers TR, O'Neill WW, Pica M, el. Patterns of coronary compromise resulting in acute right ventricular ischemic dysfunction. *Circulation* 2002;106:1104–9.

33. Berger PB, Ryan TJ. Inferior myocardial infarction. High-risk subgroups. *Circulation* 1990;81:401–11.

34. Kinch JW, Ryan TJ. Right ventricular infarction. *N Engl J Med* 1994;330:1211–7.

35. Goldstein JA. Pathophysiology and management of right heart ischemia. *J Am Coll Cardiol* 2002;40:841–53.

36. Cohn JN, Guiha NH, Broder MI, et al. Right ventricular infarction. Clinical and hemodynamic features. *Am J Cardiol* 1974;33:209–14.

37. Dell'Italia LJ, Starling MR, O'Rourke RA. Physical examination for exclusion of hemodynamically important right ventricular infarction. *Ann Intern Med* 1983;99:608–11.

38. Braat SH, Brugada P, de Zwaan C, et al. Value of electrocardiogram in diagnosing right ventricular involvement in patients with an acute inferior wall myocardial infarction. *Br Heart J* 1983;49:368–72.

39. Andersen HR, Falk E, Nielsen D. Right ventricular infarction: diagnostic accuracy of electrocardiographic right chest leads V3R to V7R investigated prospectively in 43 consecutive fatal cases from a coronary care unit. *Br Heart J* 1989;61:514–20.

40. Zehender M, Kasper W, Kauder E, et al. Right ventricular infarction as an independent predictor of prognosis after acute inferior myocardial infarction. *N Engl J Med* 1993;328:981–8.

41. Goldstein JA, Barzilai B, Rosamond TL, et al. Determinants of hemodynamic compromise with severe right ventricular infarction. *Circulation* 1990;82:359–68.

42. Coma-Canella I, Lopez-Sendon J, Gamallo C. Low output syndrome in right ventricular infarction. *Am Heart J* 1979;98:613–20.

43. Braat SH, de Zwaan C, Brugada P, et al. Right ventricular involvement with acute inferior wall myocardial infarction identifies high risk of developing atrioventricular nodal conduction disturbances. *Am Heart J* 1984;107:1183–7.

44. Bueno H, Lopez-Palop R, Bermejo J, et al. In-hospital outcome of elderly patients with acute inferior myocardial infarction and right ventricular involvement. *Circulation* 1997;96:436–41.

45. Mehta SR, Eikelboom JW, Natarajan MK, et al. Impact of right ventricular involvement on mortality and morbidity in patients with inferior myocardial infarction. *J Am Coll Cardiol* 2001;37:37–43.

46. Bowers TR, O'Neill WW, Grines C, et al. Effect of reperfusion on biventricular function and survival after right ventricular infarction. *N Engl J Med* 1998;338:933–40.

47. Thompson CR, Buller CE, Sleeper LA, et al. Cardiogenic shock due to acute severe mitral regurgitation complicating acute myocardial infarction: a report from the SHOCK Trial Registry. SHould we use emergently revascularize Occluded Coronaries in cardiogenic shocK? *J Am Coll Cardiol* 2000;36(3 Suppl A):1104–9.

48. Burch GE, DePasquale NP, Phillips JH. The syndrome of papillary muscle dysfunction. *Am Heart J* 1968;75:399–415.

49. Barbour DJ, Roberts WC. Rupture of a left ventricular papillary muscle during acute myocardial infarction: analysis of 22 necropsy patients. *J Am Coll Cardiol* 1986;8:558–65.

50. Coma-Canella I, Gamallo C, Onsurbe PM, et al. Anatomic findings in acute papillary muscle necrosis. *Am Heart J* 1989;118:1188–92.

51. Sharma SK, Seckler J, Israel DH, et al. Clinical, angiographic and anatomic findings in acute severe ischemic mitral regurgitation. *Am J Cardiol* 1992;70:277–80.

52. Calvo FE, Figueras J, Cortadellas J, et al. Severe mitral regurgitation complicating acute myocardial infarction. Clinical and angiographic differences between patients with and without papillary muscle rupture. *Eur Heart J* 1997;18:1606–10.

53. Heikkila J. Mitral incompetence complicating acute myocardial infarction. *Br Heart J* 1967;29:162–9.

54. Morrow AG, Cohen LS, Roberts WC, et al. Severe mitral regurgitation following acute myocardial infarction and ruptured papillary muscle. Hemodynamic findings and results of operative treatment in four patients. *Circulation* 1968;37(4 Suppl)II:124–32.

55. Maisel AS, Gilpin EA, Klein L, et al. The murmur of papillary muscle dysfunction in acute myocardial infarction: clinical features and prognostic implications. *Am Heart J* 1986;112:705–11.

56. Barzilai B, Davis VG, Stone PH, et al. Prognostic significance of mitral regurgitation in acute myocardial infarction. The MILIS Study Group. *Am J Cardiol* 1990;65:1169–75.

57. Lehmann KG, Francis CK, Sheehan FH, et al. Effect of thrombolysis on acute mitral regurgitation during evolving myocardial infarction. Experience from the Thrombolysis in Myocardial Infarction (TIMI) Trial. *J Am Coll Cardiol* 1993;22:714–9.

58. Wei JY, Hutchins GM, Bulkley BH. Papillary muscle rupture in fatal acute myocardial infarction: a potentially treatable form of cardiogenic shock. *Ann Intern Med* 1979;90:149–52.

59. Hochman JS, Gersh B. Acute myocardial infarction: complications. In: Topol EJ, editor. *Comprehensive Cardiovascular Medicine*. Philadelphia: Lippincott-Raven; 1998:467–510.

60. Tcheng JE, Jackman JD Jr, Nelson CL, et al. Outcome of patients sustaining acute ischemic mitral regurgitation during myocardial infarction. *Ann Intern Med* 1992;117:18–24.

61. Moursi MH, Bhatnagar SK, Vilacosta I, et al. Transesophageal echocardiographic assessment of papillary muscle rupture. *Circulation* 1996;94:1003–9.

62. Fasol R, Lakew F, Wetter S. Mitral repair in patients with a ruptured papillary muscle. *Am Heart J* 2000;139:549–54.

63. Hutchins GM. Rupture of the interventricular septum complicating myocardial infarction: pathological analysis of 10 patients with clinically diagnosed perforations. *Am Heart J* 1979;97:165–73.

64. Topaz O, Taylor AL. Interventricular septal rupture complicating acute myocardial infarction: from pathophysiologic features to the role of invasive and noninvasive diagnostic modalities in current management. *Am J Med* 1992;93:683–8.

65. Cummings RG, Reimer KA, Califf R, et al. Quantitative analysis of right and left ventricular infarction in the presence of postinfarction ventricular septal defect. *Circulation* 1988;77:33–42.

66. Crenshaw BS, Granger CB, Birnbaum Y, et al. Risk factors, angiographic patterns, and outcomes in patients with ventricular septal defect complicating acute myocardial infarction. GUSTO-I (Global Utilization of Streptokinase and TPA for Occluded Coronary Arteries) Trial Investigators. *Circulation* 2000;101:27–32.

67. Menon V, Webb JG, Hillis LD, et al. Outcome and profile of ventricular septal rupture with cardiogenic shock after myocardial infarction: a report from the SHOCK Trial Registry. SHould we emergently revascularize Occluded Coronaries in cardiogenic shocK? *J Am Coll Cardiol* 2000;36(3 Suppl A):1110–6.

68. Radford MJ, Johnson RA, Daggett WM Jr, et al. Ventricular septal rupture: a review of clinical and physiologic features and an analysis of survival. *Circulation* 1981;64:545–53.

69. Moore CA, Nygaard TW, Kaiser DL, et al. Postinfarction ventricular septal rupture: the importance of location of infarction and right ventricular function in determining survival. *Circulation* 1986;74:45–55.

70. Pretre R, Rickli H, Ye Q, et al. Frequency of collateral blood flow in the infarct-related coronary artery in rupture of the ventricular septum after acute myocardial infarction. *Am J Cardiol* 2000;85:497–9,A10.

71. Birnbaum Y, Fishbein MC, Blanche C, et al. Ventricular septal rupture after acute myocardial infarction. *N Engl J Med* 2002;347:1426–32.

72. Smyllie JH, Sutherland GR, Geuskens R, et al. Doppler color flow mapping in the diagnosis of ventricular septal rupture and acute mitral regurgitation after myocardial infarction. *J Am Coll Cardiol* 1990;15:1449–55.

73. Topaz O, Mallon SM, Chahine RA, et al. Acute ventricular septal rupture. Angiographic-morphologic features and clinical assessment. *Chest* 1989;95:292–8.

74. Lee EM, Roberts DH, Walsh KP. Transcatheter closure of a residual postmyocardial infarction ventricular septal defect with the Amplatzer septal occluder. *Heart* 1998;80:522–4.

75. Pienvichit P, Waters J. Successful closure of coronary artery perforation using makeshift stent sandwich. *Catheter Cardiovasc Interv* 2001;54:209–13.

76. Campbell RW, Murray A, Julian DG. Ventricular arrhythmias in first 12 hours of acute myocardial infarction. Natural history study. *Br Heart J* 1981;46:351–7.

77. Thompson CA, Yarzebski J, Goldberg RJ, et al. Changes over time in the incidence and case-fatality rates of primary ventricular fibrillation complicating acute myocardial infarction: perspectives from the Worcester Heart Attack Study. *Am Heart J* 2000;139:1014–21.

78. Volpi A, Cavalli A, Santoro L, et al. Incidence and prognosis of early primary ventricular fibrillation in acute myocardial infarction—results of the Gruppo Italiano per lo Studio della Sopravvivenza nell'Infarto Miocardico (GISSI-2) database. *Am J Cardiol* 1998;82:265–71.

79. Newby KH, Thompson T, Stebbins A, et al. Sustained ventricular arrhythmias in patients receiving thrombolytic therapy: incidence and outcomes. The GUSTO Investigators. *Circulation* 1998;98:2567–73.

80. Al-Khatib SM, Stebbins AL, Califf RM, et al. Sustained ventricular arrhythmias and mortality among patients with acute myocardial infarction: Results from the GUSTO-III trial. *Am Heart J* 2003;145:515–21.

81. Solomon SD, Ridker PM, Antman EM. Ventricular arrhythmias in trials of thrombolytic therapy for acute myocardial infarction. A meta-analysis. *Circulation* 1993;88:2575–81.

82. Dorian P, Cass D, Schwartz B, et al. Amiodarone as compared with lidocaine for shock-resistant ventricular fibrillation. *N Engl J Med* 2002;346:884–90.

83. Kudenchuk PJ, Cobb LA, Copass MK, et al. Amiodarone for resuscitation after out-of-hospital cardiac arrest due to ventricular fibrillation. *N Engl J Med* 1999;341:871–8.

84. Volpi A, Maggioni A, Franzosi MG, et al. In-hospital prognosis of patients with acute myocardial infarction complicated by primary ventricular fibrillation. *N Engl J Med* 1987;317:257–61.

85. Berger PB, Ruocco NA, Ryan TJ, et al. Incidence and significance of ventricular tachycardia and fibrillation in the absence of hypotension or heart failure in acute myocardial infarction treated with recombinant tissue-type plasminogen activator: results from the Thrombolysis in Myocardial Infarction (TIMI) Phase II trial. *J Am Coll Cardiol* 1993;22:1773–9.

86. Volpi A, Cavalli A, Turato R, et al. Incidence and short-term prognosis of late sustained ventricular tachycardia after myocardial infarction: results of the Gruppo Italiano per lo Studio della Sopravvivenza nell'Infarto Miocardico (GISSI-3) Data Base. *Am Heart J* 2001;142:87–92.

87. Bigger JT Jr, Dresdale FJ, Heissenbuttel RH, et al. Ventricular arrhythmias in ischemic heart disease: mechanism, prevalence, significance, and management. *Prog Cardiovasc Dis* 1977;19:255–300.

88. Braunwald E. *Heart Disease: a Textbook of Cardiovascular Medicine*. 5th ed. Philadelphia: Saunders; 1997.

89. Cheema AN, Sheu K, Parker M, et al. Nonsustained ventricular tachycardia in the setting of acute myocardial infarction: tachycardia characteristics and their prognostic implications. *Circulation* 1998;98:2030–6.

99. Al-Khatib SM, Granger CB, Huang Y, et al. Sustained ventricular arrhythmias among patients with acute coronary syndromes with no ST-segment elevation: incidence, predictors, and outcomes. *Circulation* 2002;106:309–12.

91. Moss AJ, Hall WJ, Cannom DS, et al. Improved survival with an implanted defibrillator in patients with coronary disease at high risk for ventricular arrhythmia. Multicenter Automatic Defibrillator Implantation Trial Investigators. *N Engl J Med* 1996;335:1933–40.

92. Buxton AE, Lee KL, DiCarlo L, et al. Electrophysiologic testing to identify patients with coronary artery disease who are at risk for sudden death. Multicenter Unsustained Tachycardia Trial Investigators. *N Engl J Med* 2000;342:1937–45.

93. Moss AJ, Zareba W, Hall WJ, et al. Prophylactic implantation of a defibrillator in patients with myocardial infarction and reduced ejection fraction. *N Engl J Med* 2002;346:877–83.

94. MacMahon S, Collins R, Peto R, et al. Effects of prophylactic lidocaine in suspected acute myocardial infarction. An overview of results from the randomized, controlled trials. *JAMA* 1988;260:1910–6.

95. Sadowski ZP, Alexander JH, Skrabucha B, et al. Multicenter randomized trial and a systematic overview of lidocaine in acute myocardial infarction. *Am Heart J* 1999;137:792–8.

96. Amiodarone Trials Meta-Analysis Investigators. Effect of prophylactic amiodarone on mortality after acute myocardial infarction and in congestive heart failure: meta-analysis of individual data from 6500 patients in randomised trials. *Lancet* 1997;350:1417–24.

97. Elizari MV, Martinez JM, Belziti C, et al. Morbidity and mortality following early administration of amiodarone in acute myocardial infarction. *Eur Heart J* 2000;21:198–205.

98. Myerburg RJ, Kessler KM, Castellanos A. Sudden cardiac death. Structure, function, and time-dependence of risk. *Circulation* 1992;85(1 Suppl):I2–10.

99. Huikuri HV, Castellanos A, Myerburg RJ. Sudden death due to cardiac arrhythmias. *N Engl J Med* 2001;345:1473–82.

10

Guidelines for unstable angina and non-ST-segment elevation myocardial infarction

Christopher P Cannon

Introduction

In Europe and the US, approximately 2.5–3.0 million patients are admitted to hospital every year with unstable angina and non-ST-segment elevation myocardial infarction (UA/NSTEMI). Because of the large number of patients involved, there has been intense research into the diagnosis and management of this patient population. In recent years, many advances have been seen, including numerous effective medical therapies, such as antiplatelet and cholesterol-lowering agents and beta-blockade, as well as a clearer definition of appropriate triage for cardiac procedures.

To help improve the treatment of UA/NSTEMI, two new sets of guidelines have been drawn up for the diagnosis and management of these patients, one by the American College of Cardiology (ACC) together with the American Heart Association (AHA) and the other by the European Society of Cardiology (ESC). The guidelines make recommendations about the appropriate use of medications and interventions based on evidence from randomized clinical trials.

The ACC/AHA guidelines were updated just 18 months after their initial publication [1], following the results of several landmark trials. Both guidelines make essentially the same recommendations in several areas.

Firstly, they recommend that evaluation of a patient should consist of two steps: i) an assessment of the likelihood that the patient's symptoms represent acute coronary syndromes (ACS) (as opposed to noncardiac chest pain) and ii) (if the symptoms do represent ACS) risk stratification to distinguish high-risk and low-risk patients. The ACC/AHA guidelines mention three risk categories in the risk table, but in the recommendations give guidance only based on high and low risk. The ESC guidelines divide patients into high-risk and low-risk groups.

Secondly, both guidelines recommend that some treatments be targeted only at high-risk patients, while other treatments are recommended for all patients.

Finally, both guidelines put increased emphasis on the importance of secondary prevention strategies.

Risk stratification

Both sets of guidelines highlight risk stratification as a key step in helping to target the type and intensity of medical and interventional therapies. Studies have found that high-risk patients benefit from more aggressive treatments. Factors associated with a high risk of either death or nonfatal myocardial infarction (MI) include: prolonged rest pain, ST-segment changes, elevated cardiac biomarkers (eg, troponin), diabetes, evidence of congestive heart failure, and age over 75 years. Low-risk patients present without rest pain [2], electrocardiogram changes, or evidence of heart failure. Other factors are highlighted as markers of long-term risk, such as extent of coronary artery disease, left ventricular dysfunction, and elevated markers of inflammation (see **Table 1**).

The ESC guidelines highlight troponin as a very powerful tool for both risk stratification and the targeting of therapies.

Patients with a positive tropinin benefit more from treatment with low molecular weight heparin (LMWH), glycoprotein (GP)IIb/IIIa inhibitors, and an early, invasive strategy. In comparison, in patients with a negative troponin, almost no benefit is seen with such a treatment strategy [3–7]. GPIIb/IIIa inhibitors have demonstrated a 50%–70% reduction in death and MI in troponin-positive patients, but no benefit in patients with a negative troponin [4,5].

Interestingly, a very different pattern has been seen with oral antiplatelet agents: aspirin and clopidogrel have been shown to benefit low-, intermediate-, and

Table 1. Risk assessment in the European Society of Cardiology guidelines.

Risks	Marker
Thrombotic risk (ie, acute risk)	Recurrence of chest pain ST-segment depression Dynamic ST-segment changes Elevated level of cardiac troponins Thrombus on angiography
Underlying disease (ie, long-term risk)	Clinical markers • age • history of previous myocardial infarction, prior coronary artery bypass graft, diabetes, congestive heart failure, hypertension Biologic markers • renal dysfunction (elevated creatinine or reduced creatinine clearance) • inflammatory markers, C-reactive protein elevation, fibrinogen elevation, interleukin-6 elevation Angiographic markers • left ventricular dysfunction • extent of coronary artery disease

high-risk patients, as well as those with positive or negative cardiac markers [8–10]. Thus, both aspirin and clopidogrel have been recommended for all patients regardless of their category of risk (see **Table 2**).

Acute medical therapy

Aspirin

Initial treatment should include aspirin, which leads to a 50%–70% relative risk reduction in death or MI versus placebo [11]. Current data demonstrate that aspirin is beneficial for long-term treatment at doses as low as 75 mg/day [8]. New data from the CURE trial found that lower doses of aspirin (eg, 81 mg) are associated with a 50% lower rate of major bleeding over 1 year of treatment compared with doses of 200–325 mg [12]. Thus, for acute management in hospital, an aspirin dose of 160–325 mg/day is recommended, but at hospital discharge and during follow-up the new data suggest a dose of 81 mg/day may be safer.

Table 2. Overview of antithrombotic therapy recommendations of the American College of Cardiology and American Heart Association (ACC/AHA) unstable angina and non-ST-segment elevation myocardial infarction (UA/NSTEMI) guidelines. GP: glycoprotein; IV: intravenous; LMWH: low molecular weight heparin; PCI: percutaneous coronary intervention; SC: subcutaneous. Reproduced with permission from *Circulation* 2003;107:2640–5.

Possible ACS	Likely/definite ACS	Definite ACS with catheterization and PCI or high-risk (IIa)
Aspirin	Aspirin + SC LMWH (Class IIa recommendation: enoxaparin preferred over unfractionated heparin) or IV heparin	Aspirin + SC LMWH or IV heparin + IV platelet GPIIb/IIIa antagonist
	Clopidogrel	Clopidogrel

Clopidogrel

The ACC/AHA 2002 guideline update included new class I recommendations for the use of clopidogrel in addition to aspirin. The CURE trial found that clopidogrel plus aspirin led to a 20% relative risk reduction in cardiovascular death, MI, or stroke compared with aspirin alone [9]. This benefit was seen in both low- and high-risk patients [10] at as early as 24 hours [13], with the Kaplan–Meier curves diverging after just 2 hours.

This benefit has also been seen in two other trials: in the CREDO trial of patients undergoing percutaneous coronary intervention, clopidogrel was associated with a significant 27% relative reduction in the combined risk of death, MI, or stroke at 1 year (P = 0.02) [14]. Similarly, in the CAPRIE trial, clopidogrel alone significantly reduced the risk of ischemic events compared with aspirin through 3 years of follow-up in patients with prior atherothrombotic disease [15]. There is, therefore, strong evidence from large, double-blind, randomized trials that clopidogrel plus aspirin is the optimal long-term antithrombotic regimen.

GPIIb/IIIa inhibitors

Intravenous GPIIb/IIIa inhibitors have also been shown to be beneficial in treating UA/NSTEMI [16]. The "small molecule" inhibitors eptifibatide and tirofiban have shown clear benefit in "upstream" management (ie, initiating therapy when the patient first presents to the hospital). Abciximab showed no benefit in an unselected UA/NSTEMI patient population [17], and is contraindicated in patients treated with a noninvasive strategy [1]. The ESC guidelines put more emphasis on "preparation" of the patient prior to cardiac catheterization, with early use of antithrombotic therapy.

UFH and LMWH

Unfractionated heparin (UFH) or LMWH are recommended for the treatment of UA/NSTEMI [18]. Trials comparing enoxaparin, an LMWH, with UFH have demonstrated its superiority in reducing recurrent cardiac events [19,20]. Based on these data, the 2002 ACC/AHA guideline update made a class IIA recommendation that enoxaparin is the preferred antithrombin over UFH [1].

Anti-ischemic therapy

Anti-ischemic therapy with intravenous nitrates for ongoing ischemic pain and beta-blockade early and during long-term follow-up is also recommended (see **Table 2**) [21].

Invasive versus conservative strategy

Nine randomized trials have compared the merits of an invasive strategy (involving routine cardiac

Figure 1. Evidence-based risk stratification to target therapies in UA/NSTEMI, as recommended in the ESC and ACC/AHA Guidelines. Adapted with permission from *Circulation* 2002;106:1588–91. CHF: congestive heart failure; ECG: electrocardiogram; GP: glycoprotein; LMWH: low molecular weight heparin.

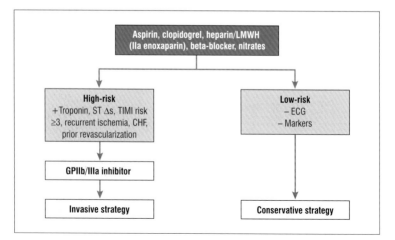

catheterization, with revascularization if feasible) with a conservative strategy (where angiography and revascularization are reserved for patients who have evidence of recurrent ischemia either at rest or on provocative testing). Of these, the most recent six have all shown a significant benefit of the invasive strategy (see **Figure 1**), especially in higher-risk patients [6,12,22].

Accordingly, the 2002 ACC/AHA guideline update added ST-segment changes and positive troponin to the list of high-risk indicators that would lead to a Class I recommendation for an early invasive strategy (see **Table 2**) [1]. The ESC guidelines have a similar recommendation for an invasive strategy for high-risk patients. With regard to timing of an invasive strategy, the ISAR-COOL study found a benefit of an immediate invasive strategy (average

Figure 2. The "weight of the evidence" showing benefit of an invasive over a conservative strategy in patients with UA/NSTEMI. Adapted with permission from *Circulation* 2002;106:1588–91.

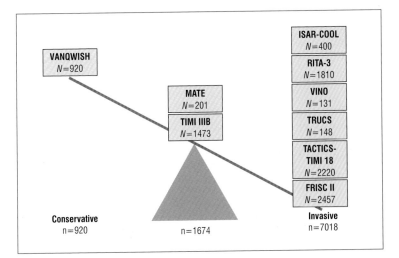

time to catheterization of 2 hours) compared with a delayed invasive strategy (average time to catheterization of 4 days) [23]. Whether an immediate invasive approach is better than catheterization 24–48 hours after admission has not yet been evaluated in a randomized study.

Summary: acute therapy for UA/NSTEMI

Five baseline therapies are now recommended for all patients: aspirin, clopidogrel, heparin or LMWH (with enoxaparin the preferred antithrombin), beta-blockers, and nitrates (see **Figure 2**) [3]. Two further treatments are best targeted at high-risk patients: an invasive strategy and a GPIIb/IIIa inhibitor.

Long-term secondary prevention

Risk modification and long-term secondary prevention have been given much greater emphasis in the new guidelines. The time of hospital discharge is a "teachable moment" for the patient, where the physician can review and optimize the medical regimen. Risk factor modification is critical, and includes discussions with the patient (as appropriate) about the importance of smoking cessation, achieving optimal weight, daily exercise, following an appropriate diet, good blood pressure control, tight glycemic control in diabetics, and lipid management (see **Box 1**).

Long-term medical therapy

Five classes of drugs are recommended in the guidelines for long-term medical therapy (see **Box 2)**. Statins and angiotensin-converting enzyme (ACE) inhibitors are recommended for long-term treatment to facilitate plaque stabilization. Beta-blockers are indicated for anti-ischemic therapy, and may help to decrease "triggers" for MI during follow-up. The combination of aspirin and clopidogrel is now recommended for antiplatelet therapy. This combination will prevent or decrease the severity of any thrombosis that would occur if a plaque were to rupture.

Thus, a multifactorial approach to long-term medical therapy is recommended to prevent the various components of atherothrombosis.

Box 1. Recommendations of the American College of Cardiology and American Heart Association (ACC/AHA) for risk factor modification.

Class I recommendations for risk factor modification

Smoking cessation

Achieve optimal weight

Daily exercise

American Heart Association diet

Hypertension control to a blood pressure <130/85 mm Hg

Tight control of hyperglycemia in diabetics

Hydroxymethylglutaryl coenzyme A reductase inhibitor for low-density lipoprotein cholesterol >130 mg/dL

Lipid-lowering agent if low-density lipoprotein cholesterol after diet is >100 mg/dL

A fibrate or niacin if high-density lipoprotein <40 mg/dL

Data from *Circulation* 2002;106:1893–900.

Box 2. Therapies recommended by the ACC/AHA guidelines for long-term management following unstable angina and non-ST-segment elevation myocardial infarction (UA/NSTEMI).

Class I recommendations for long-term medical therapy

Aspirin 75–325 mg/day

Clopidogrel 75 mg/day when aspirin is not tolerated

Combination of aspirin and clopidogrel for 9 months after UA/NSTEMI

Beta-blocker

Lipid-lowering agent and diet in patients with low-density lipoprotein cholesterol >130 mg/dL

Lipid-lowering agent if low-density lipoprotein cholesterol after diet >100 mg/dL

Angiotensin-converting-enzyme inhibitors for patients with congestive heart failure, left ventricular dysfunction (ejection fraction <0.4), hypertension, or diabetes

Data from *Circulation* 2002;106:1893-900.

Practical application of the guidelines

The practical application of the clinical trial results and the evidence-based guidelines has now become the focus of most major cardiac societies. It has been seen that there is a real gap between what physicians know and what they are doing in everyday clinical practice. An interesting survey investigating physicians' knowledge of the National Cholesterol Education Program (NCEP) guidelines found that, although they all scored well on the theory (see **Figure 3**) [24], when their patients' charts were evaluated, only 18% of these outpatients were found to be at the NCEP Adult Treatment Panel (ATP) III goal of a low-density lipoprotein (LDL) <100 mg/dL [24]. Thus, there was a huge disparity between what the physicians knew and what they were doing in practice. Underutilization of medical therapies has also been seen in international surveys of practice [27].

Analyses of outcomes by treatment received provide further evidence of the need to improve care. In a single-center study, Giugliano and colleagues found that patients who were treated according to the guidelines had an adjusted survival that was significantly better compared with those who had lower compliance with guideline recommendations [26]. Similar data have been seen in acute MI [27], and have been presented in preliminary form from the CRUSADE registry [28].

Publication and distribution of the cardiac society guidelines would appear to be an obvious step towards improving the quality of patient care. One analysis of the effect of publication of guidelines on the quality of care looked at two registries: the TIMI III Registry [29], which was carried out before the first UA guidelines were published in 1994, and the GUARANTEE Registry [30], which was carried out a year after publication of the guidelines. Following publication of the guidelines there was a slight improvement in the use of aspirin, heparin, and beta-blockers (see **Table 3**); nevertheless, only 80% of patients were receiving aspirin on admission and only 50% were receiving beta-blockers. This analysis suggested that publication of guidelines is not sufficient: specific tools are required to ensure that recommendations are implemented.

A second key part of the overall quality improvement program is the monitoring of data on performance. It has been seen that the simple act of monitoring performance, such as the use of specific therapies, can improve their use. Thus, for ACS, monitoring the rates of use of aspirin, beta-blockers, and heparin and all the other therapies (in conjunction with the use of critical pathways and other strategies) should translate into improved outcome for ACS patients.

Figure 3. Awareness is not enough! The gap between physician awareness and implementation of the NCEP Guidelines. Data from *Arch Intern Med* 2000;160:459–67.

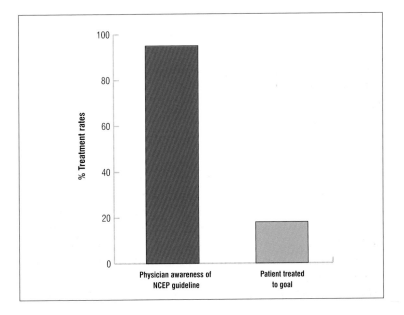

Critical pathways

Critical pathways are standardized protocols for the management of specific diseases (eg, ACS) that aim to optimize and streamline patient care [31,32]. In general, these pathways involve having standardized (or computerized) order sets, or simple pocket cards, reminders, or checklists of the appropriate therapies. In addition, when a pathway is being initiated, there should be physician and nurse education, including presentations to the relevant caregivers at grand rounds, in-services, and other educational meetings throughout the institution.

Several well conducted studies have shown that use of critical pathways can lead to improved quality of care. In the US CHAMP initiative, a nurse uses a checklist to ensure that all patients are on appropriate guideline-recommended therapies. **Figure 4** shows the results of this program on aspirin and beta-blocker use: use of both therapies increased dramatically pre-CHAMP to post-CHAMP, acutely and at follow-up [33]. Aspirin use increased from 68% before the program was launched to 94%

Table 3. Impact of publication of the first unstable angina and non-ST-segment elevation myocardial infarction (UA/NSTEMI) guideline on use of recommended therapies. Data from *Crit Path Cardiol* 2002;1:151–60.

		Pre-guideline		Post-guideline		Comparison of P values pre- to post-guideline	
		Men	Women	Men	Women	Men	Women
Number of patients		1678	1640	1788	1160		
% On admission	Aspirin	82	77	84	80	0.30	0.05
	Heparin	63	50	66	60	0.13	0.001
	Beta-blockers	41	35	53	49	0.001	0.001

1 year later. A similar increase was seen for beta-blocker and ACE inhibitor use and an enormous improvement was achieved in statin use.

The ACC-sponsored GAP (Guideline Applied in Practice) program, led by Kim Eagle in Michigan, provided important multicenter data supporting the efficacy of critical pathways. In this first GAP project, 10 hospitals participated in the quality-improvement effort. Each worked to implement pathways for MI patients, including education of hospital staff through grand round programs, development and implementation of standardized order sets, and the use of pocket cards with

Figure 4. Improvement in utilization of guideline recommended therapies with the CHAMP (Cardiac Hospitalization Atherosclerosis Management Program) program. Data from Fonarow GC, Gawlinski A, Moughrabi S, et al. Improved treatment of coronary heart disease by implementation of a Cardiac Hospitalization Atherosclerosis Management Program (CHAMP). Data from *Am J Cardiol* 2001;87:891–22.

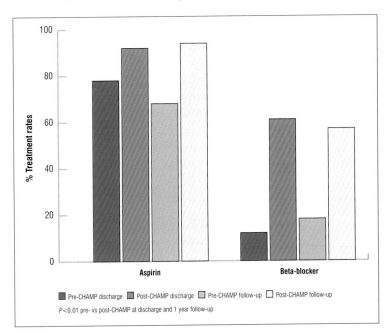

Pre-CHAMP discharge ■ Post-CHAMP discharge ■ Pre-CHAMP follow-up □ Post-CHAMP follow-up

$P<0.01$ pre- vs post-CHAMP at discharge and 1 year follow-up treatment guidelines. As shown in **Figure 5**, improvements were found in the use of guideline-recommended therapies and procedures: early use of aspirin and beta-blockers and measurement of LDL cholesterol were all improved after implementation of the GAP quality improvement effort [34]. The most interesting observation was found when they looked in the charts to see whether the checklists and order sets had actually been used for each patient's care: patients in whom pathways and tools had been used had the highest rates of treatment with the recommended therapies. This demonstrated that having tools available for clinicians to use as reminders can lead to improvements in the use of therapies.

A "re-engineering" effort to improve the standard of cardiology care in the US Veterans' Affairs health system was initiated in the late 1990s. This effort focused on using standardized approaches and pathways, information technology, and computer order sets to build a system to help clinicians administer appropriate care [35]. A key part of this effort was to monitor and publicly disclose data on the results at each of the individual hospitals. Over the course of the 4 years of the program to date, improvements have been seen in the use of key therapies like aspirin and beta-blockers, on admission and at discharge. All of these treatment rates significantly improved and reached very high levels (greater than 90%–95% for use of aspirin and beta-blockers). This provides further data that critical pathways can be implemented, in parallel with a system to monitor data, and lead to considerable improvement in treatment rates.

Conclusion

In the fast-evolving field of ACS, there is a need for rapid uptake of new clinical trial information to translate trials into practice. Publication of ACC/AHA and ESC guidelines is a key part of the effort to improve care. Critical pathways have been shown in numerous studies to improve the quality of care and to be associated with improved outcomes. Monitoring performance is key to ensuring that the efforts in education and system changes translate into tangible improvements in care. It is hoped that more

Figure 5. Improved utilization of guideline recommended therapies with the Guideline Applied in Practice (GAP) program, especially when tools such as critical pathway standardized order sets were used. Adapted with permission from *JAMA* 2002;287:1269–76.

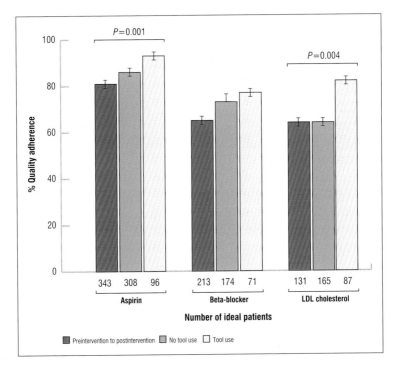

institutions will implement critical pathways and initiate quality improvement efforts and thereby improve the care for their patients.

References

1. Braunwald E, Antman EM, Beasley JW et al. ACC/AHA Guideline Update for the Management of Patients With Unstable Angina and Non-ST-Segment Elevation Myocardial Infarction-2002: Summary Article: A Report of the American College of Cardiology/American Heart Association Task Force on Practice Guidelines (Committee on the Management of Patients With Unstable Angina). *Circulation* 2002;106:1893–900.

2. Scirica BM, Cannon CP, Gibson CM et al. Assessing the effect of publication of clinical guidelines on the management of unstable angina and non-ST-elevation myocardial infarction in the TIMI III [1990–93] and the GUARANTEE [1995–96] registries. *Crit Path Cardiol* 2002;1:151–160.

3. Cannon CP. Evidence-based risk stratification to target therapies in acute coronary syndromes. *Circulation* 2002;106:1588–91.

4. Hamm CW, Heeschen C, Goldmann B et al. Benefit of abciximab in patients with refractory unstable angina in relation to serum troponin T levels. c7E3 Fab Antiplatelet Therapy in Unstable Refractory Angina (CAPTURE) Study Investigators. *N Engl J Med* 1999;340:1623–9.

5. Heeschen C, Hamm CW, Goldmann B et al. Troponin concentrations for stratification of patients with acute coronary syndromes in relation to therapeutic efficacy of tirofiban. *Lancet* 1999;354:1757–62.

6. Cannon CP, Weintraub WS, Demopoulos LA et al. Comparison of early invasive and conservative strategies in patients with unstable coronary syndromes treated with the glycoprotein IIb/IIIa inhibitor tirofiban. *N Engl J Med* 2001;344:1879–87.

7. Morrow DA, Cannon CP, Rifai N et al. Ability of minor elevations of troponin I and T to predict benefit from an early invasive strategy in patients with unstable angina and non-ST elevation myocardial infarction: results from a randomized trial. *JAMA* 2001;286:2405–12.

8. Antithrombotic Trialists' Collaboration. Collaborative meta-analysis of randomised trials of antiplatelet therapy for prevention of death, myocardial infarction, and stroke in high risk patients. *BMJ* 2002;324:71–86. Erratum in *BMJ* 2002;324:141

9. Yusuf S, Zhao F, Mehta SR et al; Clopidogrel in Unstable Angina to Prevent Recurrent Events Trial Investigators. Effects of clopidogrel in addition to aspirin in patients with acute coronary syndromes without ST-segment elevation. *N Engl J Med* 2001;345:494–502.

10. Budaj A, Yusuf S, Mehta SR et al. Benefit of clopidogrel in patients with acute coronary syndromes without ST-segment elevation in various risk groups. *Circulation* 2002;106:1622–6.

11. Theroux P, Ouimet H, McCans J et al. Aspirin, heparin or both to treat unstable angina. *N Engl J Med* 1988;319:1105–11.

12. Peters RJGZ, F., Lewis BSF, KAA. , Yusuf S, the CURE Investigators. Aspirin dose and bleeding events in the CURE study. *Eur Heart J* 2002;4 (Suppl.):510.

13. Yusuf S, Mehta SR, Zhao F et al. Early and late effects of clopidogrel in patients with acute coronary syndromes. *Circulation* 2003;107:966–72.

14. Steinhubl SR, Berger PB, Mann JT 3rd et al. Early and sustained dual oral antiplatelet therapy following percutaneous coronary intervention: a randomized controlled trial. *JAMA* 2002;288:2411–20.
15. CAPRIE Steering Committee. A randomised, blinded, trial of Clopidogrel versus Aspirin in Patients at Risk of Ischaemic Events (CAPRIE). *Lancet* 1996;348:1329–39.
16. Boersma E, Harrington RA, Moliterno DJ et al. Platelet glycoprotein IIb/IIIa inhibitors in acute coronary syndromes: a meta-analysis of all major randomised clinical trials. *Lancet* 2002;359:189–98.
17. Simmons ML; the GUSTO IV-ACS Investigators. Effect of glycoprotein IIb/IIIa receptor blocker abciximab on outcome in patients with acute coronary syndromes without early coronary revascularisation: the GUSTO IV-ACS randomised trial. *Lancet* 2001;357:1915–24.
18. Oler A, Whooley MA, Oler J et al. Adding heparin to aspirin reduces the incidence of myocardial infarction and death in patients with unstable angina. A meta-analysis. *JAMA* 1996;276:811–5.
19. Antman EM, Cohen M, Radley D et al. Assessment of the treatment effect of enoxaparin for unstable angina/non-Q-wave myocardial infarction: TIMI 11B-ESSENCE meta-analysis. *Circulation* 1999;100:1602–8.
20. Goodman S. INTERACT trial. American College of Cardiology Scientific Sessions. Atlanta, 2002.
21. Braunwald E, Antman EM, Beasley JW et al. ACC/AHA guidelines for the management of patients with unstable angina and non-ST segment elevation myocardial infarction: a report of the American College of Cardiology/American Heart Association Task Force on Practice Guidelines (Committee on the Management of Unstable Angina and Non-ST Segment Elevation Myocardial Infarction). *J Am Coll Cardiol* 2000;36:970–1056.
22. FRagmin and Fast Revascularisation during InStability in Coronary artery disease Investigators. Invasive compared with non-invasive treatment in unstable coronary-artery disease: FRISC II prospective randomised multicentre study. *Lancet* 1999;354:708–15.
23. Neumann FJ, Kastrati A, Pogatsa-Murray G, et al. Evaluation of prolonged antithrombotic treatment ("cooling-off" strategy) before intervention in patients with unstable coronary syndromes: a randomized controlled trial. *JAMA* 2003;290:1593–9.
24. Pearson TA, Laurora I, Chu H et al. The lipid treatment assessment project (L-TAP): a multicenter survey to evaluate the percentages of dyslipidemic patients receiving lipid-lowering therapy and achieving low-density lipoprotein cholesterol goals. *Arch Intern Med* 2000;160:459–67.
25. Fox KA, Goodman SG, Klein W et al. Management of acute coronary syndromes. Variations in practice and outcome; findings from the Global Registry of Acute Coronary Events (GRACE). *Eur Heart J* 2002;23:1177–89.
26. Giugliano RP, Lloyd-Jones DM, Camargo CA Jr et al. Association of unstable angina guideline care with improved survival. *Arch Intern Med* 2000;160:1775–80.
27. Chen J, Radford MJ, Wang Y et al. Do "America's best hospitals" perform better for acute myocardial infarction? *N Engl J Med* 1999;340:286–92.
28. Hoekstra JW, Pollack CV, Jr., Roe MT et al. Improving the care of patients with non-ST-elevation acute coronary syndromes in the emergency department: the CRUSADE initiative. *Acad Emerg Med* 2002;9:1146–55.
29. Stone PH, Thompson B, Anderson HV et al. Influence of race, sex, and age on management of unstable angina and non-Q-wave myocardial infarction: The TIMI III Registry. *JAMA* 1996;275:1104–12.

30. Scirica BM, Moliterno DJ, Every NR et al. Differences between men and women in the management of unstable angina pectoris (The GUARANTEE Registry). The GUARANTEE Investigators. *Am J Cardiol* 1999;84:1145–50.

31. Cannon CP, O'Gara PT. Critical pathways in acute coronary syndromes. In: Cannon CP, ed. *Management of Acute Coronary Syndromes*. Totowa: Humana Press, 1999:611–27.

32. Every NR, Hochman J, Becker R et al.; Committee on Acute Cardiac Care; Council of Clinical Cardiology; American Heart Association. Critical pathways: a review. *Circulation* 2000;101:461–5.

33. Fonarow GC, Gawlinski A, Moughrabi S et al. Improved treatment of coronary heart disease by implementation of a Cardiac Hospitalization Atherosclerosis Management Program (CHAMP). *Am J Cardiol* 2001;87:819–22.

34. Mehta RH, Montoye CK, Gallogly M et al. Improving quality of care of acute myocardial infarction: The Guideline Applied in Practice (GAP) Initiative. *JAMA* 2002;287:1269–76.

35. Jha AK, Perlin JB, Kizer KW et al. Effect of the transformation of the Veterans Affairs Health Care System on the quality of care. *N Engl J Med* 2003;348:2218–27.

11

Guidelines for ST-segment elevation myocardial infarction

Marcus D Flather, Anil K Taneja, & Umair Mallick

Introduction

This chapter provides an overview of the American College of Cardiology (ACC)/American Heart Association (AHA) and the European Society of Cardiology (ESC) guidelines for the management of patients presenting with ST-segment elevation acute coronary syndromes (ACS) [1,2]. The ACC/AHA guidelines (last updated in 1999) are based on high- and low-risk categories for the management of ST-segment elevation myocardial infarction (STEMI). The phases of management are broadly categorized into four sections:

- emergency treatment
- early (or prehospital) management
- in-hospital management
- longer-term risk modification

The guidelines generally follow the same pattern of recommendation, indicating on the one hand the reliability of information available in the published literature ("levels of evidence") and on the other hand the opinion of experts based on this information ("class of recommendation") (see **Tables 1** and **2**). The ESC guidelines have based the usefulness or efficacy of the recommended treatment on the class and level of evidence, whereas the ACC/AHA have classified it on similar class categories without separately classifying evidence.

The information in this chapter complements that provided in more detail elsewhere in this book. We have avoided providing the evidence base for recommendations, except where this is essential. The AHA/ACC and ESC guidelines vary in some details, in their style of presentation, and in the way different aspects are classified. In these situations we have taken a pragmatic view to simplify the different approaches.

According to the guidelines, the initial diagnosis of acute myocardial infarction (MI) is based on the presence of two of the factors opposite.

Table 1. The ESC's suggestion for classification of the recommended routine treatments and the level of evidence on which these recommendations are based.

Classifications	
Class I	Evidence and/or general agreement that a given treatment is beneficial, useful, and effective
Class II	Conflicting evidence and/or a divergence of opinion about the usefulness/efficacy of the treatment
Class IIa	Weight of evidence/opinion is in favor of usefulness/efficacy
Class IIb	Usefulness/efficacy is less well established by evidence/opinion
Class III	Evidence or general agreement that the treatment is not useful/effective and in some cases may be harmful
Level of evidence	
Level A	Data derived from at least two randomized clinical trials
Level B	Data derived from a single randomized clinical trial and/or meta-analysis or from nonrandomized studies
Level C	Consensus opinion of the experts based on trials and clinical experience

- history of cardiac-sounding chest pain/discomfort

- electrocardiogram (ECG) changes of acute MI including ST-segment elevation (or depression), (presumed) new left bundle branch block (LBBB), and the development of Q-waves on the ECG

- elevated levels of markers of myocardial necrosis, for example creatine kinase (CK)–MB and troponins (ECG and perfusion scintigraphy may also be helpful to rule out acute MI, but are not currently part of the routine diagnosis)

The guidelines broadly recommend four phases of care:

- immediate or emergency care: to relieve pain and prevent or treat cardiac arrest, followed by a rapid diagnosis and early risk stratification

- early care: this could be initiated by paramedics or on reaching the hospital. The aim is to stabilize the patient and start reperfusion therapy where indicated as soon as possible to prevent loss of myocardial tissue and complications

Table 2. ACC/AHA format for classes of management.

Class I	Conditions for which there is evidence and/or general agreement that a given procedure or treatment is beneficial, useful, and effective
Class II	Conditions for which there is conflicting evidence and/or a divergence of opinion about the usefulness/efficacy of a procedure or treatment
Class IIa	Weight of evidence/opinion is in favor of usefulness/efficacy
Class IIb	Usefulness/efficacy is less well established by evidence/opinion
Class III	Conditions for which there is evidence and/or general agreement that a procedure/treatment is not useful/effective and in some cases may be harmful

- in-hospital care: this consists of the main part of the hospital care, post-emergency care, and the prevention and management of complications

- long-term risk modification for secondary prevention

Emergency/immediate care

This phase involves prompt initial diagnosis and early risk stratification to identify patients requiring early reperfusion therapy or other interventions. The other early priority should be to relieve pain and alleviate anxiety (see **Table 3**). An ECG should be obtained within a few minutes of presentation with suspected ACS.

Repeated ECG recordings should be taken and compared with the initial ECGs. In some cases the ECG can take up to 4 hours to show changes [3,4]. Patients should also have continuous cardiac monitoring to detect arrhythmias. CK-MB and troponin should be requested immediately and repeated after a few hours (troponin may take up to 8 hours to rise after ACS). CK-MB is often repeated daily for the first 2–3 days.

Relief of pain, breathlessness, and anxiety

Relief of pain is of utmost importance not only to alleviate patients' suffering, but also because pain increases sympathetic activation leading to vasoconstriction and increased cardiac workload. A number of measures can be taken to relieve pain, breathlessness, and anxiety:

- intravenous opiates can be administered, eg, 4–8 mg morphine (with additional doses of 2 mg at 5 minute intervals) or diamorphine, where available (2.5–5.0 mg with additional doses of 2.5 mg if needed). This should be accompanied by an antiemetic. Naloxone may be used to reverse opioid-induced respiratory depression

- oxygen (2–4 L/min); caution needs to be taken in patients with a history of chronic obstructive pulmonary disease

- intravenous beta-blockers or nitrates if opioids fail to relieve pain

- sedatives may be helpful

Management of cardiac arrest

At least 50% of all patients who experience acute MI die within the first few hours, before reaching hospital [5,6]. Most of these deaths are due to fatal

Table 3. Recommendations for prehospital and early care. ACE: angiotensin-converting enzyme; ECG: electrocardiogram; EMS: emergency medical services; MI: myocardial infarction.

ACC/AHA recommendations for prehospital and early care		
Prehospital care	Class I	Availability of emergency service telephone access Availability of an EMS system staffed by persons trained to treat cardiac arrest with defibrillation (if indicated) and to triage patients with ischemic-type chest discomfort
	Class IIa	Availability of a first-responder defibrillation program in a tiered-response system. Healthcare providers educate patients and families about signs and symptoms of acute MI, accessing EMS, and medications
	Class IIb	12-lead telemetry Prehospital thrombolysis in special circumstances (eg, transport time >90 min)
Early care	Class I	Supplemental oxygen, intravenous access, and continuous ECG monitoring should be established in all patients with acute ischemic-type chest discomfort An ECG should be obtained and interpreted within 10 minutes of arrival in the emergency department in all patients with suspected acute ischemic-type chest discomfort

ESC recommendations for the prehospital and early-phase management of ST-segment elevation MI		
Recommendations	**Class**	**Level of evidence**
Aspirin	I	A
Beta-blocker	IIb	A
ACE inhibitor	IIa	A
Nitrates	IIb	A
Calcium antagonists	III	B
Magnesium	III	A

arrhythmias, which can often be prevented by appropriate and prompt resuscitation, defibrillation, drug treatment, and monitoring. Basic life support should be started in the absence of trained personnel. Trained personnel should give advanced life support. Management of arrhythmias is covered in the next section of this chapter.

Prehospital or early in-hospital management

In cases of ST-segment elevation ACS (or typical cardiac chest pain and LBBB), the primary objective is to restore coronary flow and myocardial tissue reperfusion by mechanical or pharmacological means. In this phase, the emphasis should be on prehospital emergency care (see **Table 3**) to facilitate a rapid reperfusion strategy.

Aspirin

Aspirin is recommended for all patients presenting with ST-segment elevation ACS and should be given as early as possible (see **Table 4**). Aspirin should not be given to patients with a known bleeding peptic ulcer, hypersensitivity, bleeding disorders, or severe hepatic disease. Aspirin should be used with caution in patients with asthma. Clopidogrel should be given to patients intolerant to aspirin [7]. A loading dose of 300 mg and maintenance dose of 75–150 mg daily are recommended for all patients presenting with suspected acute MI. Chewable aspirin is absorbed faster than aspirin that is swallowed and is especially useful after MI and the use of opiates.

Nitrates (including nitroglycerin)

Patients with ischemic-type chest pain should receive sublingual nitroglycerin unless their initial systolic blood pressure is <90 mm Hg. Nitroglycerin should also be avoided in patients with marked bradycardia (<50 bpm) or tachycardia and should be used with caution in patients with right ventricular (RV) infarction. Nitroglycerin acts by reducing the workload for the heart and by dilating coronary arteries. ACC/AHA and ECS guidelines do not recommend the routine use of nitrates in the acute phase for patients with ST-segment elevation ACS (see **Table 4**). The ACC/AHA guidelines recommend nitrates:

- in patients with left ventricular (LV) dysfunction

- in patients with recurrent ischemia, post–acute MI, or raised blood pressure

and with caution in cases with RV or inferior infarct and in hypotensive patients (systolic blood pressure of 90 mm Hg or mean of 80 mm Hg).

Table 4. ACC/AHA recommendations for oxygen, aspirin, and nitroglycerin. CHF: congestive heart failure; IV: intravenous; MI: myocardial infarction.

Class	Aspirin	IV nitroglycerin	Oxygen
I	A dose of 160–325 mg on day 1 of acute MI and continued indefinitely on a daily basis thereafter	For the first 24–48 hours in patients with acute MI and CHF, large anterior infarction, persistent ischemia, or hypertension Continued use (beyond 48 hours) in patients with recurrent angina or persistent pulmonary congestion	Overt pulmonary congestion Arterial oxygen desaturation <90%
IIa	–	None	Routine administration to all patients with uncomplicated MI during the first 2–3 hours
IIb	Other antiplatelet agents such as dipyridamole, ticlopidine, or clopidogrel may be substituted if true aspirin allergy is present or if the patient is unresponsive to aspirin	For the first 24–48 hours in all patients with acute MI who do not have hypotension, bradycardia, or tachycardia Continued use (beyond 48 hours) in patients with a large or complicated infarction	Routine administration of supplemental oxygen to patients with uncomplicated MI beyond 3–6 hours
III	–	Patients with systolic pressure <90 mm Hg or severe bradycardia (<50 bpm)	–

Beta-blockers

Beta-blockers should be given to patients in the early phase of ST-segment elevation ACS to relieve pain, myocardial ischemia, and ultimately to reduce morbidity and mortality [8,9]. The CIBIS-II trial [10], MERIT-HF trial [11], CAPRICORN trial [12], Norwegian study on timolol [13] and a meta-analysis [9] have shown a 20%–25% reduction in mortality and re-infarction with the use of beta blockers in patients who have recovered from an acute MI. Beta-blockers are thought to limit infarct size and reduce the occurrence of fatal arrhythmias and pain [14,15].

In addition to reducing myocardial oxygen demand by decreasing heart rate, beta-blockers also reduce arterial blood pressure and myocardial contractility. Beta-blockers should ideally be given intravenously (either 5–10 mg of atenolol divided into two doses, or 15 mg of metoprolol divided into three doses) followed by an oral regimen. Oral beta-blockers have a slower onset of action than intravenous beta-blockers. Beta-blockers are recommended by both ACC/AHA and ESC guidelines in the absence of contraindications (see **Box 1** and **Table 5**).

Box 1. Potential contraindications to beta-blockers.

Heart rate <60 bpm

Systolic arterial pressure <100 mm Hg

Moderate left ventricular failure

Signs of peripheral hypoperfusion

PR interval >0.24 seconds

Second- or third-degree atrioventricular block

Severe chronic obstructive pulmonary disease

History of asthma

Severe peripheral vascular disease

Reperfusion therapy

Reperfusion of the infarct-related artery should be undertaken as soon as possible in ST-segment elevation ACS. This can be achieved by pharmacological (fibrinolysis) or mechanical (percutaneous coronary intervention [PCI]) methods.

The revascularization policy recommendations are presented in **Figure 1** and **Table 6**.

Fibrinolytic (thrombolytic) therapy

Emergency departments should evaluate ACS patients with a clinical review and ECG within 10 minutes of presentation and, if indicated, fibrinolytic therapy should be given within 30 minutes of presentation ("door-to-needle time" <30 minutes). Plasminogen activators are fibrinolytic agents that cause dissolution of the fibrin thrombus occluding the infarct-related artery, leading to coronary reperfusion. Fibrinolytic therapy reduces the risk of death in patients with ACS and

Table 5. ACC/AHA recommendations for early therapy with beta-adrenoceptor blocking agents. LV: left ventricular.

Class	Recommendation
I	Patients without a contraindication to beta-adrenoceptor blocker therapy who can be treated within 12 hours of onset of infarction, irrespective of administration of concomitant thrombolytic therapy or performance of primary angioplasty
	Patients with continuing or recurrent ischemic pain
	Patients with tachyarrhythmias, such as atrial fibrillation with a rapid ventricular response
	Non-ST-segment elevation myocardial infarction
IIb	Patients with moderate LV failure (the presence of bibasilar rales without evidence of low cardiac output) or other contraindications to beta-adrenoceptor blocker therapy, provided they can be closely monitored
III	Patients with severe LV failure

ST-segment elevation or LBBB especially when given early, but a reduction in mortality has been observed when treatment is given up to 12 hours after symptom onset [16–28].

The Fibrinolytic Therapy Trialists' (FTT) analysis evaluated patients presenting within 24 hours of symptom onset with STEMI or new LBBB [16]. For every 1,000 patients treated within 6 hours, 30 deaths could be prevented and between 7 and 12 hours, 20 deaths could be prevented. There was no convincing evidence of benefit beyond 12 hours [16].

Figure 1.
Recommendations for
a reperfusion policy.
CABG: coronary artery
bypass grafting; MI:
myocardial infarction;
PCI: percutaneous
coronary intervention;
Acc tPA: accelerated tissue
plasminogen activator.

There has been debate over the use of fibrinolysis in the elderly [44]. A recent re-analysis of the FTT study indicates that in approximately 3,300 patients aged >75 years presenting within 12 hours of

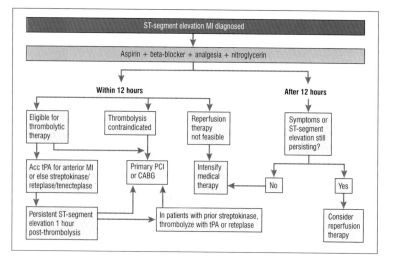

ACC/AHA recommendations for reperfusion therapy (fibrinolysis or primary percutaneous coronary intervention) for ST-segment elevation MI

The constellation of clinical features that must be present (although not necessarily at the same time) to serve as standard indications for administration of thrombolytic therapy to patients with acute MI are as follows:

Class	Recommendation
I	ST-segment elevation (>0.1 mV, two or more contiguous leads), time to therapy 12 hours or less, age <75 years Bundle branch block (obscuring ST-segment analysis) and history suggesting acute MI
IIa	ST-segment elevation, age ≥75 years Comment: In persons >75 years, the overall risk of mortality from infarction is high without and with therapy. Although the proportionate reduction in mortality is less than in patients <75 years, the absolute reduction results in 10 lives saved per 1,000 patients treated in those >75 years. The relative benefit of therapy is reduced [27]
IIb	ST-segment elevation, time to therapy >12–24 hours Blood pressure on presentation >180 mm Hg systolic and/or >110 mm Hg diastolic associated with high-risk MI Comment: there is only a small trend for benefit of therapy in cases presenting >12–24 hours, but thrombolysis may be considered for selected patients with ongoing ischemic pain and extensive ST-segment elevation. Blood pressure can be reduced by beta-blockers or nitrates before thrombolyzing
III	ST-segment elevation, time to therapy >24 hours, ischemic pain resolved

ESC guidelines for the reperfusion policy					
Class	Level	Categories	**Type of reperfusion recommended**		
			Thrombolysis	Primary PCI	Rescue PCI
I	A	Patient with ST-segment elevation MI or new LBBB on the ECG and presenting within 12 hours	Where primary PCI not possible within 90 minutes	Preferred, if done by expert team within <90 minutes of presentation	–
	B	Patient with ST-segment elevation MI or new LBBB on the ECG and presenting within 12 hours	Prehospital initiation	–	In cases with large infarcts who fail thrombolysis
	C	Patient with ST-segment elevation MI or new LBBB on the ECG and presenting within 12 hours	–	In shock when thrombolysis is contraindicated	–
IIa	B	Patients with ST-segment elevation MI or new LBBB on the ECG but presenting late (>4 hours of symptom onset)	Tenecteplase or alteplase preferred	–	–

Table 6. Recommendations for reperfusion therapy. ECG: electrocardiogram; LBBB: left bundle branch block; MI: myocardial infarction; PCI: percutaneous coronary intervention.

symptom onset (with either ST-segment elevation or LBBB) mortality rates were reduced from 29.4% to 26% ($P = 0.03$) [29].

Prehospital fibrinolysis should be instituted where possible, since a further proportional mortality reduction of about 15% was observed with prehospital fibrinolysis when compared to in-hospital fibrinolysis [30,31]. There are several effective fibrinolytic agents; the relative merits of each are discussed in detail in **Chapter 6**.

Fibrinolysis is associated with an elevated risk of bleeding and a small, but definite, excess risk of intracerebral hemorrhage. Bleeding risks are also related to the level of concomitant antithrombotic therapy including heparin, direct thrombin inhibitors, or glycoprotein (GP)IIb/IIIa inhibitors. ACC/AHA guidelines and ESC recommendations are summarized in **Tables 6** and **7** (agents with doses), respectively. The contraindications to fibrinolytic therapy are listed in **Table 8**.

Repeat administration of fibrinolytic agents

In cases with evidence of reocclusion or reinfarction with recurrence of ST-segment elevation or LBBB, further fibrinolysis is indicated if interventional reperfusion is unavailable [32]. However, re-fibrinolysis is no longer appropriate in countries where transfer for PCI can occur. Alteplase (tissue plasminogen activator [tPA]) and its variants can be administered, but carry a higher risk of bleeding complications. The factors influencing risk of bleeding are low body weight, age >75 years, female gender, prior cardiovascular accident, and high blood pressure [33–35].

Primary percutaneous transluminal coronary intervention

Primary PCI is associated with lower risks of death, MI, and bleeding, including stroke, and provides early visualization of coronary anatomy that is helpful in the management of ST-segment elevation ACS. Early primary PCI can be divided into:

- primary PCI: angioplasty and/or stenting without prior thrombolysis

- PCI combined with pharmacological reperfusion therapy

- rescue PCI: angioplasty and/or stenting performed in cases with occluded coronary flow despite fibrinolytic therapy

ESC guidelines recommend primary PCI for cases presenting within the first 90 minutes of acute MI, especially in centers with interventional resources. The DANAMI-2 [36] and PRAGUE-2 [38] studies showed that transfer of patients for primary PCI to a tertiary referral center within 3 hours of admission is safe and provides better results than fibrinolysis [36].

There is no clear role for PCI combined with fibrinolysis, although this approach may be used in

Table 7. ESC task force recommendations for the dose regimens of fibrinolytic agents. IV: intravenous.

Fibrinolytic agent	Initial treatment	Antifibrin cotherapy
Streptokinase	1.5 million units in 100 mL of 5% dextrose or normal saline over 30–60 minutes	None or IV heparin for 24–48 hours
Alteplase	15 mg IV bolus, followed by 0.75 mg/kg over 30 minutes and then 0.5 mg/kg over next 60 minutes Maximum dose not to exceed 100 mg	IV heparin for 24–48 hours
Reteplase	10 U + 10 U IV bolus given 30 minutes apart	IV heparin for 24–48 hours
Tenecteplase	Single IV bolus 30 mg if <60 kg, thereafter, for every extra 10 kg weight, dose recommended is additional 5 mg to a maximum of 50 mg	IV heparin for 24–48 hours

Contraindications for fibrinolysis	
Absolute contraindications	Previous hemorrhagic stroke at any time: other strokes (including ischemic) or cerebrovascular events within 1 year
	Known intracranial neoplasm
	Active internal bleeding (does not include menses)
	Suspected aortic dissection
	ESC guidelines (2003) also recommend the following to be included in the list of absolute contraindications
	• central nervous system damage (recommended to be a relative contraindication by ACC/AHA 1999)
	• known bleeding disorder (recommended to be a relative contraindication by ACC/AHA 1999)
	• gastrointestinal bleeding within the last month
	• recent major trauma/surgery/head injury (within the preceding 3 weeks)
Cautions/relative contraindications	Severe uncontrolled hypertension on presentation (blood pressure >180/110 mm Hg) (an absolute contraindication in low-risk patients with myocardial infarction)
	History of prior cerebrovascular accident or known intracerebral pathology not covered in contraindications (ESC task force recommends this as an absolute contraindication)
	Current use of anticoagulants in therapeutic doses (INR $\geq$2–3)
	Known bleeding diathesis (ESC task force recommends this as an absolute contraindication)
	Recent trauma (within 2–4 weeks), including head trauma (ESC task force recommends this as an absolute contraindication)
	Noncompressible vascular punctures
	Recent internal bleeding (within 2–4 weeks)
	For streptokinase/anistreplase: prior exposure (especially within 5 days to 2 years) or prior allergic reaction
	Pregnancy
	Active peptic ulcer
	History of chronic hypertension
	ESC task force recommends the following as relative contraindications:
	• infective endocarditis
	• advanced liver disease
	• within 1 week of postpartum
	• transient ischemic attack in preceding 6 months

Table 8. Contraindications and cautions for the use of fibrinolytic therapy in ST-segment elevation acute coronary syndromes (recommended by both the ACC/AHA and the ESC). INR: international normalized ratio.

selected cases [39–41]. Investigations are underway to evaluate this further. Rescue PCI may be performed in patients with apparent acute coronary occlusion following fibrinolysis. GPIIb/IIIa inhibitors may be used in primary PCI. ESC guidelines suggest the use of abciximab for primary angioplasty, as shown in the CADILLAC trial [42]. Recommendations from the ACC/AHA guidelines on PCI are summarized in **Table 9**.

Heparin and thrombin inhibitors

Heparin is routinely recommended for patients given tPA as an infusion over 24–48 hours [43,44]. There is no clear evidence of benefit of routine heparin with streptokinase [45]. Intravenous heparin improves coronary flow from hours to days later in patients treated with tPA. Heparin does not have any effect on clot lysis [46]. Low molecular weight

Table 9. ACC/AHA recommendations for percutaneous intervention (coronary artery bypass graft rate <5% among all patients undergoing the procedure). LBBB: left bundle branch block; MI: myocardial infarction; PTCA: percutaneous transluminal coronary angioplasty.

Class	Recommendation
I	As an alternative to thrombolytic therapy in patients with acute MI and ST-segment elevation or new or presumed new LBBB who can undergo angioplasty of the infarct-related artery within 12 hours of onset of symptoms or >12 hours if ischemic symptoms persist, if performed in a timely fashion by persons skilled in the procedure (an individual who performs >75 PTCA procedures per year) and supported by experienced personnel in an appropriate laboratory environment (a center that performs >200 PTCA procedures per year and has cardiac surgical capability) In patients who are within 36 hours of an acute ST-segment elevation/Q-wave or new LBBB MI who develop cardiogenic shock, are <75 years of age, and revascularization can be performed within 18 hours of onset of shock
IIa	As a reperfusion strategy in candidates for reperfusion who have a contraindication to thrombolytic therapy
IIb	In patients with acute MI who do not present with ST-segment elevation but who have reduced flow of the infarct-related artery (less than TIMI grade 2) and when angioplasty can be performed within 12 hours of symptom onset
III	This classification applies to patients with acute MI who: • undergo elective angioplasty of a noninfarct-related artery at the time of acute MI • are >12 hours after symptom onset and have no evidence of myocardial ischemia • have received fibrinolytic therapy and have no symptoms of myocardial ischemia • are eligible for thrombolysis and are undergoing primary angioplasty performed by a low-volume operator in a laboratory without surgical capability

heparin may be a better agent than unfractionated heparin when given with fibrinolytic therapy [47], but evidence from further trials is awaited. Studies with direct thrombin inhibitors (such as bivalirudin, argatroban, and hirudin) show that they may also be useful as adjunctive treatments to fibrinolysis [48–50]. The HERO-II trial showed good safety and slightly better efficacy with bivalirudin versus unfractionated heparin when given with streptokinase [51]. ESC guidelines recommend a heparin IV bolus of 60 U/kg with a maximum of 4,000 U intravenous infusion or 12 U/kg for 24–48 hours with a maximum of 1,000 U/hour with a target activated partial thromboplastin time (aPTT) of 50–70 seconds. aPTT should be monitored at 3, 6, 12, and 24 hours after the start of treatment. The recommendations from the ACC/AHA guidelines are summarized in **Table 10**.

Other potential treatments

Glycoprotein IIb/IIIa inhibitors

There are two potential strategies for the use of GPIIb/IIIa inhibitors in patients with ST-segment elevation ACS: combination therapy (with modified dose regimens of fibrinolytics and GPIIb/IIIa receptor blockers) and adjunctive GPIIb/IIIa blockade during primary angioplasty. These strategies are discussed in depth in **Chapter 4**. At present, there is no evidence to support the routine use of GPIIb/IIIa inhibitors with thrombolytic treatment in view of the high risk and incidence of bleeding. The present data, however, support the use of abciximab in primary angioplasty and stenting in combination with low-dose heparin.

Angiotensin-converting enzyme inhibitors

After the early (reperfusion) phase of management, ESC guidelines recommend the use of angiotensin-converting enzyme (ACE) inhibitors in patients with impaired LV ejection fraction or heart failure. The GISSI-3, ISIS-4, and Chinese studies have reported modest but definite reductions in mortality at 6 weeks with the use of ACE inhibitors [52,53]. ACE inhibitors may therefore be given routinely to patients within 24–36 hours from the onset of symptoms, or as a more selective policy to patients with heart failure or larger infarcts [54]. The best approach is to start with small doses titrating to therapeutic doses over 24–48 hours, with careful monitoring of blood pressure. In general, treatment should be used with caution in patients with systolic blood pressures <100 mm Hg. The ACC/AHA recommendations are summarized in **Table 11**.

Table 10. ACC/AHA recommendations for the use of unfractionated heparin (UFH). AF: atrial fibrillation; aPTT: activated partial thromboplastin time; IV: intravenous; LMWH: low molecular weight heparin; MI: myocardial infarction; PTCA: percutaneous transluminal coronary angioplasty; SC: subcutaneous; SK: streptokinase.

Class	Recommendation
I	Patients undergoing percutaneous or surgical revascularization. For PTCA, monitoring of activated clotting time is recommended, with a goal of 300–350 seconds during the procedure.
IIa	IV in patients undergoing reperfusion therapy with alteplase. The recommended regimen is 60 U/kg as a bolus at initiation of alteplase infusion, then an initial maintenance dose of approximately 12 U/kg/h (with a maximum of 4,000 U bolus and 1,000 U/h infusion for patients weighing >70 kg), adjusted to maintain aPTT at 1.5–2.0 times control (50–70 seconds) for 48 hours. Continuation of heparin infusion beyond 48 hours should be considered in patients at high risk for systemic or venous thromboembolism. IV UFH or SC LMWH for patients with non-ST-segment elevation MI. SC UFH (eg, 7,500 U twice a day) or LMWH (eg, enoxaparin 1 mg/kg twice a day) in all patients not treated with thrombolytic therapy who do not have a contraindication to heparin. In patients who are at high risk for systemic emboli (large or anterior MI, AF, previous embolus, or known left ventricular thrombus), IV heparin is preferred. IV in patients treated with nonselective thrombolytic agents (SK, anistreplase, urokinase) who are at high risk for systemic emboli (large or anterior MI, AF, previous embolus, or known left ventricular thrombus).
IIb	Patients treated with nonselective thrombolytic agents, not at high risk, SC heparin, 7,500–12,500 U twice a day until completely ambulatory.
III	Routine IV heparin within 6 hours to patients receiving a nonselective fibrinolytic agent (SK, anistreplase, urokinase) who are not at high risk for systemic emboli.

Calcium antagonists

There is no evidence to support prophylactic use of calcium antagonists in the acute phase of STEMI. Diltiazem may be a useful substitute if a beta-blocker is contraindicated, but this is not strictly evidence based. Verapamil may be useful for rate reduction, but has a negative inotropic effect that may depress myocardial function. Nifedipine should be avoided in view of its tachycardic effect in patients in the acute phase of MI.

Glucose–insulin–potassium infusion

Glucose–insulin–potassium (GIK) infusions may provide metabolic protection for patients with acute myocardial ischemia. A meta-analysis of ~2,000 patients suggested that it may result in a 28% reduction in hospital mortality [55]. Some recent studies have also shown promising evidence of a benefit, but the studies have not been large enough to support the routine use of GIK infusions. Results of further large on-going trials are awaited.

Table 11. ACC/AHA recommendations for use of angiotensin-converting enzyme (ACE) inhibitors. LV: left ventricular; MI: myocardial infarction.

Class	Recommendation
I	Patients within the first 24 hours of a suspected acute MI with ST-segment elevation in two or more anterior precordial leads or with clinical heart failure in the absence of hypotension (systolic blood pressure <100 mm Hg) or known contraindications to ACE inhibitors. Patients with MI and LV ejection fraction <40% or patients with clinical heart failure on the basis of systolic pump dysfunction during and after convalescence from acute MI.
IIa	All other patients within the first 24 hours of a suspected or established acute MI, provided significant hypotension or other clear-cut contraindications are absent. Asymptomatic patients with mildly impaired LV function (ejection fraction 40%–50%) and a history of old MI.
IIb	Patients who have recently recovered from MI but have normal or mildly abnormal global LV function.

Magnesium

The MAGIC trial confirmed the lack of benefit of magnesium in acute MI [56]. Magnesium may have a role in the treatment of ventricular arrhythmias (including torsade de pointes).

Management of high-risk patients or those with complications

The management of mechanical and electrical complications is discussed in detail in **Chapter 9**. In this chapter, the summary recommendations from the guidelines on the use of coronary artery surgery, intra-aortic balloon pumps, and pacing in ST-segment elevation ACS are outlined.

Coronary artery bypass surgery

ESC guidelines recommend coronary artery bypass grafting (CABG) during the acute phase of MI in:

- patients with failed PCI
- patients with sudden occlusion of a coronary artery during catheterization
- patients who are difficult cases for PCI or in whom PCI is not feasible
- selected patients with cardiogenic shock
- patients undergoing surgery for ventricular septal defect or mitral regurgitation (secondary to a infarct)

Recommendations of the ACC/AHA are outlined in **Table 12**.

Intra-aortic balloon pump insertion

This is a useful approach for stabilizing patients with intractable ischemia or with continued hypoperfusion. It should only be used in centers with facilities to place and manage the balloon pump. ACC/AHA guidelines for this procedure are summarized in **Table 13**.

Pacing

Pacing is indicated in patients with symptomatic bradycardia or heart block. First-degree heart block does not require any treatment. Type I second-degree heart block (Mobitz I or Wenkebach) rarely causes adverse hemodynamic effects but, if these do occur, they should be treated with atropine first. Failing improvement with atropine, pacing needs to be considered. Type II second-degree heart block (Mobitz II) and complete heart block (third-degree heart block) need insertion of a pacing electrode. Atrioventricular (AV) sequential pacing should be offered to patients with severe hemodynamic disturbances. A pacing wire could be inserted in patients with bifascicular or trifascicular block.

New LBBB or hemi-block in the presence of anterior ST-segment elevation on the ECG indicates extensive

Table 12. ACC/AHA recommendations for emergency or urgent coronary artery bypass graft surgery. PTCA: percutaneous transluminal coronary angioplasty.

Class	Recommendation
I	Failed angioplasty with persistent pain or hemodynamic instability in patients with coronary anatomy suitable for surgery Acute myocardial infarction with persistent or recurrent ischemia refractory to medical therapy in patients with coronary anatomy suitable for surgery who are not candidates for catheter intervention At the time of surgical repair of postinfarction ventricular septal defect or mitral valve insufficiency
IIa	Cardiogenic shock with coronary anatomy suitable for surgery
IIb	Failed PTCA and small area of myocardium at risk; hemodynamically stable
III	When the expected surgical mortality rate equals or exceeds the mortality rate associated with appropriate medical therapy

anterior infarct and calls for pacing wire insertion. Transcutaneous pacing may be used if transvenous pacing facilities are not available. The ACC/AHA recommendations for this procedure are listed in **Table 14**.

Permanent pacing after acute myocardial infarction

A requirement for temporary pacing in acute MI does not by itself constitute an indication for permanent pacing. The unfavorable long-term prognosis of patients who have experienced an acute MI that has caused conduction disturbances is related primarily to the extent of associated myocardial injury. Consequently, these patients are at greater risk for death from heart failure and ventricular tachyarrhythmia than from progressive heart block. Indications for permanent pacing after acute MI in patients experiencing conduction disturbances are related primarily to the degree and type of AV block and do not necessarily depend on

Table 13. ACC/AHA recommendations for intra-aortic balloon counterpulsation. MI: myocardial infarction; PTCA: percutaneous transluminal coronary angioplasty.

Class	Recommendation
I	Cardiogenic shock not quickly reversed with pharmacological therapy as a stabilizing measure for angiography and prompt revascularization
	Acute mitral regurgitation or ventricular septal defect complicating MI as a stabilizing therapy for angiography and repair/revascularization
	Recurrent intractable ventricular arrhythmias with hemodynamic instability
	Refractory post-MI angina as a bridge to angiography and revascularization
IIa	Signs of hemodynamic instability, poor left ventricular function, or persistent ischemia in patients with large areas of myocardium
IIb	In patients with successful PTCA after failed thrombolysis or those with three-vessel coronary disease to prevent reocclusion
	In patients known to have large areas of myocardium at risk, with or without active ischemia

the presence of symptoms. The ACC/AHA recommendations for this procedure are summarized in **Table 15**.

Management of arrhythmias

Arrhythmias and conduction disturbances are very common and carry a high mortality rate in the early hours of an MI. Ventricular arrhythmias and complete AV block require prompt correction and management.

Table 14. ACC/AHA recommendations for temporary transvenous pacing. AFB: anterior fascicular block; AV: atrioventricular; BBB: bundle branch block; LAFB: left anterior fascicular block; LBBB: left bundle branch block; LPFB: left posterior fascicular block; RBBB: right bundle branch block.

Class	Recommendation
I	Asystole
	Symptomatic bradycardia (includes sinus bradycardia with hypotension and type I second-degree AV block with hypotension not responsive to atropine)
	Bilateral BBB (alternating BBB or RBBB with alternating LAFB/LPFB) (any age)
	New or indeterminate age bifascicular block (RBBB with AFB or LPFB, or LBBB) with first-degree AV block
	Mobitz type II second-degree AV block
IIa	RBBB and LAFB or LPFB (new or indeterminate)
	RBBB with first-degree AV block
	New or indeterminate LBBB
	Incessant ventricular tachycardia, for atrial or ventricular overdrive pacing
	Recurrent sinus pauses (>3 seconds) not responsive to atropine
	(Note also the recommendations for transcutaneous standby pacing)
IIb	Bifascicular block of indeterminate age
	New or indeterminate age isolated RBBB
III	First-degree heart block
	Type I second-degree AV block with normal hemodynamics
	Accelerated idioventricular rhythm
	BBB or fascicular block known to exist before acute MI

The hemodynamic status of patients with arrhythmia is important in deciding the type and urgency of treatment. All patients with acute MI must have continuous cardiac monitoring. The underlying factors giving rise to these arrhythmias vary from electrolyte and acid–base imbalance to continuing ischemia and pump failure.

Ventricular arrhythmias

No specific therapy is indicated for the ventricular ectopics, multiform complexes, accelerated idioventricular rhythm, or the R-on-T phenomenon. However, close monitoring is advised.

Nonsustained runs of ventricular tachycardia may be well tolerated without the need for any specific treatment, but prolonged episodes are associated with hypotension and cardiac failure, thus leading to ventricular fibrillation. Longer episodes of nonsustained ventricular tachycardia should be treated with beta-blockers (metoprolol or atenolol) as the first line of management, unless contraindicated.

Table 15. ACC/AHA recommendations for permanent pacing after acute myocardial infarction. AV: atrioventricular; BBB: bundle branch block; LAFB: left anterior fascicular block.

Class	Recommendation
I	Persistent second-degree AV block in the His-Purkinje system with bilateral BBB or complete heart block after acute myocardial infarction
	Transient advanced (second- or third-degree) AV block and associated BBB
	Symptomatic AV block at any level
IIb	Persistent advanced (second- or third-degree) block at the AV node level
III	Transient AV conduction disturbances in the absence of intraventricular conduction defects
	Transient AV block in the presence of isolated LAFB
	Acquired LAFB in the absence of AV block
	Persistent first-degree AV block in the presence of BBB that is old or of indeterminate age

Table 16. ACC/AHA recommendations for treatment of ventricular tachycardia (VT)/ventricular fibrillation (VF). CABG: coronary artery bypass graft; PTCA: percutaneous transluminal coronary angioplasty.

Sustained ventricular tachycardia and ventricular fibrillation should be treated with intravenous lidocaine/lignocaine or amiodarone. Amiodarone is considered superior in such cases, especially for recurrent sustained ventricular tachycardia

Class	Recommendation
I	VF should be treated with an unsynchronized electric shock with an initial energy of 200 J; if unsuccessful, a second shock of 200–300 J should be given, and, if necessary, a third shock of 360 J.
	Sustained (>30 seconds or causing hemodynamic collapse) polymorphic VT should be treated with an unsynchronized electric shock using an initial energy of 200 J; if unsuccessful, a second shock of 200–300 J should be given, and, if necessary, a third shock of 360 J.
	Episodes of sustained monomorphic VT associated with angina, pulmonary edema, or hypotension (blood pressure <90 mm Hg) should be treated with a synchronized electric shock of 100 J initial energy. Increasing energies may be used if not initially successful.
	Sustained monomorphic VT not associated with angina, pulmonary edema, or hypotension (blood pressure <90 mm Hg) should be treated with one of the following regimens (see section on recommended doses of drugs for ventricular arrhythmias for dosing): • lidocaine: initial bolus; supplemental boluses to a maximum of 3 mg/kg total • procainamide: 20–30 mg/min loading infusion, up to 12–17 mg/kg; this may be followed by an infusion • amiodarone: 150 mg infused over 10 minutes followed by a constant infusion and then a maintenance infusion • synchronized electrical cardioversion starting at 50 J (brief anesthesia is necessary)
	Comment: knowledge of the pharmacokinetics of these agents is important because dosing varies considerably, depending on age, weight, and hepatic and renal function.
IIa	Infusions of antiarrhythmic drugs may be used after an episode of VT/VF, but should be discontinued after 6–24 hours and the need for further arrhythmia management assessed.
	Electrolyte and acid–base disturbances should be corrected to prevent recurrent episodes of VF when an initial episode of VF has been treated.
IIb	Drug-refractory polymorphic VT should be managed by aggressive attempts to reduce myocardial ischemia, including therapies such as beta-adrenoceptor blockade, intra-aortic balloon pumping, and emergency PTCA/CABG surgery.
	Amiodarone, 150 mg infused over 10 minutes followed by a constant infusion of 1.0 mg/min for up to 6 hours and then a maintenance infusion at 0.5 mg/min, may also be helpful.
III	Treatment of isolated ventricular premature beats, couplets, runs of accelerated idioventricular rhythm, and nonsustained VT.
	Prophylactic administration of antiarrhythmic therapy when using thrombolytic agents.

requiring cardioversion, or in patients with ventricular fibrillation. In the absence of a defibrillator, a precordial thump could be tried in patients with ventricular fibrillation. Lidocaine/lignocaine should not be given to a patient who is in shock. The ACC/AHA guidelines for ventricular arrhythmia treatment are shown in **Table 16**.

Table 17. Recommended doses of drugs for ventricular arrhythmias. VF: ventricular fibrillation; VT: ventricular tachycardia.

Drug	Doses recommended by ESC task force	Doses recommended by ACC/AHA task force	Route and indication
Lignocaine/lidocaine	Initial bolus of 1 mg/kg followed by 0.5 mg/kg after 8–10 minutes to a maximum of 4 mg/kg or continuous infusion of 1–3 mg/min	Initial bolus of 1–1.5 mg/kg (75–100 mg) with additional boluses of 0.5–0.75 mg/kg (25–50 mg) every 5–10 minutes to a maximum of 3 mg/kg. Followed by a maintenance infusion of 1–4 mg/min, reduced after 24 hours (to 1–2 mg/min)	Intravenous for sustained VT or VF or prolonged nonsustained VT or wide complex tachycardia of uncertain type
Amiodarone	5 mg/kg in the first hour followed by 900–1,200 mg in 24 hours	500 mg per 24 hours given as rapid infusion of 150 mg over 10 minutes, followed by early maintenance infusion of 1 mg/min for 6 hours and later maintenance infusion of 0.50 mg/min	Intravenous for VF, pulseless VT, and sustained or prolonged nonsustained VT
Procainamide	Not mentioned	Loading dose of 10–15 mg/kg (500–1,250 mg), at rate of 20 mg/min (over 30–60 minutes) followed by maintenance of 1–4 mg/min	Intravenous for cases with contraindication or failure with lignocaine
Bretylium	Not mentioned	Bolus of 5 mg/kg for VF. Supplemental doses of 10 mg/kg after every 5 minutes to a maximum of 30–35 mg/kg. In stable VT, loading dose should be diluted to 50 mL with 5% dextrose over 8–10 minutes. Recommended infusion rate is 1–2 mg/min	Resistant VF/pulseless VT and hemodynamically unstable VT after lignocaine/defibrillation have failed

Supraventricular arrhythmias

Atrial fibrillation occurs in ~20% of patients presenting with acute MI and is more common in patients with associated LV dysfunction. Short episodes are self-limiting. Patients with longer or continuous episodes, who have a controlled ventricular rate, do not require any specific antiarrhythmic treatment. Beta-blockers and digoxin are recommended for rate control, but amiodarone has been shown to be more effective in terminating the arrhythmia. Doses and indications of antiarrhythmics recommended for management of ventricular arrhythmias are shown in **Table 17**.

Verapamil is not recommended for patients with supraventricular arrhythmia, but intravenous adenosine could be used in other supraventricular tachycardias except atrial flutter. Counter shock should be employed if arrhythmia is poorly tolerated. The ACC/AHA recommendations regarding the management of atrial fibrillation in patients presenting with STEMI are shown in **Table 18**.

Table 18. ACC/AHA recommendations for treatment of atrial fibrillation. LV: left ventricular.

Class	Recommendation
I	Electrical cardioversion for patients with severe hemodynamic compromise or intractable ischemia
	Rapid digitalization to slow a rapid ventricular response and improve LV function
	Intravenous beta-adrenoceptor blockers to slow a rapid ventricular response in patients without clinical LV dysfunction, bronchospastic disease, or atrioventricular block
	Heparin should be given
IIa	Either diltiazem or verapamil (intravenous) to slow a rapid ventricular response if beta-adrenoceptor blocking agents are contraindicated or ineffective

Sinus bradycardia and heart block

Heart blocks and sinus bradycardia are common in patients with an inferior infarct. Atropine is recommended in doses of 0.3–0.5 mg for this condition and can be repeated up to a maximum of 1.5–2.0 mg.

If associated with hypotension or hemodynamic instability, temporary pacing should be considered. Details of guidelines recommended for pacing and recommendations on the use of atropine for sinus brachycardia and heartblock are included in **Table 19**.

At discharge from hospital

Both ACC/AHA and ESC guidelines give recommendations for the preparation of patients with a diagnosis of MI for discharge, based on principles of risk assessment, rehabilitation, and secondary prevention. Stratification of individual patients into high or low risk should be categorized for urgency and type of investigations indicated; these include:

Table 19. ACC/AHA recommendations for atropine. AV: atrioventricular.

Class	Recommendation
I	Symptomatic sinus bradycardia (generally, heart rate <50 bpm associated with hypotension, ischemia, or escape ventricular arrhythmia)
	Ventricular asystole
	Symptomatic AV block occurring at the AV nodal level (second-degree type I or third-degree with a narrow-complex escape rhythm)
III	AV block occurring at an infranodal level (usually associated with anterior myocardial infarction with a wide-complex escape rhythm)
	Asymptomatic sinus bradycardia

- performing noninvasive and invasive evaluations of these patients to assess the degree of myocardial perfusion and viability (see **Table 20**)
- measurement of infarct size
- assessment of LV function to measure risk of ventricular arrhythmias and to perform risk stratification
- exercise stress testing
- radionuclide imaging scans
- echocardiography
- 24-hour ambulatory ECG monitoring

Table 20. ACC/AHA recommendations for noninvasive evaluation of low-risk patients. ECG: electrocardiogram.

Assessment of myocardial viability, stunning, and hibernation by myocardial perfusion scintigraphy or

Class	Recommendation
I	Stress ECG: • before discharge for prognostic assessment or functional capacity (submaximal at 4–6 days or symptom limited at 10–14 days) • early after discharge for prognostic assessment and functional capacity (14–21 days) • late after discharge (3–6 weeks) for functional capacity and prognosis if early stress was submaximal Exercise, vasodilator stress nuclear scintigraphy, or exercise stress echo when baseline abnormalities on the ECG compromise interpretation
IIa	Dipyridamole or adenosine stress perfusion nuclear scintigraphy or dobutamine echo before discharge for prognostic assessment in patients judged to be unable to exercise Exercise two-dimensional echo or nuclear scintigraphy (before or early after discharge for prognostic assessment)
III	Stress testing within 2–3 days of acute myocardial infarction Either exercise or pharmacological stress testing at any time to evaluate patients with unstable postinfarction angina pectoris At any time to evaluate patients with acute myocardial infarction who have uncompensated congestive heart failure, cardiac arrhythmia, or noncardiac conditions that severely limit their ability to exercise Before discharge to evaluate patients who have already been selected for cardiac catheterization. In this situation, an exercise test may be useful after catheterization to evaluate function or identify ischemia in distribution of a coronary lesion of borderline severity

stress echocardiography is recommended initially and (if required) by positron emission tomography or by magnetic resonance imaging. Invasive investigations include coronary angiography and possible percutaneous transluminal coronary angiography as an adjunct to thrombolysis or after failed thrombolysis during the initial management (see **Table 21**). Long-term anticoagulation may be needed in selected cases (see **Table 22**).

For secondary prevention, long-term aspirin, statins, ACE inhibitors, and beta-blockers are routinely recommended. Lifestyle changes are required, including an increase in physical activity, appropriate diet, smoking cessation, stress management, and adherence to medication (see **Table 23**).

Encouraging patients to participate in the formal cardiac rehabilitation programs facilitates these changes and should be a routine policy; this should take into account the patient's physical, psychological, and socioeconomic needs. The ESC guidelines specifically recommend use of the Mediterranean diet (low in saturated fat; high in

Table 21. ACC/AHA recommendations for early coronary angiography in patients not undergoing primary percutaneous transluminal coronary angioplasty (PTCA).

Class	Recommendation
I	None
IIa	Patients with cardiogenic shock or persistent hemodynamic instability
IIb	Patients with evolving large or anterior infarcts treated with thrombolytic agents in whom it is believed that the artery is not patent and adjuvant PTCA is planned
III	Routine use of angiography and subsequent PTCA within 24 hours of administration of thrombolytic agents

polyunsaturated fat, fruits, and vegetables) [57]. There is no evidence for a role of antioxidants in postinfarction patients [58]. Guidelines also emphasize the need for optimum glycemic control and control of blood pressure.

Class	Recommendation
I	For secondary prevention of MI in post-MI patients unable to take daily aspirin (see also section on aspirin)
	Post-MI patients in persistent atrial fibrillation
	Patients with LV thrombus
IIa	Post-MI patients with extensive wall motion abnormalities
	Patients with paroxysmal atrial fibrillation
IIb	Post-MI patients with severe LV systolic dysfunction with or without CHF

Table 22. Indications for long-term anticoagulation after acute myocardial infarction (MI). CHF: congestive heart failure; LV: left ventricular; MI: myocardial infarction.

Therapy	First 24 hours	After first 24 hours	Discharge
Dietary advice	–	Education on low-fat diet	Recommend low-fat diet
Smoking	Reinforce cessation	Reinforce cessation	Referral to smoking cessation classes if desired
Exercise	Education	Hallway ambulation	Recommend regular aerobic exercise
Pre-discharge ETT	For uncomplicated patient plan on 4–5 days	Perform predischarge ETT	Catheterize patients with significant ischemia
Measure LVEF	–	Echocardiography or MUGA prior to d/c if no LV gram	ACE inhibitors if LVEF ≤40% or in-hospital CHF
Cardiac rehabilitation	–	Start exercise	Refer to rehab program near their home

Table 23. Nonpharmacological therapy. ETT: exercise tolerance test; LVEF: left ventricular ejection fraction; ACE: angiotensin-converting enzyme; MUGA: multiple update gated acquisition; CHF: congestive heart failure. Adapted from: ACC/AHA Pocket Guidelines for The Management of Patients with Acute Myocardial Infarction (A Report of the ACC/AHA Task Force on Practice Guidelines) April, 2000.

References

1. Ryan TJ, Antman EM, Brooks NH, et al. 1999 update: ACC/AHA guidelines for the management of patients with acute myocardial infarction. A report of the American College of Cardiology/American Heart Association Task Force on Practice Guidelines (Committee on Management of Acute Myocardial Infarction). Available at http://www.acc.org/clinical/guidelines/miguide.pdf and http://www.americanheart.org. Accessed on October 2, 2003.

2. Van de Werf, Ardissino D, Betriu A, et al. The Task Force on the Management of Acute Myocardial Infarction of the European Society of Cardiology. Management of acute myocardial infarction in patients presenting with ST-segment elevation. *Eur Heart J* 2003;24:28–66

3. Adams J, Trent R, Rawles J; The GREAT Group. Earliest electrocardiographic evidence of myocardial infarction: implications for thrombolytic therapy. *Br Med J* 1993;307:409–13.

4. Grijseels EW, Deckers JW, Hoes AW, et al. Prehospital infarction. Evaluation of previously developed algorithms and new proposals. *Eur Heart J* 1995;16:325–32.

5. Herlitz J, Blohm M, Hartford M, et al. Delay time in suspected acute myocardial infarction and the importance of its modification. *Clin Cardiol* 1989;12:370–4.

6. National Heart, Lung and Blood Institute. Morbidity and Mortality: Chartbook on Cardiovascular, Lung, and Blood Diseases. Bethesda, MD:US Department of health and human services, Public health service, National Institutes of health; May 1992.

7. CAPRIE Steering Committee. A randomized, blinded trial of clopidogrel versus aspirin in patients at risk of ischaemic events (CAPRIE). *Lancet* 1996;348:1329–39.

8. Yusuf S, Lessem J, Jha P, et al. Primary and secondary prevention of myocardial infarction and strokes: an update of randomly allocated controlled trials. *J Hypertens* 1993;11(Suppl 4):S61–S73.

9. Freemantle N, Cleland J, Young P, et al. Beta blockade after myocardial infarction: systematic review and meta regression analysis. *Br Med J* 1999;318:1730–7.

10. The CIBIS-II investigators. The Cardiac Insufficiency Bisprolol Study II. (CIBIS-II): a randomised trial. *Lancet* 1999;353:9–13.

11. The MERIT-HF investigators. Effect of metoprolol CR/XL in chronic heart failure: Metoprolol CR/XL Randomised Intervention Trial in Congestive Heart Failure (MERIT-HF). *Lancet* 1999;353:2001–7.

12. The CAPRICORN investigators. Effect of carvedilol on outcome after myocardial infarction in patients with leftventricular dysfunction: the CAPRICORN randomised trial. *Lancet* 2001;357:1385–90.

13. Pedersen TR. The Norwegian Multicenter Study of Timolol after Myocardial Infarction. *Circulation* 1983;67:149–153.

14. Gunnar RM, Bourdillon PDV, Dixon DW, et al. Guidelines for the early management of patients with acute myocardial infarction: a report of the American College of cardiology/American Heart Association Task Force on Assessment of Diagnostic and Therapeutic Cardiovascular Procedures (Subcommittee to Develop Guidelines for the Early Management of Patients with Acute Myocardial Infarction). *J Am Coll Cardiol* 1990;16:249–52.

15. Epstein AE, Hallstrom AP, Rogers WJ, et al. Mortality following ventricular arrhythmia suppression by encainide, flecainide, and moricizine after myocardial infarction: the original design concept of the Cardiac Arrhythmia Suppression Trial (CAST). *JAMA* 1993;270:2451–5.

16. Fibrinolytic Therapy Trialists' (FTT) Collaborative Group. Indications for fibrinolytic therapy in suspected acute myocardial infarction: collaborative overview of early mortality and major morbidity results from all randomized trials of more than 1000 patients. *Lancet* 1994;343:311–22.

17. ISIS-2 (Second International Study of Infarct Survival) Collaborative Group. Randomised trial of intravenous streptokinase, oral aspirin, both, or neither among 17,187 cases of suspected acute myocardial infarction: ISIS-2. *Lancet* 1988;2:349–60.

18. ISIS-3 (Third International Study of Infarct Survival) Collaborative Group. ISIS-3: a randomised comparison of streptokinase vs tissue plasminogen activator vs anistreplase and of aspirin plus heparin vs aspirin alone among 41,299 cases of suspected acute myocardial infarction. *Lancet* 1992;339:753–70.

19. Gruppo Italiano per lo Studio della Streptochinasi nell'Infarto Miocardico (GISSI). Effectiveness of intravenous thrombolytic treatment in acute myocardial infarction. *Lancet* 1986;1:397–402.

20. The International Study Group. In-hospital mortality and clinical course of 20,891 patients with suspected acute myocardial infarction randomised between alteplase and streptokinase with or without heparin. *Lancet* 1990;336:71–5.

21. The GUSTO Investigators. An international randomized trial comparing four thrombolytic strategies for acute myocardial infarction. *N Engl J Med* 1993; 329:673–82.

22. Neuhaus KL, Feuerer W, Jeep-Tebbe S et al. Improved thrombolysis with a modified dose regimen of recombinant tissue-type plasminogen activator. *J Am Coll Cardiol* 1989;14:1566–9.

23. A comparsion of reteplase with alteplase for acute myocardial infarction. The Global Use of Strategies to Open Occluded Coronary Arteries (GUSTO III) Investigators. *N Engl J Med* 1997;337:1118–23.

24. Randomised, double-blind comparison of reteplase doublebolus administration with streptokinase in acute myocardial infarction (INJECT): trial to investigate equivalence. International Joint Efficacy Comparison of Thrombolytics. *Lancet* 1995;346:329–36.

25. The Continuous Infusion versus Double-Bolus Administration of Alteplase (COBALT) Investigators. A comparison of continuous infusion of alteplase with double-bolus administration for acute myocardial infarction. *N Engl J Med* 1997;337:1124–30.

26. Single-bolus tenecteplase compared with front-loaded alteplase in acute myocardial infarction: the ASSENT-2 double-blind randomised trial. Assessment of the Safety and Efficacy of a New Thrombolytic Investigators. *Lancet* 1999;354:716–22.

27. Tebbe U, Michels R, Adgey J et al; Comparison Trial of Saruplase and Streptokinase (COMPASS) Investigators. Randomized, double-blind study comparing saruplase with streptokinase therapy in acute myocardial infarction: the COMPASS Equivalence Trial. *J Am Coll Cardiol* 1998;31:487–93.

28. Intravenous NPA for the treatment of infarcting myocardium early. In TIME-II, a double-blind comparison of singlebolus lanoteplase vs accelerated alteplase for the treatment of patients with acute myocardial infarction. *Eur Heart J* 2000;21:2005–13.

29. White H. Thrombolytic therapy in the elderly. *Lancet* 2000;356:2028–30.

30. White HD, Van de Werf FJ. Thrombolysis for acute myocardial infarction. *Circulation* 1998;97:1632–46.

31. Morrison LJ, Verbeek PR, McDonald AC, et al. Mortality and prehospital thrombolysis for acute myocardial infarction: a meta-analysis. *JAMA* 2000;283:2686–92.

32. Barbash GI, Birnbaum Y, Bogaerts KM, et al. Treatment of reinfarction after thrombolytic therapy for acute myocardial infarction: an analysis of outcome and treatment choices in the global utilization of streptokinase and tissue plasminogen activator for occluded coronary arteries (GUSTO I) and assessment of the safety of a new thrombolytic (ASSENT 2) studies. *Circulation* 2001;103:954–60.

33. Gore JM, Granger CB, Simoons ML, et al. Stroke after thrombolysis. Mortality and functional outcomes in the GUSTO-I trial. Global Use of Strategies to Open Occluded Coronary Arteries. *Circulation* 1995;92:2811–8.

34. Simoons ML, Maggioni AP, Knatterud G, et al. Individual risk assessment for intracranial haemorrhage during thrombolytic therapy. *Lancet* 1993;342:1523–8.

35. Maggioni AP, Franzosi MG, Santoro E, et al. The risk of stroke in patients with acute myocardial infarction after thrombolytic and antithrombotic treatment. Gruppo Italiano per lo Studio della Soprav-vivenza nell'Infarto Miocardico II (GISSI-2), and The International Study Group. *N Engl J Med* 1992;327:1–6.

36. Andersen HR, Nielsen TT, Rasmussen K, et al. A comparison of coronary angioplasty with fibrinolytic therapy in acute myocardial infarction. *N Engl J Med* 2003;349:733–42.

37. Keeley EC, Boura JA, Grines CL. Primary angioplasty versus intravenous thrombolytic therapy for acute myocardial infarction: a quantitative review of 23 randomised trials. *Lancet* 2003;361:13–20.

38. Widimsky P, Budesinsky T, Vorac D, et al; 'PRAGUE' Study Group Investigators. Long distance transport for primary angioplasty vs immediate thrombolysis in acute myocardial infarction. Final results of the randomized national multicentre trial—PRAGUE-2. *Eur Heart J* 2003;24:94–104

39. Topol EJ, Califf RM, George BS, et al. A randomized trial of immediate versus delayed elective angioplasty after intravenous tissue plasminogen activator in acute myocardial infarction. *N Engl J Med* 1987;317:581–8.

40. The TIMI Research Group. Immediate versus delayed catheterization and angioplasty following thrombolytic therapy for acute myocardial infarction. TIMI II A results. *JAMA* 1988;260:2849–58.

41. Simoons ML, Arnold AE, Betriu A, et al. Thrombolysis with tissue plasminogen activator in acute myocardial infarction: no additional benefit from immediate percutaneous coronary angioplasty. *Lancet* 1988;1:197–203.

42. Stone GW, Grines CL, Cox DA, et al; Controlled Abciximab and Device Investigation to Lower Late Angioplasty Complications (CADILLAC) Investigations. Comparison of angioplasty with stenting, with or without abciximab, in acute myocardial infarction. *N Engl J Med* 2002;346:957–66.

43. Hsia J, Hamilton WP, Kleiman N, et al. A comparison between heparin and low-dose aspirin as adjunctive therapy with tissue plasminogen activator for acute myocardial Infarction. Heparin-Aspirin Reperfusion Trial (HART) Investigators. *N Engl J Med* 1990;323:1433–7.

44. de Bono D, Simoons ML, Tijssen J, et al. Effect of early intravenous heparin on coronary patency, infarct size, and bleeding complications after alteplase thrombolysis: results of a randomized double blind European Cooperative Study Group trial. *Br Heart J* 1992;67:122–8.

45. The GUSTO Angiographic Investigators. The effects of tissue plasminogen activator, streptokinase, or both on coronary artery patency, ventricular function, and survival after acute myocardial infarction. *N Engl J Med* 1993;22:1615–22.

46. Topol EJ, George BS, Kereiakes DJ, et al. A randomized controlled trial of intravenous tissue plasminogen activator and early intravenous heparin in acute myocardial infarction. *Circulation* 1989;79:281–6.

47. Wallentin L. The ASSENT-3 PLUS trial. Presented at the 75th Scientific Sessions of the American Heart Association in Chicago, November 2002.

48. Cannon CP, McCabe CH, Henry TD, et al. A pilot trial of recombinanat desulfatohirudin compared with heparin in conjunction with tPA and aspirin for acute myocardial infarction: results of the Thrombolysis in Myocardial Infarction (TIMI) 5 trial. *J Am Coll Cardiol* 1994;23:993–1003.

49. Jang IK, Brown DF, Giugliano RP, et al. A multicenter, randomized study of argatroban versus heparin as adjunct to tissue plasminogen activator (TPA) in acute myocardial infarction: myocardial infarction with novastan and TPA. (MINT) study. *J Am Coll Cardiol* 1999;33:1879–85.

50. White HD, Aylward PE, Frey MJ, et al. Randomized, doubleblind comparison of hirulog versus heparin in patients receiving streptokinase and aspirin for acute myocardial infarction (HERO). Hirulog Early Reperfusion/Occlusion (HERO) Trial Investigators. *Circulation* 1997;96:2155–61.

51. White H; The Hirulog and Early Reperfusion or Occlusion (HERO)-2 Trial Investigators. Thrombin-specific anticoagulation with bivalirudin versus heparin in patients receiving fibrinolytic therapy for acute myocardial infarction: the HERO-2 randomised trial. *Lancet* 2001;358:1855–63.

52. Gruppo Italiano per lo Studio della Sopravvivenza nell'infarto Miocardico. GISSI-3: Effects of lisinopril and transdermal glyceryl trinitrate singly and together on 6-week mortality and ventricular function after acute myocardial infarction. *Lancet* 1994;343:1115–22.

53. ISIS-4 (Fourth International Study of Infarct Survival) Collaborative Group. ISIS-4: a randomised factorial trial assessing early oral captopril, oral mononitrate, and intravenous magnesium in 58,050 patients with suspected acute myocardial infarction. *Lancet* 1995;345:669–85.

54. Flather MD, Yusuf S, Køber L, et al, for the ACE-Inhibitor Myocardial Infarction Collaborative Group. Long-term ACE-inhibitor therapy in patients with heart failure or left-ventricular dysfunction: a systematic overview of data from individual patients. ACE-Inhibitor Myocardial Infarction Collaborative Group. *Lancet* 2000;355:1575–81

55. Fath-Ordoubadi F, Beatt KJ. Glucose-insulin-potassium therapy of acute myocardial infarction: an overview of randomized placebo-controlled trials. *Circulation* 1997;96:1152–6.

56. Early administration of intravenous magnesium to high-risk patients with acute myocardial infarction in the Magnesium in Coronaries (MAGIC) Trial: a randomised controlled trial. *Lancet* 2002;360:1189–96.

57. De Lorgeril M, Salen P, Martin JL, et al. Mediterranean diet, traditional risk factors, and the rate of cardiovascular complications after myocardial infarction: final report of the Lyon Diet Heart Study. *Circulation* 1999;99:779–85

58. Gruppo Italiano per lo Studio della Sopravvivenza nell'Infarto miocardico. Dietary supplementation with n-3 polyunsaturated fatty acids and vitamin E after myocardial infarction: results of the GISSI-Prevenzione trial. *Lancet* 1999;354:447–55.

12

Future perspectives

Ravish Sachar & Eric J Topol

Introduction

Coronary artery disease (CAD) remains the leading cause of death in the western world. Given the aging population, coupled with the epidemics of obesity and diabetes, the worldwide prevalence of ischemic heart disease is predicted to increase considerably in the future. In 2001, the annual US spending on healthcare was $1.42 trillion (14% of the gross domestic product), with the largest segment supporting cardiovascular diseases – this figure is projected to increase.

The increase in spending has been and will be fueled not only by the growing number of patients with ischemic heart disease seeking treatment, but also by the explosion in the use of expensive technology, such as drug-eluting coronary stents and implantable defibrillators. Thus, in order to diminish the financial burden on the health care system, it is paramount that targeted and more efficient therapies be developed.

Over the last two decades, there have been dramatic advances in the treatment of acute coronary syndromes (ACS). Until recently, the serum markers of myocardial necrosis that we relied upon for the diagnosis and treatment of ACS consisted merely of creatine kinase and its myocardial band isoenzyme (CK-MB). While newer treatment strategies developed over the last two decades have yielded excellent results in terms of clinical outcomes, we continue to treat most patients without individualized strategies and subject them to polypharmacy with a standardized cocktail of drugs.

Moving forward, research efforts will continue to deliver improvements in the diagnosis, acute treatment, and chronic management of patients with ACS. Concepts such as cardiac biomarkers, genetic screening to predict future clinical outcomes and therapeutic responsiveness, and stem cell therapy for damaged myocardium should continue to improve outcomes for selected patients with ACS. It is likely that this type of targeted, individualized treatment will ultimately help to reduce the economic costs of health care.

ACS can be broadly classified into ST-segment elevation myocardial infarction (STEMI) and non-ST-segment elevation myocardial infarction (NSTEMI). The first part of this chapter largely focuses on the use of novel cardiac biomarkers in the diagnosis and management of patients with ACS, including NSTEMI; exciting developments in the field of pharmacogenomics are discussed in the second part of the chapter; finally, future trends in the treatment of STEMI are addressed in the third part of this chapter.

This chapter is not meant to be a comprehensive review of all the novel strategies that may find a role in the future treatment of ACS; important areas such as stem cell therapy have not been addressed. Rather, it takes a look at the general direction in which the treatment of ACS may be headed.

Cardiac biomarkers in ACS and NSTEMI

Over the past decade, a growing body of evidence has supported an early invasive strategy as the optimal approach for reducing the incidence of reinfarction and death in patients with ACS, even in high-risk patients without STEMI [1–4]. However, patients with ACS are heterogeneous, with a spectrum of risk.

High-risk criteria include prolonged chest pain at rest, ST-segment depression, and myonecrosis, as evidenced by cardiac biomarkers such as CK-MB and cardiac troponins T and I. There is little debate that these patients benefit from an early invasive strategy. Among patients considered to be at low or intermediate risk, however, practice patterns differ – some favor an early invasive strategy for all patients with suspected ACS, while others favor initial aggressive medical therapy, followed by invasive evaluation only if deemed necessary based upon the results of noninvasive studies.

Proponents of an early invasive strategy for all patients argue that optimal risk stratification requires coronary anatomic data obtained through cardiac catheterization. Those favoring initial aggressive medical therapy cite the potentially higher risk and lack of evidence of benefit with an early invasive strategy [5,6], especially among low-risk patients [1,2]. Several classification systems have been developed to help identify those patients who would benefit from an early invasive strategy. These are largely based upon clinical presentation, and attempt to stratify patients at higher short- and long-term risk.

The most widely utilized classification scheme stratifies patients based upon presentation with stable or unstable angina. Symptoms in patients with stable angina are thought to be due to high-grade coronary stenoses, while symptoms among patients with unstable angina are attributed to plaque instability or rupture. Other classification systems, such as the TIMI risk score, are also largely based on presenting symptoms and comorbidities.

All such classification systems share a common goal: to identify patients with coronary plaque that is prone to rupture. The problem with using demographic and routine clinical parameters alone to risk-stratify patients lies in their lack of accuracy in predicting short-term outcomes.

Furthermore, one half of all cardiac deaths are sudden and are not heralded by prior symptoms; thus, relying on symptoms alone to prevent future events will miss a large number of at-risk patients. To this end, a variety of diagnostic modalities have been developed, both invasive and noninvasive, to help with the identification of the patient with vulnerable plaque. At any given time, however, a substantial proportion of patients with atherosclerotic CAD, whether stable or unstable, will have heightened inflammatory activity reflected by abnormal biomarker proteins.

Until recently, the initial laboratory evaluation of patients presenting with ACS consisted entirely of CK-MB measurement. Over the past decade, cardiac troponins have rapidly gained acceptance as being a more sensitive marker than CK-MB for detecting myocardial injury. Beyond measuring the degree of myocardial necrosis, however, several other factors are responsible for making patients with CAD vulnerable to future cardiac events. Such factors include inflammation, hemodynamic stress, and genetic predisposition. Novel cardiac biomarkers have been developed to measure the impact of each of these factors (see **Table 1**).

The future management of ACS will probably employ a multimarker strategy to more accurately risk-stratify patients and guide treatment. By adequately collating all available data, including physical examination and history, electrocardiogram results, and cardiac biomarkers, each patient's therapy could be individualized.

Markers of inflammation

Inflammation has been firmly established as pivotal for the development of future clinical events in both asymptomatic and symptomatic patients. It is now widely accepted that inflammation plays a central role in not only the development and progression of atherosclerosis, but also in the subsequent plaque instability and thrombosis that result in the clinical manifestation of this systemic process as an acute syndrome. Among patients presenting with ACS, inflammation probably worsens cardiac outcomes by not only increasing the likelihood of future plaque rupture in other areas of the coronary vasculature, but also by increasing the degree of distal thromboembolization (and consequent myocardial injury) during any given plaque rupture [7].

C-reactive protein

High-sensitivity C-reactive protein (hsCRP) is the most widely studied inflammatory biomarker. It is a strong predictor of short- and long-term

Table 1. Cardiac biomarkers. BNP: B-type natriuretic peptide; hsCRP: high-sensitivity C-reactive protein; ICAM: intercellular adhesion molecule; Lp-PLA2: lipoprotein-associated phospholipase A2; TNF: tumor necrosis factor; VCAM: vascular cell adhesion molecule; VEGF: vascular endothelial growth factor.

Markers of inflammation	Markers of myocardial necrosis	Markers of hemodynamic stress
hsCRP	Creatine kinase-MB	BNP
Interleukin-6	Troponin I	N-terminal Pro-BNP
VCAM-1	Troponin T	
ICAM-1		
Myeloperoxidase		
P-selectin		
Soluble CD40 ligand		
TNF-α		
Lp-PLA2		
White blood cells		
VEGF		
von Willebrand factor		

cardiovascular risk among healthy men and women, and among patients with prior events [8–10]. CRP measured in the acute phase after myocardial infarction (MI) is associated with infarct size [11], and is independently associated with long-term mortality after acute MI [12].

Serum hsCRP is also highly predictive of adverse cardiac events after coronary revascularization [13], and has recently been implicated in cholesterol embolization after cardiac catheterization [14]. Its value as a predictor is independent of, and additive to, the predictive value of serum low-density lipoprotein (LDL) levels [10]. As such, it should be routinely measured in all patients presenting with ACS. While CRP is produced mainly by the liver in response to interleukin (IL)-6 [15], recent evidence suggests that it is also produced by smooth muscle cells in the arterial wall [16] and is deposited in atheromatous plaque. As such, it plays a key role in the progression of atherosclerosis, rather than simply being a marker of inflammation [17,18].

Data further suggest that CRP induces endothelial dysfunction and insulin resistance, enables the expression of vascular cellular adhesion molecule (VCAM)-1 and intercellular adhesion molecule (ICAM)-1 in endothelial cells, promotes the production of monocyte chemoattractant protein (MCP)-1 by endothelial cells, and mediates the opsonization of oxidized LDL by macrophages, thus enabling foam cell formation [19–22].

CD40 ligand

Another promising biomarker for risk stratification is soluble CD40 ligand (CD40L), which is part of the CD40–CD40L system. Although it is found on a wide variety of cells, including leukocytes, endothelial cells, and smooth muscle cells, more than 90% of the body's store is derived from platelets. Soluble CD40L is shed from activated platelets. This system plays an important role in the development of ACS by (among other mechanisms) inducing the expression of matrix-degrading proteinases and the procoagulant tissue factor on macrophages [23].

Soluble CD40L levels predict adverse outcomes in healthy women, and have further been shown to portend adverse short-term outcomes among patients presenting with ACS [24]. Not only is soluble CD40L released from activated platelets, but it is also likely to be responsible for further platelet activation [25].

Myeloperoxidase

The role of polymorphonuclear neutrophils in mediating ACS has been highlighted by emerging reports on the ability of myeloperoxidase (MPO) to predict adverse clinical outcomes among patients presenting with ACS [26,28]. This powerful predictive ability is independent of other biomarkers such as troponin T, soluble CD40L, or CRP (see **Table 2**).

Other markers of inflammation

Other markers of inflammation that have been shown to portend an adverse prognosis include the cellular adhesion molecules VCAM-1 and ICAM-1

Table 2. Independent predictors of death or nonfatal myocardial infarction at 6 months among patients presenting with acute coronary syndromes (reproduced with permission from *Circulation* 2003; 108:1440–5). hsCRP: high-sensitivity C-reactive protein; MPO: myeloperoxidase; VEGF: vascular endothelial growth factor.

Biomarker	Adjusted hazard ratio	95% confidence interval	*P* value
Troponin T >0.01 µg/L	1.99	1.16–3.64	0.023
hsCRP tertiles	1.25	1.02–1.68	0.044
VEGF >300 µg/L	1.87	1.03–3.51	0.041
Soluble CD40 ligand >5 µg/L	2.78	1.57–4.91	<0.001
MPO >350 µg/L	2.11	1.21–3.67	0.008

[9,29], P-selectin [30], vascular endothelial growth factor (VEGF) [27], and IL-6 [31]. Tumor necrosis factor (TNF)-α also appears to play an important role in atherosclerosis and inflammation [15], but its short half-life may limit its role in acute patient care.

Recently, a blood test for the inflammatory marker lipoprotein-associated phospholipase A2 (Lp-PLA2) has been approved by the US Food and Drug Administration after being found to predict the risk of coronary disease [32]. However, its appropriate application in clinical practice will require additional prospective studies with extended follow-up.

Point-of-care testing

It is very likely that in the near future, some of these markers may play a role in the management of ACS patients as part of a point-of-care multimarker diagnostic kit. Currently, the three most attractive candidates for use in such a strategy are CRP, soluble CD40L, and MPO.

As point-of-care testing for inflammation becomes a reality, these markers may not only aid with risk stratification, but also help to guide therapy. For example, treatment with glycoprotein (GP)IIb/IIIa inhibitors during ACS appears to be specifically beneficial to patients with elevated levels of soluble CD40L [25]. Furthermore, in the FRISC II trial, an early invasive strategy was associated with a significant reduction in 1-year mortality among patients with elevated levels of IL-6. On the other hand, an early invasive strategy did not result in a reduction in mortality among those *without* elevated IL-6 levels [33]. Finally, even an elevated white blood cell count, a relatively crude marker of inflammation, appears to be associated with a greater benefit of revascularization [34].

Markers of myocardial necrosis

Beyond being markers for myocardial necrosis, elevated levels of cardiac troponins suggest the presence of intracoronary thrombus and high-risk angiographic characteristics at the site of the culprit lesion [35–37].

Furthermore, abnormal tissue perfusion has been associated with elevated levels of troponin T, suggesting thromboembolization with subsequent platelet aggregation [38]. Small elevations in cardiac troponin I and T levels have been shown to be predictive of future adverse clinical outcomes [39], and their predictive value is superior to that of CK–MB alone [40].

Establishing elevated serum troponin levels is essential for guiding therapy among ACS patients, as these patients derive particular benefit from treatment with low molecular weight heparins and GPIIb/IIIa inhibitors, as well as from early invasive therapy [41–45].

Markers of hemodynamic stress

B-type natriuretic peptide (BNP) is a cardiac neurohormone that is elevated in response to left ventricular pressure overload. Initial studies have demonstrated that serum levels are elevated in patients with congestive heart failure [46]. When measured in patients presenting with chest pain, elevated serum levels have been found to be indicative of concomitant left ventricular dysfunction and prognostic of adverse short- and medium-term cardiac outcomes [47–49]. Furthermore, the N-terminal fragment of the BNP prohormone has been found to be strongly predictive of long-term mortality in patients presenting with ACS [24,50]. When used as part of a multimarker strategy, BNP levels provide incremental prognostic information over and above troponin I and CRP levels [51], but have not yet been coupled with treatment strategies based upon such levels.

Assessing vulnerable plaque

The majority of ACS are due to plaque rupture, fissure, or erosion and subsequent thrombus formation at the site of the vulnerable plaque. Future management of patients with ACS may include point-of-care evaluation for the presence and extent of vulnerable plaque (see **Table 2**) by noninvasive methods. This may involve radiological studies, such as magnetic resonance imaging (MRI) and ultrafast computed tomography (UFCT), or invasive methods during catheterization, such as intravascular ultrasound (IVUS), thermography, and optical coherence tomography (OCT). While currently not possible, data derived by these methods could, in the future, guide both acute and chronic therapy.

Magnetic resonance imaging and ultrafast computed tomography

Enormous improvements in computer processor speeds have improved the precision of MRI and UFCT for detecting and quantifying the size and extent of vulnerable plaque. MRI is already being used to detect plaque progression and regression [52,53]. Inadequate resolution, the Achilles' heel of MRI, may be adequately addressed with the use of intravascular MRI coils [54].

Intravascular ultrasound

The IVUS criteria by which to identify vulnerable plaque have been outlined by several groups. These criteria tend to utilize ultrasound evidence of a thin fibrous cap, a large lipid core as suggested by a high ratio of echolucent material, and positive remodeling at the lesion site [55–57].

Small studies have found a higher incidence of subsequent adverse coronary events among patients with IVUS-defined features of vulnerable plaque [58]. With the current state of technology, however, postmortem histopathological studies have shown a low sensitivity of IVUS in detecting vulnerable plaque [59].

Optical coherence tomography

The principles of OCT are similar to those of IVUS and, with improvements, this technology may eventually be a sensitive method of differentiating water-based tissue from lipid-based tissue [60]. At this time, however, it remains investigational.

Thermography

Thermography takes advantage of temperature differences in inflamed areas of the vasculature to identify vulnerable plaque [61]. Using this technique, pilot studies have found higher median temperatures at the culprit lesion site in patients with unstable angina or ACS as compared with patients with stable angina [62].

While these methods hold promise for the future, it must be emphasized that they all remain investigational at this point for the detection of vulnerable plaque. Whether or not they will find a place in the routine diagnosis and treatment of ACS remains to be seen.

Metabolomics

"Metabolomics", also referred to as "metabonomics", refers to the study of the whole metabolic profile of a patient's serum, just as proteomics and genomics refer to the protein and genetic profiles of patients, respectively. Exciting work in this field has recently shown that proton nuclear magnetic resonance (^{1}H–NMR) spectroscopy of human serum can be used to diagnose the presence and severity of CAD – one study reported >90% specificity for diagnosing the presence of three-vessel disease [63].

Furthermore, the ^{1}H–NMR spectra of serum in patients with hypertension was found to be different among those with systolic blood pressure >130 mm Hg as compared with those with lower blood pressures. This finding was attributed, in part, to differences in lipoprotein particle composition between patients [64]. While this technology is in its infancy and its use in the management of patients remains speculative, it highlights the potential role for novel technologies in the noninvasive diagnosis of CAD.

Pharmacogenomics

Over the past decade, it has become evident that individuals' responses to pharmacotherapy vary considerably. This is highlighted by the observation that, despite treatment with the best pharmacological agents we currently have available, a large number of ACS patients still go on to suffer coronary events (see **Table 3**) [65]. A proportion of these events are probably due to an inadequate response to drug therapy as a result of genetic polymorphisms that result in allelic variation and drug resistance. In this arena, technologies enabling the rapid identification of single-nucleotide polymorphisms (SNPs) could potentially be used to predict individual responses to therapeutic strategies, guide treatment, and improve therapeutic efficiency.

Variations in platelet surface glycoproteins due to genetic differences between patients are relatively common [66–68]. While the clinical implications of such inherited differences are not yet completely

Table 3. The benefit and lack of benefit of selected pharmacotherapy for the prevention of adverse cardiac outcomes (reproduced with permission from *Prog Cardiovasc Dis* 2002;44:479–98).

Trial	Drug	Event rate (0%)		Benefit/100	Lack of benefit/100
		Placebo	Treated		
HOPE	Ramipril	17.8	14.0	3.8	96.2
APTC	Aspirin	14.0	10.0	4.0	96.0
FTT	Thrombolytics	11.5	9.6	1.9	98.1
4S	Simvastatin	28.0	19.0	9.0	91.0
EPIC	Abciximab	12.8	8.3	4.5	95.5
CURE	Clopidogrel	11.5	9.3	2.2	97.8

understood, they may result in heterogeneous responses to antiplatelet agents and a propensity for ACS [69–73]. For example, aspirin resistance is well documented [74–76], has been associated with gene polymorphisms [67], and has recently been reported to impart significant future cardiac risk in the setting of a randomized controlled trial [77].

Similarly, considerable interindividual responses to thienopyridine treatment have been documented [78,79], and one study found that up to 29% of patients undergoing PCI did not completely respond to clopidogrel [80]. Additionally, the recently reported P2Y12 haplotype, which is present in 14% of healthy individuals, appears to confer resistance to thienopyridines [81].

The detection of thienopyridine resistance is clinically important as it may predict the dreaded complication of subacute thrombosis after stent implantation [82]. Finally, SNPs have been found that interfere with response to statin therapy, the cornerstone of our current long-term treatment of patients with CAD [83]. The importance of understanding the variability in interindividual response to statin therapy cannot be overstated.

In the future, the application of nanotechnology, with gold nanosensors attached to oligonucleotide probes, may allow the creation of point-of-care diagnostic systems for patients presenting with ACS [84,85]. While such systems will not be available for several years, they may become invaluable in rapidly identifying the subset of patients who will not benefit from traditional antiplatelet drugs and statins. Individualizing treatment in this manner could further help to prevent drug toxicities and identify patients at higher risk for adverse drug–drug interactions.

Future perspectives in the treatment of patients with STEMI

The treatment of STEMI has been revolutionized by the introduction of thrombolytic therapy and primary PCI. The data supporting the benefits of these two strategies are incontrovertible. Over the past few years, however, we appear to have reached a plateau in our ability to reduce short-term mortality after acute STEMI. As we move forward, research focused on three key areas may help us to improve clinical outcomes after STEMI:

- emboli prevention and tissue-level perfusion
- facilitated PCI
- Centers of Excellence

Emboli prevention and tissue-level perfusion

Over the past decade, considerable data have amassed to highlight the importance and adverse consequences of distal embolization during PCI in ACS and during elective procedures. The recognition of the significance of atheroembolization represents a paradigm shift in our understanding and treatment of CAD.

Thrombus and atheromatous debris that embolize from the epicardial vessels to the distal microvasculature not only inhibit flow and tissue-level perfusion, but also amplify the inflammatory cascade by acting as foci for further platelet aggregation and thrombus formation [7]. After PCI, patients with evidence of microvascular obstruction and myocardial necrosis have adverse clinical outcomes as compared with patients with intact tissue level perfusion [86–89]. Accordingly, increasingly diffuse atheromatous disease (as assessed by the length of the lesion, the number of vessels involved, and the presence of degenerated saphenous vein grafts) and the invasiveness of the procedure have both been identified as predictors of distal embolization and adverse outcomes [90,91].

Glycoprotein IIb/IIIa inhibitors

The rapid acceptance of GPIIb/IIIa inhibitors as necessary adjunctive pharmacotherapy during PCI has been based upon the ability of these agents to reduce periprocedural MI [87,88,92]. GPIIb/IIIa inhibitors have been found to have maximal beneficial effect in patients who show signs of myocardial necrosis, as assessed by cardiac enzymes [93]. It is now generally accepted that patients who have myocardial necrosis have probably already embolized; in these patients, GPIIb/IIIa inhibitors reduce adverse outcomes by attenuating further platelet aggregation and thrombus formation in the distal microvasculature [7].

Emboli prevention devices

While adjunctive pharmacotherapy can attenuate the consequences of distal embolization after it has occurred, prevention of distal embolization remains the optimal scenario. Several emboli prevention devices have now been developed. These devices were initially developed for use in the carotid arteries to prevent intracerebral embolization and in degenerated saphenous vein grafts, and have been shown to be safe and effective in these scenarios [94,95].

There are two basic types of devices: occlusion balloons and filter wires. While the adoption of such devices for use in the native coronary vasculature during AMI has been slow, two devices have now been approved:

- the PercuSurge GuardWire™ (Medtronic Corporation, MN, USA)

- the FilterWire EX™ Embolic Protection System (Boston Scientific, MA, USA)

While these devices represent a large step forward as compared with PCI without distal protection during AMI, they are bulky and significantly increase procedure time. Furthermore, they can only be used in large proximal vessels for lesions that are not ostial and do not have any large side branches nearby. Finally, the distal occlusion devices can result in distal ischemia, which some patients may not tolerate, and the filter systems allow some particulate matter to slip through.

Other types of devices have been developed, such as the Proxis™ proximal occlusion balloon catheter (Velocimed Inc., MN, USA). When inflated, this stops flow in the vessel distal to the occlusion, allowing percutaneous intervention without the risk of thrombus and atheromatous debris embolizing to the distal vasculature. However, flow from side branches negates the effect of this device in native coronary arteries, and thus the utility of this device is limited to aorto-coronary grafts.

These restrictions limit use of the current generation of distal emboli prevention devices to a minority of lesions in native coronary arteries. Newer-generation devices are likely to be smaller and more user friendly, and thereby applicable in a larger number of anatomical and clinical scenarios.

Facilitated percutaneous coronary intervention

Facilitated PCI refers to the combination of pharmacological and mechanical reperfusion strategies to achieve improved patency rates. Early studies that combined thrombolytic therapy with routine angioplasty for AMI reported no benefit of this strategy as compared with thrombolytics alone, and one trial suggested worse outcomes due to higher rates of reinfarction and death [96–98].

These adverse outcomes have been attributed to the potential paradoxical hypercoagulable state induced by thrombolytics. Accordingly, it has been suggested that combining GPIIb/IIIa inhibitors with reduced-dose thrombolytics, followed by routine PCI, may be a better strategy for achieving improved patency rates in the epicardial vessels and in the microcirculation.

Pilot studies combining thrombolytic therapy with GPIIb/IIIa inhibitors without routine PCI have achieved promising results [99–101]. The GUSTO-V trial, which randomized 16,588 patients with AMI to standard-dose reteplase alone (n = 8,260) versus half-dose reteplase plus abciximab (n = 8,328), showed a significant benefit of combination therapy for the combined endpoint of death or nonfatal MI (7.4% vs 8.8%; $P = 0.011$). This outcome was primarily driven by a reduction in nonfatal MI, and no short- or long-term mortality benefit was seen. Subset analyses, however, revealed a trend toward a mortality benefit with the combination strategy among patients <75 years of age and among those with anterior MI [102].

The large, ongoing FINESSE trial has been designed to study pretreatment with GPIIb/IIIa inhibitors with or without thrombolytic therapy prior to PCI for AMI. This trial has three arms: routine pretreatment with abciximab alone; routine pretreatment with half-dose thrombolytic therapy with abciximab; or no pretreatment. The results of this trial are eagerly awaited – they will help to assess whether pretreatment with combination therapy is beneficial, and will further address whether thrombolytics are helpful at any dose, and whether there is any benefit of giving abciximab in the ambulance or in the emergency room. A pilot trial has suggested that early initiation of the GPIIb/IIIa inhibitor tirofiban in the emergency room compared with at the time of catheterization results in improved angiographic outcomes [103].

Centers of Excellence

Data that have accumulated over the past decade highlight the superiority of catheter-based reperfusion therapy over fibrinolytic therapy for the treatment of AMI [104]. These trials were largely conducted in tertiary care centers. Accordingly, for STEMI patients presenting to such centers with well-established PCI programs, the decision to treat with primary angioplasty is not difficult. However, it is debatable whether the benefit of primary angioplasty can be extrapolated to all hospitals, including smaller community hospitals with lower volumes, less experienced operators, and fewer facilities.

Proponents of allowing primary angioplasty for acute MI in all hospitals cite the C-PORT trial, where 11 community hospitals in Maryland and Massachusetts randomized patients to primary angioplasty versus fibrinolytic therapy. They found a significant benefit among those patients randomized to angioplasty in terms of death, reinfarction, or stroke at 30 days [105]. However, the staff in the enrolling hospitals had to attend comprehensive in-service programs, the catheterization laboratories were equipped to very high standards, and the percutaneous interventions were performed by high-volume operators. In reality, not all community hospitals can comply with the same high standards; thus, the clinical outcomes in patients treated at similar hospitals may not be as good as suggested by this trial.

Current protocols followed by emergency medical personnel mandate the treatment of patients with acute MI at the nearest emergency room. As such, patients with acute MI often present to the emergency rooms of hospitals that are not equipped for primary angioplasty. Several trials have examined whether it is better for such patients to be treated with fibrinolytic therapy at the first hospital to which they are admitted, or to delay treatment and transfer the patient to a facility that is equipped for primary angioplasty [106–110].

A meta-analysis by Dalby and colleagues reviewed the data from six trials that compared early thrombolytic therapy versus transport for primary PCI. They found a 42% reduction in the combined endpoints of death, stroke, and MI among patients who were transported [111]. Furthermore, acute MI patients with contraindications to thrombolytic therapy have significantly better outcomes when treated with primary PCI as compared with medical therapy alone, underscoring the importance of primary PCI facilities for this patient population [112]. The data thus far are compelling that transfer for catheter-based reperfusion results in superior outcomes, despite the time delay that is inherent in such a strategy.

One reason for this appears to be that the linear relationship between adverse outcomes and the elapsed time from symptom onset to treatment among patients treated with fibrinolytic therapy does not hold true for those treated with primary PCI. While delays in reperfusion therapy undoubtedly result in more damaged myocardium with either strategy, the significance of the delay is far less when the patient is treated with primary angioplasty than with fibrinolytic therapy [113–116]. Thus, when presenting to a facility without primary PCI facilities, patients with acute MI may have better outcomes if they are transferred to another center that does have such facilities, as long as this can be done within a reasonable time frame. The exact amount of time that can elapse after which the advantage of delayed PCI over immediate thrombolysis begins to abate remains to be delineated.

Another probable reason for improved outcomes in referral hospitals is operator experience. Operator and hospital primary angioplasty volume is an important predictor of patient outcomes [117,118]. Furthermore, larger centers tend to be more reliably equipped with the wide variety of interventional tools that may be needed during treatment of an acute MI, such as emboli prevention devices and mechanical thrombectomy devices.

Conclusions

Over the past decade, advances in the standard of care for ACS have resulted in dramatic improvements in clinical outcomes. These advances have been in both the diagnosis and treatment of patients presenting with ACS. Inflammatory biomarkers such as hsCRP, soluble CD40L, and

MPO are proving to be invaluable in assessing the extent of myocardial damage and the presence of inflammation. We are rapidly moving towards an era where a number of such markers will be used concomitantly as part of a multimarker strategy affording accurate risk stratification and allowing therapeutic guidance.

Advances in the field of pharmacogenomics will allow us to determine, ahead of time, the therapeutic efficacy of pharmacotherapy on patients, and thereby allow us to individualize therapy and minimize our present reliance on drug cocktails. We can envision a future where such tests may be performed at the point-of-care using high-throughput DNA technology, allowing therapeutic decisions to be made at the time of presentation.

For patients presenting with STEMI, routine pretreatment with adjunctive pharmacotherapy (such as GPIIb/IIIa inhibitors and half-dose thrombolytics) before PCI and the development of better emboli prevention devices will increase our ability to perform primary PCI without compromising the distal microvasculature and thereby reduce adverse clinical outcomes.

Finally, it remains to be seen whether political and economic forces will allow a national policy of Centers of Excellence for the treatment of AMI. The implementation of such a policy would undoubtedly be logistically challenging. However, based on current evidence, such a system would result in improvements in short- and long-term clinical outcomes.

The challenge for the future will lie in finding the optimal set of diagnostic and treatment modalities to accurately identify and treat those patients who are at high risk for future adverse clinical outcomes. Much more investment is required, in terms of clinical trials, before we will be able to fine-tune our health care apparatus to individualize therapy and achieve these goals. If we succeed, however, the result will be targeted and efficacious therapy for patients. This will not only improve clinical outcomes, but will do so in an economically efficient manner. As the financial burden on the health care system continues to increase, the importance of such cost-effective treatment strategies cannot be overstated.

References

1. FRagmin and Fast Revascularisation during InStability in Coronary artery disease (FRISC II) Investigators. Invasive compared with non-invasive treatment in unstable coronary-artery disease: FRISC II prospective randomised multicentre study. *Lancet* 1999;354:708–15.
2. Cannon CP, Weintraub WS, Demopoulos LA, et al. Comparison of early invasive and conservative strategies in patients with unstable coronary syndromes treated with the glycoprotein IIb/IIIa inhibitor tirofiban. *N Engl J Med* 2001;344:1879–87.
3. Fox KA, Poole-Wilson PA, Henderson RA, et al. Interventional versus conservative treatment for patients with unstable angina or non-ST-elevation myocardial infarction: the British Heart Foundation RITA 3 randomised trial. Randomized Intervention Trial of unstable Angina. *Lancet* 2002;360:743–51.
4. Cho L, Bhatt DL, Marso SP, et al. An invasive strategy is associated with decreased mortality in patients with unstable angina and non-ST-elevation myocardial infarction: GUSTO IIb trial. *Am J Med* 2003;114:106–11.
5. Boden WE, O'Rourke RA, Crawford MH, et al. Outcomes in patients with acute non-Q-wave myocardial infarction randomly assigned to an invasive as compared with a conservative management strategy. Veterans Affairs Non-Q-Wave Infarction Strategies in Hospital (VANQWISH) Trial Investigators. *N Engl J Med* 1998;338:1785–92.
6. Thrombolysis in Myocardial Ischemia. Effects of tissue plasminogen activator and a comparison of early invasive and conservative strategies in unstable angina and non-Q-wave myocardial infarction. Results of the TIMI IIIB Trial. *Circulation* 1994;89:1545–56.
7. Topol EJ, Yadav JS. Recognition of the importance of embolization in atherosclerotic vascular disease. *Circulation* 2000;101:570–80.
8. Ridker PM, Cushman M, Stampfer MJ, et al. Inflammation, aspirin, and the risk of cardiovascular disease in apparently healthy men. *N Engl J Med* 1997;336:973–9.
9. Ridker PM, Hennekens CH, Buring JE, et al. C-reactive protein and other markers of inflammation in the prediction of cardiovascular disease in women. *N Engl J Med* 2000;342:836–43.
10. Ridker PM, Rifai N, Rose L, et al. Comparison of C-reactive protein and low-density lipoprotein cholesterol levels in the prediction of first cardiovascular events. *N Engl J Med* 2002;347:1557–65.
11. de Beer FC, Hind CR, Fox KM, et al. Measurement of serum C-reactive protein concentration in myocardial ischaemia and infarction. *Br Heart J* 1982;47:239–43.
12. Kinjo K, Sato H, Ohnishi Y, et al. Impact of high-sensitivity C-reactive protein on predicting long-term mortality of acute myocardial infarction. *Am J Cardiol* 2003;91:931–5.

13. Chew DP, Bhatt DL, Robbins MA, et al. Incremental prognostic value of elevated baseline C-reactive protein among established markers of risk in percutaneous coronary intervention. *Circulation* 2001;104:992–7.

14. Fukumoto Y, Tsutsui H, Tsuchihashi M, et al. The incidence and risk factors of cholesterol embolization syndrome, a complication of cardiac catheterization: a prospective study. *J Am Coll Cardiol* 2003;42:211–6.

15. Heinrich PC, Castell JV, Andus T. Interleukin-6 and the acute phase response. *Biochem J* 1990;265:621–36.

16. Calabro P, Willerson JT, Yeh ET. Inflammatory cytokines stimulated C-reactive protein production by human coronary artery smooth muscle cells. *Circulation* 2003;108:1930–2.

17. Torzewski J, Torzewski M, Bowyer DE, et al. C-reactive protein frequently colocalizes with the terminal complement complex in the intima of early atherosclerotic lesions of human coronary arteries. *Arterioscler Thromb Vasc Biol* 1998;18:1386–92.

18. Yasojima K, Schwab C, McGeer EG, et al. Generation of C-reactive protein and complement components in atherosclerotic plaques. *Am J Pathol* 2001;158:1039–51.

19. Pasceri V, Willerson JT, Yeh ET. Direct proinflammatory effect of C-reactive protein on human endothelial cells. *Circulation* 2000;102:2165–8.

20. Pasceri V, Cheng JS, Willerson JT, et al. Modulation of C-reactive protein-mediated monocyte chemoattractant protein-1 induction in human endothelial cells by anti-atherosclerosis drugs. *Circulation* 2001;103:2531–4.

21. Zwaka TP, Hombach V, Torzewski J. C-reactive protein-mediated low density lipoprotein uptake by macrophages: implications for atherosclerosis. *Circulation* 2001;103:1194–7.

22. Bhatt DL, Topol EJ. Need to test the arterial inflammation hypothesis. *Circulation* 2002;106:136–40.

23. Mach F, Schonbeck U, Bonnefoy JY, et al. Activation of monocyte/macrophage functions related to acute atheroma complication by ligation of CD40: induction of collagenase, stromelysin, and tissue factor. *Circulation* 1997;96:396–9.

24. Varo N, De Lemos JA, Libby P, et al. Soluble CD40L: risk prediction after acute coronary syndromes. *Circulation* 2003 (Epub ahead of print).

25. Heeschen C, Dimmeler S, Hamm CW, et al. Soluble CD40 ligand in acute coronary syndromes. *N Engl J Med* 2003;348:1104–11.

26. Zhang R, Brennan ML, Fu X, et al. Association between myeloperoxidase levels and risk of coronary artery disease. *JAMA* 2001;286:2136–42.

27. Baldus S, Heeschen C, Meinertz T, et al. Myeloperoxidase serum levels predict risk in patients with acute coronary syndromes. *Circulation* 2003;108:1440–5.

28. Buffon A, Biasucci LM, Liuzzo G, et al. Widespread coronary inflammation in unstable angina. *N Engl J Med* 2002;347:5–12.

29. Ridker PM, Hennekens CH, Roitman-Johnson B, et al. Plasma concentration of soluble intercellular adhesion molecule 1 and risks of future myocardial infarction in apparently healthy men. *Lancet* 1998;351:88–92.

30. Ridker PM, Buring JE, Rifai N. Soluble P-selectin and the risk of future cardiovascular events. *Circulation* 2001;103:491–5.

31. de Lemos JA, Hennekens CH, Ridker PM. Plasma concentration of soluble vascular cell adhesion molecule-1 and subsequent cardiovascular risk. *J Am Coll Cardiol* 2000;36:423–6.

32. Packard CJ, O'Reilly DS, Caslake MJ, et al. Lipoprotein-associated phospholipase A2 as an independent predictor of coronary heart disease. West of Scotland Coronary Prevention Study Group. *N Engl J Med* 2000;343:1148–55.

33. Lindmark E, Diderholm E, Wallentin L, et al. Relationship between interleukin 6 and mortality in patients with unstable coronary artery disease: effects of an early invasive or noninvasive strategy. *JAMA* 2001;286:2107–13.

34. Bhatt DL, Chew DP, Lincoff AM, et al. Effect of revascularization on mortality associated with an elevated white blood cell count in acute coronary syndromes. *Am J Cardiol* 2003;92:136–40.

35. Panteghini M, Cuccia C, Pagani F, et al. Coronary angiographic findings in patients with clinical unstable angina according to cardiac troponin I and T concentrations in serum. *Arch Pathol Lab Med* 2002;126:448–51.

36. Frey N, Dietz A, Kurowski V, et al. Angiographic correlates of a positive troponin T test in patients with unstable angina. *Crit Care Med* 2001;29:1130–6.

37. deFilippi CR, Tocchi M, Parmar RJ, et al. Cardiac troponin T in chest pain unit patients without ischemic electrocardiographic changes: angiographic correlates and long-term clinical outcomes. *J Am Coll Cardiol* 2000;35:1827–34.

38. Wong GC, Morrow DA, Murphy S, et al. Elevations in troponin T and I are associated with abnormal tissue level perfusion: a TACTICS-TIMI 18 substudy. Treat Angina with Aggrastat and Determine Cost of Therapy with an Invasive or Conservative Strategy-Thrombolysis in Myocardial Infarction. *Circulation* 2002;106:202–7.

39. Heidenreich PA, Alloggiamento T, Melsop K, et al. The prognostic value of troponin in patients with non-ST elevation acute coronary syndromes: a meta-analysis. *J Am Coll Cardiol* 2001;38:478–85.

40. Rao SV, Ohman EM, Granger CB, et al. Prognostic value of isolated troponin elevation across the spectrum of chest pain syndromes. *Am J Cardiol* 2003;91:936–40.

41. Lindahl B, Venge P, Wallentin L. Troponin T identifies patients with unstable coronary artery disease who benefit from long-term antithrombotic protection. Fragmin in Unstable Coronary Artery Disease (FRISC) Study Group. *J Am Coll Cardiol* 1997;29:43–8.

42. Morrow DA, Antman EM, Tanasijevic M, et al. Cardiac troponin I for stratification of early outcomes and the efficacy of enoxaparin in unstable angina: a TIMI-11B substudy. *J Am Coll Cardiol* 2000;36:1812–7.

43. Heeschen C, Hamm CW, Goldmann B, et al. Troponin concentrations for stratification of patients with acute coronary syndromes in relation to therapeutic efficacy of tirofiban. PRISM Study Investigators. Platelet Receptor Inhibition in Ischemic Syndrome Management. *Lancet* 1999;354:1757–62.

44. Newby LK, Ohman EM, Christenson RH, et al. Benefit of glycoprotein IIb/IIIa inhibition in patients with acute coronary syndromes and troponin t-positive status: the paragon-B troponin T substudy. *Circulation* 2001;103:2891–6.

45. Morrow DA, Cannon CP, Rifai N, et al. Ability of minor elevations of troponins I and T to predict benefit from an early invasive strategy in patients with unstable angina and non-ST elevation myocardial infarction: results from a randomized trial. *JAMA* 2001;286:2405–12.

46. Omland T, Aakvaag A, Vik-Mo H. Plasma cardiac natriuretic peptide determination as a screening test for the detection of patients with mild left ventricular impairment. *Heart* 1996;76:232–7.

47. de Lemos JA, Morrow DA, Bentley JH, et al. The prognostic value of B-type natriuretic peptide in patients with acute coronary syndromes. *N Engl J Med* 2001;345:1014–21.

48. Richards AM, Nicholls MG, Espiner EA, et al. B-type natriuretic peptides and ejection fraction for prognosis after myocardial infarction. *Circulation* 2003;107:2786–92.

49. Omland T, Aakvaag A, Bonarjee VV, et al. Plasma brain natriuretic peptide as an indicator of left ventricular systolic function and long-term survival after acute myocardial infarction. Comparison with plasma atrial natriuretic peptide and N-terminal proatrial natriuretic peptide. *Circulation* 1996;93:1963–9.

50. Omland T, Persson A, Ng L, O'Brien R, et al. N-terminal pro-B-type natriuretic peptide and long-term mortality in acute coronary syndromes. *Circulation* 2002;106:2913–8.

51. Sabatine MS, Morrow DA, de Lemos JA, et al. Multimarker approach to risk stratification in non-ST elevation acute coronary syndromes: simultaneous assessment of troponin I, C-reactive protein, and B-type natriuretic peptide. *Circulation* 2002;105:1760–3.

52. James SK, Lindahl B, Siegbahn A, et al. N-terminal pro-brain natriuretic peptide and other risk markers for the separate prediction of mortality and subsequent myocardial infarction in patients with unstable coronary artery disease: a Global Utilization of Strategies To Open occluded arteries (GUSTO)-IV substudy. *Circulation* 2003;108:275–81.

53. Choudhury RP, Fayad ZA, Aguinaldo JG, et al. Serial, noninvasive, in vivo magnetic resonance microscopy detects the development of atherosclerosis in apolipoprotein E-deficient mice and its progression by arterial wall remodeling. *J Magn Reson Imaging* 2003;17:184–9.

54. Worthley SG, Helft G, Fuster V, et al. A novel nonobstructive intravascular MRI coil: in vivo imaging of experimental atherosclerosis. *Arterioscler Thromb Vasc Biol* 2003;23:346–50.

55. Schoenhagen P, Ziada KM, Kapadia SR, et al. Extent and direction of arterial remodeling in stable versus unstable coronary syndromes: an intravascular ultrasound study. *Circulation* 2000;101:598–603.

56. von Birgelen C, Klinkhart W, Mintz GS, et al. Plaque distribution and vascular remodeling of ruptured and nonruptured coronary plaques in the same vessel: an intravascular ultrasound study in vivo. *J Am Coll Cardiol* 2001;37:1864–70.

57. Nakamura M, Nishikawa H, Mukai S, et al. Impact of coronary artery remodeling on clinical presentation of coronary artery disease: an intravascular ultrasound study. *J Am Coll Cardiol* 2001;37:63–9.

58. Yamagishi M, Terashima M, Awano K, et al. Morphology of vulnerable coronary plaque: insights from follow-up of patients examined by intravascular ultrasound before an acute coronary syndrome. *J Am Coll Cardiol* 2000;35:106–11.

59. Peters RJ, Kok WE, Havenith MG, et al. Histopathologic validation of intracoronary ultrasound imaging. *J Am Soc Echocardiogr* 1994;7:230–41.

60. Jang IK, Bouma BE, Kang DH, et al. Visualization of coronary atherosclerotic plaques in patients using optical coherence tomography: comparison with intravascular ultrasound. *J Am Coll Cardiol* 2002;39:604–9.

61. Stefanadis C, Toutouzas K, Vaina S, et al. Thermography of the cardiovascular system. *J Interv Cardiol* 2002;15:461–6.

62. Stefanadis C, Diamantopoulos L, Vlachopoulos C, et al. Thermal heterogeneity within human atherosclerotic coronary arteries detected in vivo: A new method of detection by application of a special thermography catheter. *Circulation* 1999;99:1965–71.

63. Brindle JT, Antti H, Holmes E, et al. Rapid and noninvasive diagnosis of the presence and severity of coronary heart disease using 1H-NMR-based metabonomics. *Nature Med* 2002;8:1439–44.

64. Brindle JT, Nicholson JK, Schofield PM, et al. Application of chemometrics to 1H NMR spectroscopic data to investigate a relationship between human serum metabolic profiles and hypertension. *Analyst* 2003;128:32–6.

65. Mukherjee D, Topol EJ. Pharmacogenomics in cardiovascular diseases. *Prog Cardiovasc Dis* 2002;44:479–98.
66. Quinn MJ, Topol EJ. Common variations in platelet glycoproteins: pharmacogenomic implications. *Pharmacogenomics* 2001;2:341–52.
67. Macchi L, Christiaens L, Brabant S, et al. Resistance in vitro to low-dose aspirin is associated with platelet PlA1 (GP IIIa) polymorphism but not with C807T(GP Ia/IIa) and C-5T Kozak (GP Ibalpha) polymorphisms. *J Am Coll Cardiol* 2003;42:1115–9.
68. Kunicki TJ, Newman PJ. The molecular immunology of human platelet proteins. *Blood* 1992;80:1386–404.
69. Nurden AT. Platelet glycoprotein IIIa polymorphism and coronary thrombosis. *Lancet* 1997;350:1189–91.
70. Weiss EJ, Bray PF, Tayback M, et al. A polymorphism of a platelet glycoprotein receptor as an inherited risk factor for coronary thrombosis. *N Engl J Med* 1996;334:1090–4.
71. Walter DH, Schachinger V, Elsner M, et al. Platelet glycoprotein IIIa polymorphisms and risk of coronary stent thrombosis. *Lancet* 1997;350:1217–9.
72. Bottiger C, Kastrati A, Koch W, et al. Polymorphism of platelet glycoprotein IIb and risk of thrombosis and restenosis after coronary stent placement. *Am J Cardiol* 1999;84:987–91.
73. Kastrati A, Schomig A, Seyfarth M, et al. PlA polymorphism of platelet glycoprotein IIIa and risk of restenosis after coronary stent placement. *Circulation* 1999;99:1005–10.
74. Gum PA, Kottke-Marchant K, Poggio ED, et al. Profile and prevalence of aspirin resistance in patients with cardiovascular disease. *Am J Cardiol* 2001;88:230–5.
75. Buchanan MR, Brister SJ. Individual variation in the effects of ASA on platelet function: implications for the use of ASA clinically. *Can J Cardiol* 1995;11:221–7.
76. Helgason CM, Tortorice KL, Winkler SR, et al. Aspirin response and failure in cerebral infarction. *Stroke* 1993;24:345–50.
77. Gum PA, Kottke-Marchant K, Welsh PA, et al. A prospective, blinded determination of the natural history of aspirin resistance among stable patients with cardiovascular disease. *J Am Coll Cardiol* 2003;41:961–5.
78. Gurbel PA, Bliden KP, Hiatt BL, et al. Clopidogrel for coronary stenting: response variability, drug resistance, and the effect of pretreatment platelet reactivity. *Circulation* 2003;107:2908–13.
79. Jaremo P, Lindahl TL, Fransson SG, et al. Individual variations of platelet inhibition after loading doses of clopidogrel. *J Intern Med* 2002;252:233–8.
80. Muller I, Besta F, Schulz C, et al. Prevalence of clopidogrel non-responders among patients with stable angina pectoris scheduled for elective coronary stent placement. *Thromb Haemost* 2003;89:783–7.
81. Fontana P, Dupont A, Gandrille S, et al. Adenosine diphosphate–induced platelet aggregation is associated with P2Y12 gene sequence variations in healthy subjects. *Circulation* 2003;108:989–95.
82. Barragan P, Bouvier JL, Roquebert PO, et al. Resistance to thienopyridines: clinical detection of coronary stent thrombosis by monitoring of vasodilator-stimulated phosphoprotein phosphorylation. *Catheter Cardiovasc Interv* 2003;59:295–302.
83. Maitland-van der Zee AH, Klungel OH, Stricker BH, et al. Genetic polymorphisms: importance for response to HMG-CoA reductase inhibitors. *Atherosclerosis* 2002;163:213–22.
84. Jain KK. Nanodiagnostics: application of nanotechnology in molecular diagnostics. *Expert Rev Mol Diagn* 2003;3:153–61.

85. Maxwell DJ, Taylor JR, Nie S. Self-assembled nanoparticle probes for recognition and detection of biomolecules. *J Am Chem Soc* 2002;124:9606–12.
86. Elliott JM, Berdan LG, Holmes DR, et al. One-year follow-up in the Coronary Angioplasty Versus Excisional Atherectomy Trial (CAVEAT I). *Circulation* 1995;91:2158–66.
87. Topol EJ, Ferguson JJ, Weisman HF, et al. Long-term protection from myocardial ischemic events in a randomized trial of brief integrin beta3 blockade with percutaneous coronary intervention. EPIC Investigator Group. Evaluation of Platelet IIb/IIIa Inhibition for Prevention of Ischemic Complication. *JAMA* 1997;278:479–84.
88. The EPILOG Investigators. Platelet glycoprotein IIb/IIIa receptor blockade and low-dose heparin during percutaneous coronary revascularization. *N Engl J Med* 1997;336:1689–96.
89. Lincoff AM, Tcheng JE, Califf RM, et al. Sustained suppression of ischemic complications of coronary intervention by platelet GP IIb/IIIa blockade with abciximab: one-year outcome in the EPILOG trial.Evaluation in PTCA to Improve Long-term Outcome with abciximab GP IIb/IIIa blockade. *Circulation* 1999;99:1951–8.
90. Abdelmeguid AE, Topol EJ, Whitlow PL, et al. Significance of mild transient release of creatine kinase-MB fraction after percutaneous coronary interventions. *Circulation* 1996;94:1528–36.
91. Abdelmeguid AE, Ellis SG, Sapp SK, et al. Defining the appropriate threshold of creatine kinase elevation after percutaneous coronary interventions. *Am Heart J* 1996;131:1097–105.
92. The EPISTENT Investigators. Randomised placebo-controlled and balloon-angioplasty-controlled trial to assess safety of coronary stenting with use of platelet glycoprotein-IIb/IIIa blockade. Evaluation of Platelet IIb/IIIa Inhibitor for Stenting. *Lancet* 1998;352:87–92.
93. Hamm CW, Heeschen C, Goldmann B, et al. Benefit of abciximab in patients with refractory unstable angina in relation to serum troponin T levels. c7E3 Fab Antiplatelet Therapy in Unstable Refractory Angina (CAPTURE) Study Investigators. *N Engl J Med* 1999;340:1623–9.
94. Baim DS, Wahr D, George B, et al. Randomized trial of a distal embolic protection device during percutaneous intervention of saphenous vein aorto-coronary bypass grafts. *Circulation* 2002;105:1285–90.
95. Cremonesi A, Manetti R, Setacci F, et al. Protected carotid stenting: clinical advantages and complications of embolic protection devices in 442 consecutive patients. *Stroke* 2003;34:1936–41.
96. Topol EJ, Califf RM, George BS, et al. A randomized trial of immediate versus delayed elective angioplasty after intravenous tissue plasminogen activator in acute myocardial infarction. *N Engl J Med* 1987;317:581–8.
97. Williams DO, Braunwald E, Knatterud G, et al. One-year results of the Thrombolysis in Myocardial Infarction investigation (TIMI) Phase II Trial. *Circulation* 1992;85:533–42.
98. SWIFT trial of delayed elective intervention v conservative treatment after thrombolysis with anistreplase in acute myocardial infarction. SWIFT (Should We Intervene Following Thrombolysis?) Trial Study Group. *Br Med J* 1991;302:555–60.
99. Group TS. Trial of abciximab with and without low-dose reteplase for acute myocardial infarction. Strategies for Patency Enhancement in the Emergency Department (SPEED) Group. *Circulation* 2000;101:2788–94.
100. Antman EM, Giugliano RP, Gibson CM, et al. Abciximab facilitates the rate and extent of thrombolysis: results of the thrombolysis in myocardial infarction (TIMI) 14 trial. The TIMI 14 Investigators. *Circulation* 1999;99:2720–32.

101. Brener SJ, Zeymer U, Adgey AA, et al. Eptifibatide and low-dose tissue plasminogen activator in acute myocardial infarction: the integrilin and low-dose thrombolysis in acute myocardial infarction (INTRO AMI) trial. *J Am Coll Cardiol* 2002;39:377–86.

102. Topol EJ. Reperfusion therapy for acute myocardial infarction with fibrinolytic therapy or combination reduced fibrinolytic therapy and platelet glycoprotein IIb/IIIa inhibition: the GUSTO V randomised trial. *Lancet* 2001;357:1905–14.

103. Lee DP, Herity NA, Hiatt BL, et al. Adjunctive platelet glycoprotein IIb/IIIa receptor inhibition with tirofiban before primary angioplasty improves angiographic outcomes: results of the TIrofiban Given in the Emergency Room before Primary Angioplasty (TIGER-PA) pilot trial. *Circulation* 2003;107:1497–501.

104. Weaver WD, Simes RJ, Betriu A, et al. Comparison of primary coronary angioplasty and intravenous thrombolytic therapy for acute myocardial infarction: a quantitative review. *JAMA* 1997;278:2093–8.

105. Aversano T, Aversano LT, Passamani E, et al. Thrombolytic therapy vs primary percutaneous coronary intervention for myocardial infarction in patients presenting to hospitals without on-site cardiac surgery: a randomized controlled trial. *JAMA* 2002;287:1943–51.

106. Widimsky P, Budesinsky T, Vorac D, et al. Long distance transport for primary angioplasty vs immediate thrombolysis in acute myocardial infarction. Final results of the randomized national multicentre trial—PRAGUE-2. *Eur Heart J* 2003;24:94–104.

107. Widimsky P, Groch L, Zelizko M, et al. Multicentre randomized trial comparing transport to primary angioplasty vs immediate thrombolysis vs combined strategy for patients with acute myocardial infarction presenting to a community hospital without a catheterization laboratory. The PRAGUE study. *Eur Heart J* 2000;21:823–31.

108. Grines CL, Westerhausen DR Jr, Grines LL, et al. A randomized trial of transfer for primary angioplasty versus on-site thrombolysis in patients with high-risk myocardial infarction: the Air Primary Angioplasty in Myocardial Infarction study. *J Am Coll Cardiol* 2002;39:1713–9.

109. Bonnefoy E, Lapostolle F, Leizorovicz A, et al. Primary angioplasty versus prehospital fibrinolysis in acute myocardial infarction: a randomised study. *Lancet* 2002;360:825–9.

110. Andersen HR, Nielsen TT, Rasmussen K, et al. A comparison of coronary angioplasty with fibrinolytic therapy in acute myocardial infarction. *N Engl J Med* 2003;349:733–42.

111. Dalby M, Bouzamondo A, Lechat P, et al. Transfer for Primary Angioplasty Versus Immediate Thrombolysis in Acute Myocardial Infarction. A Meta-Analysis. *Circulation* 2003;108:1809–14.

112. Grzybowski M, Clements EA, Parsons L, et al. Mortality Benefit of Immediate Revascularization of Acute ST-Segment Elevation Myocardial Infarction in Patients With Contraindications to Thrombolytic Therapy: A Propensity Analysis. *JAMA* 2003;290:1891–1898.

113. Brodie BR, Stone GW, Morice MC, et al. Importance of time to reperfusion on outcomes with primary coronary angioplasty for acute myocardial infarction (results from the Stent Primary Angioplasty in Myocardial Infarction Trial). *Am J Cardiol* 2001;88:1085–90.

114. Brodie BR, Stuckey TD, Wall TC, et al. Importance of time to reperfusion for 30-day and late survival and recovery of left ventricular function after primary angioplasty for acute myocardial infarction. *J Am Coll Cardiol* 1998;32:1312–9.

115. Milavetz JJ, Giebel DW, Christian TF, et al. Time to therapy and salvage in myocardial infarction. *J Am Coll Cardiol* 1998;31:1246–51.

116. Zijlstra F, Patel A, Jones M, et al. Clinical characteristics and outcome of patients with early (<2 h), intermediate (2–4 h) and late (>4 h) presentation treated by primary coronary angioplasty or thrombolytic therapy for acute myocardial infarction. *Eur Heart J* 2002;23:550–7.
117. Magid DJ, Calonge BN, Rumsfeld JS, et al. Relation between hospital primary angioplasty volume and mortality for patients with acute MI treated with primary angioplasty vs thrombolytic therapy. *JAMA* 2000;284:3131–8.
118. Canto JG, Every NR, Magid DJ, et al. The volume of primary angioplasty procedures and survival after acute myocardial infarction. National Registry of Myocardial Infarction 2 Investigators. *N Engl J Med* 2000;342:1573–80.

Abbreviations

ACC	American College of Cardiology
ACE	angiotensin-converting enzyme
ACLS	advanced cardiac life support
ACS	acute coronary syndromes
ACT	activated clotting time
ADP	adenosine diphosphate
AHA	American Heart Association
aPTT	activated partial thromboplastin time
AT_2	angiotensin II
ATT	Antithrombotic Therapy Trialists
AV	atrioventricular
BBB	bundle branch block
BNP	B-type natriuretic peptide or brain natriuretic peptide
BP	blood pressure
CABG	coronary artery bypass graft
CAD	coronary artery disease
CD40L	CD40 ligand
CHF	congestive heart failure
CI	confidence interval
CK	creatine kinase
CK-MB	creatine kinase isoenzyme MB
COX	cyclo-oxygenase
CRP	C-reactive protein
cTnI	cardiac troponin I
cTnT	cardiac troponin T
CTS	cardiothoracic surgery
DES	drug-eluting stents
DTI	direct thrombin inhibitor
ECG	electrocardiogram
EF	ejection fraction
ESC	European Society of Cardiology
FTT	Fibrinolytic Therapy Trialists

GAP	Guidelines Applied in Practice
GIK	glucose–insulin–potassium
GP	glycoprotein
HDL	high-density lipoprotein
hsCRP	high-sensitivity C-reactive protein
IABP	intra-aortic balloon pump
ICAM	intercellular adhesion molecule
ICD	implantable cardioverter defibrillator
IL	interleukin
IMA	internal mammary artery
INR	international normalized ratio
IRA	infarct-related artery
IV	intravenous
IVUS	intravascular ultrasound
JCAHO	Joint Commission on Accreditation of Healthcare Organizations
LA	left atrium
LAD	left anterior descending
LBBB	left bundle branch block
LDL	low-density lipoprotein
LMWH	low molecular weight heparin
Lp-PLA2	lipoprotein-associated phospholipase A2
LV	left ventricular
LVEF	left ventricular ejection fraction
MCP	monocyte chemoattractant protein
MI	myocardial infarction
MPO	myeloperoxidase
MR	mitral regurgitation
MRI	magnetic resonance imaging
NMR	nuclear magnetic resonance
NRMI	National Registry of Myocardial Infarction (US)
NSTEMI	non-ST-segment elevation myocardial infarction
OCT	optical coherence tomography
OR	odds ratio
PCI	percutaneous coronary intervention
PCWP	pulmonary capillary wedge pressure
PTCA	percutaneous transluminal coronary angioplasty
RA	right atrium
RCA	right coronary artery

RRR	relative risk ratio
RV	right ventricular
SC	subcutaneous
SK	streptokinase
SNP	single-nucleotide polymorphism
STEMI	ST-segment elevation myocardial infarction
SVG	saphenous vein graft
SVR	systemic vascular resistance
TEE	transesophageal echocardiography
TF	tissue factor
TFPI	tissue factor pathway inhibitor
TNF	tumor necrosis factor
tPA	tissue plasminogen activator
TVR	target-vessel revascularization
UA	unstable angina
UFCT	ultrafast computed tomography
UFH	unfractionated heparin
VCAM	vascular cellular adhesion molecule
VEGF	vascular endothelial growth factor
VF	ventricular fibrillation
VSD	ventricular septal defect
VSR	ventricular septal rupture
VT	ventricular tachycardia

Trial acronyms

4S	Scandinavian Simvastatin Survival Study
ACUITY	Acute Catheterization and Urgent Intervention Thrombotic Strategy
ADMIRAL	Abciximab Before Direct Angioplasty and Stenting in Myocardial Infarction Regarding Acute and Long-term Follow-up
ADVANCE-MI	Addressing the Value of Primary Angioplasty After Combination Therapy or Eptifibatide Monotherapy in Acute Myocardial Infarction
Air PAMI	Air Primary Angioplasty in Myocardial Infarction
AIRE	Acute Infarction Ramipril Efficacy

ASSENT	Assessment of the Safety and Efficacy of a New Thrombolytic Regimen
CADILLAC	Controlled Abciximab and Device Investigation to Lower Late Angioplasty Complications
CAPRIE	Clopidogrel versus Aspirin in Patients at Risk of Ischaemic Events
CAPTIM	Comparison of Angioplasty and Prehospital Thrombolysis in Acute Myocardial Infarction
CARE	Cholesterol and Recurrent Events
COMMIT	Clopidrogel Metoprolol Myocardial Infarction Trial
C-PORT	Cardiovascular Patient Outcomes Research Team
CREDO	Clopidogrel for the Reduction of Events During Observation
CRUISE	Coronary Revascularization Using Integrilin and Single Bolus Enoxaparin
CRUSADE	Can Rapid Risk Stratification of Unstable Angina Patients Suppress Adverse Outcomes with Early Implementation of the ACC/AHA Guidelines?
CURE	Clopidogrel in Unstable Angina to Prevent Recurrent Events
DANAMI	Danish Multicenter Randomized Trial on Thrombolytic Therapy versus Acute Coronary Angioplasty in Acute Myocardial Infarction
DIGAMI	Diabetic Patients with Acute Myocardial Infarction
EHS-ACS	Euro Heart Survey Acute Coronary Syndromes
ELITE	Evaluation of Losartan in the Elderly
ENACT	European Network for Acute Coronary Treatment
EPIC	Evaluation of c7E3 for the Prevention of Ischemic Complications
EPILOG	Evaluation in PTCA to Improve Long-term Outcome with Abciximab GPIIb/IIIa Blockade
EPISTENT	Evaluation of Platelet IIb/IIIa Inhibitor for Stenting
ESSENCE	Efficacy and Safety of Subcutaneous Enoxaparin in Non-Q-wave Coronary Events
EUROPA	European trial on Reduction of Cardiac Events with Perindopril in Stable Coronary Artery Disease
FINESSE	Facilitated Intervention with Enhanced Reperfusion Speed to Stop Events
FRISC	Fragmin and Fast Revascularisation during Instability in Coronary Artery Disease

Index